EMPOWERED MEDICINE

A Guide for Consumers

Christi Larson, Pharm. D.

For information about this title or to order other books and/or electronic
media, contact the publisher:

Smart Leaf Press
5301 S. Superstition Mountain Drive
Suite 104, #155
Gold Canyon, AZ 85118

Or visit:
www.empoweredmedicine.com

Printed in the United States of America

Note to Readers

The information presented in this book is for informational and educational purposes only. The information presented in this book should not be considered to be a substitute for the direct medical advice of your doctor, nor is it meant to encourage the diagnosis or treatment of any illness, disease, or other medical problem by laypersons. Always consult your doctor before making any changes to your medical care.

TABLE OF CONTENTS

CHAPTER 1

CHOLESTEROL

The Empowered Medicine Guide to Cholesterol

How to Use This Chapter

Navigating the cholesterol guidelines can be daunting at first, even for health professionals. That is because there are 2 main sets of guidelines that health professionals look to when making decisions about cholesterol management. These 2 guidelines differ on some big points. The first set of guidelines are the 2013 ACC/AHA Lipid Guidelines. The second set of guidelines are the 2017 AACE/ACE Lipid Guidelines. Confusing? Just know there is a set of 2013 guidelines and 2017 guidelines.

In this chapter I will first go over each guideline separately. Then at the end we will review the medications that are often prescribed to treat high cholesterol.

Throughout the chapter you will be prompted to enter some of your own data (such as your last lipid panel numbers). Entering this data and following the directions along the way will help you and your doctor determine which medications are recommended for you.

If you wish, use Appendix I and II in the back to log your own information for easy calculations and sharing with your doctor. Also, at the end of this chapter you will find a section called 'The Bottom Line'. This box sums up the main points of the chapter.

Cholesterol: The Basics

When learning about high cholesterol, you may hear a term called 'hyperlipidemia' used. Hyperlipidemia is just a fancy word for high cholesterol. '*Hyper*' literally means *high*, '*lipid*' means *fat* and '*emia*' means in the *blood*. So '**hyperlipidemia**' means '**a high amount of fats in the blood**'.

Saying '*hyperlipidemia*' rather than '*high cholesterol*' is much more accurate because there is more to the fats floating around in your blood than just 'high cholesterol'. As we will learn in a bit, the term '*dyslipidemia*' is an even better description because it has now been learned that some of the population who may be at high risk for heart attack and stroke don't have high cholesterol (high LDL-C), they may actually have low cholesterol (low LDL-C).[7] '*Dys*' means *abnormal*. So '**dyslipidemia**' means '**abnormal fats in the blood**'.

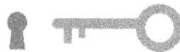

Key to Success

'**Hyper**'	+	'lipid'	+	'emia'	=	'**High**'	'fat' 'in the blood'
'**Dys**'	+	'lipid'	+	'emia'	=	'**Abnormal**'	'fat' 'in the blood'

What Causes a Heart Attack or Stroke?

There are approximately 550,000 new heart attacks and 200,000 recurrent heart attacks every year. The average age at first heart attack is 65 years old for men and 72 years old for women.[1] *A heart attack happens when the arteries that bring oxygen-rich blood to the muscles of the heart become clogged. A stroke happens when the arteries that bring oxygen-rich blood to the brain become clogged.*

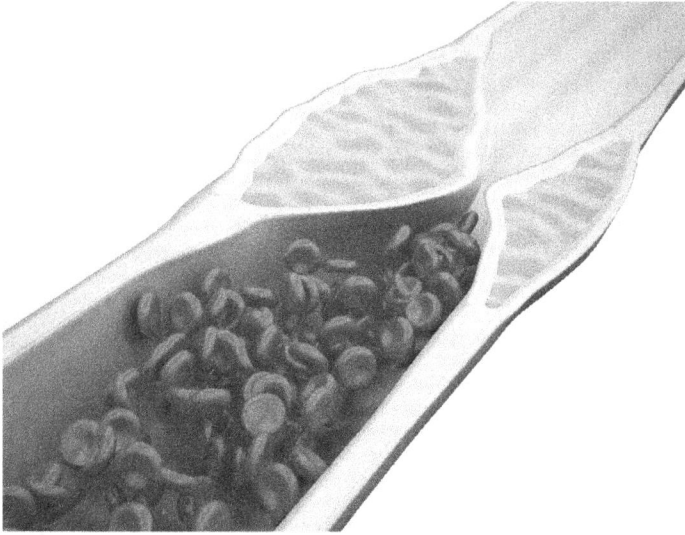

Figure 1: *Clogged Artery*

'Arteriosclerotic cardiovascular disease (ASCVD)' or just **'cardiovascular disease'** refer to the clogging of the arteries throughout the body, particularly in the heart and brain. When the cells of the heart are deprived of oxygen long enough, fatal arrhythmias (deadly irregular heart beat or rhythms) or a heart attack (heart can't work right because of the lack of oxygen) can happen. When the cells of the brain are deprived of oxygen, a stroke can happen.

Throughout this chapter I will reference either, **'cardiovascular events' or 'arteriosclerotic cardiovascular disease (ASCVD')**. Both of these terms refer to a group of events that are known to be caused by the blockage of blood flow to various areas of the body (namely heart attack, angina, stroke, transient ischemic attack (TIA) and peripheral arterial disease).

So what does cholesterol have to do with all of this?

Cholesterol's Role in Cardiovascular Disease

Over the last several decades the message has been the same. It has generally been believed that:

1. The fat and cholesterol you eat causes fat to be deposited onto the walls of the arteries.

2. High cholesterol (particularly LDL-C) in the blood leads to more fat deposits in the arteries.

3. Fat deposits in the arteries clog the arteries and lead to an increased risk of death from cardiovascular disease.

4. Statin drugs (see list of statin drugs below) lower cholesterol levels which leads to a decrease in one's risk of death from heart disease and stroke.

However, statistical data does not entirely support all of these theories. It appears that cardiovascular disease may be a little more complex than that.

Table 1: **Examples of Statin Drugs Approved in the U.S.**

• Atorvastatin (Lipitor®)
• Fluvastatin (Lescol®)
• Lovastatin (Mevacor®, Altocor®)
• Pitavastatin (Livalo®)
• Pravastatin (Pravachol®)
• Simvastatin (Zocor®)
• Rosuvastatin (Crestor®)

Before we talk about why some of these theories are in question, let's look at the tests your doctor can order to help determine if you are at risk for cardiovascular disease.

In order for your doctor to determine if you are at risk for heart attack or stroke, he/she may order a blood lipid panel for you to have done at a lab. This will involve drawing some blood. You will need to fast (eat or drink nothing except for water) approximately 8 to 12 hours prior to the test. In addition to your total cholesterol level **(TC)**, a basic lipid panel measures low density lipoprotein cholesterol (**LDL-C**), high density lipoprotein cholesterol (**HDL-C**) and triglycerides **(TG)**. Your doctor may also order other labs which we will go over below. All of these values come together to paint a picture of your cardiovascular fitness and can tell you different things about the state of your health. Here's a rundown:

Table 2: **Labs Ordered for the Diagnosis and Monitoring of Dyslipidemia**

<u>**Commonly Ordered**</u> **types of blood lipid tests that may be drawn at a lab:**

- **Total cholesterol**-The total cholesterol, including 'good' and 'bad' cholesterol, in your blood stream.
- **LDL-C AKA 'bad' cholesterol**-This type of cholesterol is believed to play a big role in the formation of blockages in the arteries; however it's now recognized that LDL-C alone may not be the best measure of one's risk for heart attack or stroke.
- **HDL-C AKA 'good' cholesterol**-This type of cholesterol helps keep blockages from forming in the arteries. You want this number to be at least 40 mg/dL or as high as possible (> 60 mg/dL is best). Things that can make this number go up include increased physical activity, weight loss, quitting tobacco, and statin drugs.
- **VLDL-C**-There is no easy way to measure VLDL-C so it is usually estimated as a percentage of your triglycerides. High VLDL-C has been implicated in the production of artery-clogging plaques. You can help lower VLDL-C by lowering triglycerides.
- **Triglycerides (TG)**-Your body converts calories you don't eat into triglycerides; a type of fat in the blood. Eating more calories than your body can use on a regular basis can lead to high triglycerides. High triglycerides indicate a higher risk of cardiovascular disease. High triglycerides are commonly found in those with metabolic syndrome and diabetes. Metabolic syndrome is a group of conditions found in one person that include abdominal obesity, high blood pressure, dyslipidemia, and increased blood clotting. Metabolic syndrome appears

to be a product of insulin-resistance and is a precursor to type 2 diabetes.

- **Apo B**-Apo B represents the number of blockage-forming particles in the blood, similar to LDL-P.
- **LDL-P**-LDL-P represents the number of blockage-forming particles in the blood, similar to Apo B.
- **Non-HDL-C**-*Equal to total cholesterol minus HDL-C*. This represents the number of ALL blockage-forming particles in the blood. This is nice because it does not require another test outside of a basic lipid panel.

Less-Commonly Ordered types of blood lipid tests that may be drawn at a lab:

- **hsCRP**-This is a measurement of how much inflammation is taking place in the body. Inflammation has been associated with a higher risk of cardiovascular disease. HsCRP can be used to help determine the intensity of therapy one should pursue.
- **Lipoprotein-associated phospholipase A2 (Lp-PLA2)**-This number, along with hsCRP, indicates inflammation in the body. This inflammation has been linked to cardiovascular disease. Both of these numbers can be used to help determine how intense therapy should be.
- **Uric acid**-Increased serum uric acid levels are linked to insulin resistance syndrome, obesity, dyslipidemia, and high blood pressure. It has been linked to death due to cardiovascular disease, but according to guidelines, there is insufficient evidence to use it to identify those at risk for cardiovascular disease.
- **TG-rich remnants (RLP-TG)**-This is a marker for atherosclerosis and the development of cardiovascular disease. However, it is not commonly ordered.
- **Lipoprotein (a)**-This lab is not usually ordered but has been linked to a higher risk of cardiovascular disease. This number may be largely determined by genetics and race.
- **Homocysteine levels**-Although linked to cardiovascular disease, studies suggest that therapies that lower homocysteine levels such as vitamin B6, B12, and folic acid do not necessarily decrease one's risk of cardiovascular disease. Therefore, these levels are not often ordered.
- **Coronary artery calcification (CAC)**-(**This is actually not a**

---

blood test, but is a measurement taken using images from a CT scan)-Measures the accumulation of calcium on the walls of the coronary artery one of the main blood vessels that carry oxygen-rich blood to the heart. This number is linked to the development of cardiovascular disease, particularly heart attacks. This number may be useful in determining if a more aggressive approach to treatment might be in order.

- **Carotid intima media thickness (CIMT)-(This is actually not a blood test, but is a measurement taken using images from an ultrasound)**-Measures the thickness of the layers of the carotid arteries – the blood vessels that carry oxygen-rich blood to the brain. This number is linked to cardiovascular disease, particularly stroke. This number may also be useful in determining if a more aggressive approach to treatment might be in order.

Attempts have been made to determine if one is at a higher risk of cardiovascular events based on certain cholesterol levels alone (particularly LDL-C). You have undoubtedly heard by now that higher levels of cholesterol put you at a higher risk of heart attack, stroke, and death. As we will see, this is not as cut and dry as it sounds.

Is High Cholesterol Better?

When the media or healthcare talk about 'high cholesterol', they usually mean 'high total cholesterol' or 'high LDL-C'. Saying that 'high cholesterol is better' sounds absolutely crazy given all of the information put out by the medical community, food industry, and drug companies today. They maintain that we should lower our LDL cholesterol (LDL-C) to avoid a heart attack. *But some studies support the theory that low cholesterol puts one at a higher risk of death in older patients.*

Data from a 30-year follow up with participants from the famous Framingham Heart Study revealed that *in patients over the age of 50 years old, lower levels of cholesterol were associated with a higher rate of death.*[2] A research group from the Henry Ford Heart and Vascular Institute in Detroit, Michigan, had similar results. They looked at 500 patients admitted for heart attack. LDL-C was measured within the first 24 hours. Half of the 500 patients had LDL-C less than 105 mg/mL (LDL-C less than 100 mg/dL is thought to be optimal).[4] Three years later, *among the half with the lowest LDL-C levels, 26 patients had died. Only 12 of the patients with the highest LDL-C levels died*.[4]

Basically, the data from the Framingham Study shows that *LDL-C levels were not a good predictor of death* in this study. LDL-C levels may not be a good predictor of who develops heart disease, either. In 2015, the World Journal of Cardiology published data that compared cholesterol levels between patients with and without heart disease. As it turns out, the curves (on a graph of the data) for the patients with and without heart disease overlapped, except for those with very low or very high LDL-C. This indicates that cholesterol levels were not very good at predicting those who would develop heart disease and those who would not because *people who did or didn't have heart disease had fairly similar LDL-C levels*.[3]

The idea that one's risk of hospitalization and death can be reduced by lowering cholesterol is being challenged. Dr. Harlan Krumholz of the Department of Cardiovascular Medicine at Yale University commented on this, reporting that *older people with low cholesterol die twice as often from heart attack as do older people with high LDL-C*.[5]

All of this evidence aside, there are studies that suggest statins reduce cardiovascular events and/or mortality (death) and lower LDL-C in older people with and without cardiovascular disease.[8-18] When trying to make sense of these studies, keep in mind that some of the studies that showed a benefit from treatment with a statin were funded by manufacturers that make statins. That doesn't necesarily mean we can't accept the results of these studies as true, but it does indicate that caution should be used when evaluating them.

If LDL-C Alone Doesn't Measure Risk, What Does?

Many in the medical community are convinced there is more to cardiovascular risk than LDL-C alone. Based on recent studies, there is evidence to explain why **LDL-C alone may not be the best marker to evaluate one's risk of cardiovascular disease.**[7]

It has been proposed that the cholesterol particles in our blood are much like cars driving down a narrow road. LDL-C measures the amount of cholesterol contained in the LDL particles. So LDL-C measures the 'number of passengers in the cars'.

LDL-P (number of LDL particles) measures the 'number of cars' on the road. **Studies suggest that it is the number of cars on the road (LDL-P), not the number of passengers in the cars (LDL-C) that better predicts one's risk of developing cardiovascular disease.**[7] Logic says that the more cars on the road, the more likely some of them will crash into the walls (of the arteries). Once LDL particles start 'sticking' to the sides of the arteries, blockages can form. As mentioned above, blockages can cut off the oxygen-rich blood supply, causing a heart attack or a stroke.

With all of this in mind, when one gets their LDL-C measured and their LDL-C is low, they may believe that they are at low risk for cardiovascular disease. However, this may not be the case. Measuring the LDL-P may help more accurately determine if they are at high risk. *People with low LDL-C and high LDL-P may be at very high risk for cardiovascular disease* because their LDL-P is elevated even though their LDL-C is low.[7]

People with high LDL-C but low LDL-P may be at a low risk for cardiovascular disease.[7] Unfortunately, these people are very likely to be prescribed a statin because of their high LDL-C. Statins are not without side effects. Liver dysfunction, nerves problems, and serious muscle conditions are potential side effects of statins.

Table 3: **Summary of Blood Lipid Findings**

Cholesterol		Potential Risk
LDL-C ↑	**LDL-P↓**	Low risk
LDL-C↓	**LDL-P↓**	Low risk
LDL-C↑	**LDL-P↑**	High risk
LDL-C↓	**LDL-P↑**	High risk

Apo B and non-HDL-cholesterol (non-HDL-C)

Measuring Apo B has been proposed to help determine one's risk of cardiovascular disease. Lipoprotein particles in the blood that contain Apo B are most likely to stick to the walls of the arteries and cause a blockage. Each of these clot-containing particles carries only one Apo B molecule; so the total Apo B level reflects the total number of circulating clot-causing particles.

Apo B is basically telling us how many LDL particles (LDL-P) there are. Apo B does not require fasting to be tested. It has been standardized and can be used during therapy to help monitor your progress. This makes Apo B an easy test to get done and to interpret.

Key to Success

Measuring the LDL-P may more accurately determine if you are at high risk for cardiovascular disease. *People with low LDL-C and high LDL-P may be at very high risk for cardiovascular disease* because their LDL-P is elevated even though their LDL-C is low.[7]

People with high LDL-C but low LDL-P are likely at a low risk of cardiovascular disease.[7]

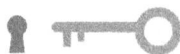

The Lipid Guidelines

Now let's look at the lipid guidelines. There are two main sets of guidelines that health providers look to when diagnosing and treating dyslipidemia. There are the *2013 American College of Cardiology/American Heart Association (ACC/AHA) guidelines* and the *2017 American Association of Clinical Endocrinologists/ American College of Endocrinology (AACE/ACE) guidelines*. First, we will look at each set of guidelines separately. Later, we will use both guidelines to help determine how one should proceed with their high cholesterol therapy.

2013 ACC/AHA Lipid Guidelines

After reviewing data from other studies, authors from one study said, "We conclude that the expectation that coronary heart disease could be prevented or eliminated by simply reducing cholesterol appears unfounded."[3]

Despite information that suggests LDL-C (in the absence of other markers) may not be the best tool for assessing cardiovascular risk, the 2 main organizations that have put out guidelines for lipid management still base many of their recommendations largely on LDL-C alone. However, the 2013 ACC/AHA recommendations did shift from trying to target certain LDL-C goals to a focus on defining groups of people who should take statins. The guidelines attribute the decrease in cardiovascular events in studies to the lowering of LDL-C by statins; however, some argue that one cannot jump to this conclusion. So it's unclear if the decrease in cardiovascular events was due to the lowering of LDL-C by statins or if there was more going on (effects on Apo B, etc.).

As mentioned at the beginning of this chapter, you will have the chance to fill in some of your own data as you read this chapter and determine which group of medications may be best for you. First, we will look at the steps you would follow if you were to follow the

2013 ACC/AHA guidelines. If you'd like to record your data on an easy-to-use worksheet that you can take to your doctor's office, **use the worksheet in Appendix I**.

2013 ACC/AHA Steps to Determining Risk and Dyslipidemia Treatment

Before we begin, please complete each of the following statements:

I have been diagnosed with heart failure	☐ Yes	☐ No
I currently undergo hemodialysis for kidney failure	☐ Yes	☐ No

If you answered 'Yes' to either of the statements above, do not continue with these assessments. They have not been studied in people with heart failure or hemodialysis. It's best to consult your doctor to discuss what medications you should consider to treat dyslipidemia. However, if you want to read about the different medications used to treat dyslipidemia toward the end of this chapter, please continue to the section titled 'Medications'.

For those who answered 'No' to both of these questions, please continue with the assessment below.

2013 ACC/AHA *Step 1*: Determine if You are in One of the Four Groups That Should Take a Statin:

There is insufficient data to make recommendations for beginning statin therapy in people without cardiovascular disease, ages 21-39 years. Also, according to the 2013 guidelines, there is not enough evidence to recommend statin therapy in people > 75 years old, although evidence supports continuing statins in people > 75 who have already been taking and tolerating them.[6] If a statin is started in someone > 75 years old, a medium-intensity statin is recommended.[6]

The following table shows scenarios where it is recommended by the 2013 panel to start taking a statin.

TO COMPLETE STEP 1: Place a check mark to the right of each statement that applies:

Table 4: **Four Groups of People Who Should Take a Statin According to 2013 ACC/AHA Lipid Guidelines**[6]

1	I have been diagnosed with cardiovascular disease, including angina, previous heart attack or stroke.	■
2	My LDL-C is 190 mg/dL or above.	■
3	I have type 2 diabetes **AND** I am between 40 and 75 years old **AND** my LDL-C 70-189 mg/dL **AND** I do **NOT** have cardiovascular disease.	■
4	I do **NOT** have cardiovascular disease or diabetes **AND** I am 40 to 75 years old **AND** my 10-year risk of heart attack or stroke greater than 7.5% (according to the 2013 risk calculator explained below).	■

If you did not check any of the boxes in STEP 1, congratulations! You do not need to take a statin according to the 2013 guidelines.

If you checked any of the boxes in rows 1, 2, or 3 above, skip ahead to STEP 3.

If you checked the box in row 4, move on to STEP 2.

2013 ACC/AHA *Step 2*: Determine Your Risk Using the 2013 ACC/AHA Risk Calculator

You can see Group #4 above includes anyone ages 40 to 75 years old with an LDL-C of 70-189 mg/dL, and a 7.5% chance of having a heart attack, stroke, or other form of cardiovascular disease in the next 10 years *according to the 2013 risk calculator*.

The 2013 cardiovascular risk calculator has been controversial. Some are concerned because persons over 70 years old using this system can qualify for a statin. The authors of the 2013 guidelines insist that most cardiovascular events happen after age 70, stating there is much potential for decreasing events in this group of people. [6] However, there is concern because some studies show an association with low LDL-C and an increased risk of cardiovascular events in older adults.[2,3,4,5]

There has also been much debate about the factors that have been added or omitted to the 2013 risk calculator. Finally, there has been discussion over how accurate the calculator is, considering it does not contain questions about weight, family history, heart health, LDL-P, or Apo B levels.

The calculator calculates one's risk of cardiovascular disease based on answers to the following questions:

Table 5: **2013 ACC/AHA Cardiovascular Risk Calculator Questions**[6]

1. What is the patient's *age*?
2. Does the patient have *diabetes mellitus*?
3. Is the patient *male or female*?
4. What is the patient's *race*?
5. Does the patient *smoke*?
6. What is the patient's *total cholesterol*?
7. What is the patient's *HDL cholesterol*?
8. What is the patient's *systolic blood pressure* (the top number)?
9. Is the patient being *treated for high blood pressure*?

You can find this calculator online by going to www.cvriskcalculator.com. Type in your information and you will receive your score. Remember, less than 7.5% is good. If your score is equal to or over 7.5%, the guidelines suggest you should use a statin if you fall into group 4.

The authors of the 2013 guidelines do mention that ***adverse effects, drug-drug interactions, and patient preferences should also be considered before prescribing a statin.***

You and your doctor might want to think about other factors as well. Consider using information from the risk assessment combined with items such as your LDL-P, non-HDL-C, Apo B level, cardiovascular health, weight, and family history to determine if a moderate to high dose statin is for you. As mentioned before, statins are capable of certain side effects including muscle and liver damage, neurological damage, and increased risk of type 2 diabetes.

2013 ACC/AHA *Step 2*: Determine your cardiovascular risk using the 2013 ACC/AHA Risk Calculator

You can visit: www.cvriskcalculator.com to obtain your risk score. Write your risk score in below for reference.

My CV Risk Score According to the 2013 ACC/AHA Risk Calculator	My Risk Score is _____ %

Key to Success

Adverse effects, drug-drug interactions, and patient preferences should be considered before prescribing a statin.

You and your doctor might also want to think about other factors as well. *Consider using information from the risk assessment combined with items such as your LDL-P, non-HDL-C, Apo B level, cardiovascular health, weight, and family history to determine if a moderate to high dose statin is for you. Also remember that statins carry the risk of certain side effects.*

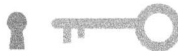

2013 ACC/AHA *Step 3*: Determine What Statin is Right for You:

If you meet one of the 4 criteria above, the 2013 ACC/AHA guidelines say you should take a statin if you can.

The authors of the 2013 ACC/AHA guidelines tell us ***that to get a true reduction in the number of cardiovascular events, moderate or high doses of statin drugs must be used (see Table 6)***. Note that at higher doses, side effects may be more common.

The authors also say that in the trials, a decrease in cardiovascular events was observed over a large range of LDL-C levels over 70 mg/dL.[6] In other words, according to them, it wasn't just those with the highest LDL-C levels who demonstrated a decrease in heart disease-related death.

The 2013 guidelines note that the addition of other therapies (like niacin) to statins can help lower LDL–C, but they did not reduce cardiovascular events any further in studies. Therefore, other medications besides statins are not generally recommended in the 2013 guidelines because it is believed that the benefit of using them does not outweigh the potential for side effects.

Table 6: **Low, Moderate, and High-Intensity Statin Drugs**[6]

Low-intensity Statins	Moderate-intensity Statins	High-intensity Statins
Lowers LDL-C by less than 30%	Lowers LDL-C by 30-50%	Lowers LDL-C by more than 50%
Simvastatin 10 mg	Atorvastatin 10-20 mg	Atorvastatin 40-80 mg
Pravastatin 10-20 mg	Rosuvastatin 5-10 mg	Rosuvastatin 20-40 mg
Lovastatin 20 mg	Simvastatin 20-40 mg	
Fluvastatin 20-40 mg	Pravastatin 40-80 mg	
Pitavastatin 1 mg	Lovastatin 40 mg	
	Fluvastatin XL 80 mg	
	Fluvastatin 40 mg twice daily	
	Pitavastatin 2-4 mg	

Here is a breakdown of how to figure out which statin to use (from the 2013 Guidelines). [6]

Those *with* cardiovascular disease

- **Take a high-intensity statin if:**
  - Age is less than or equal to 75 years old.
- **Take a medium-intensity statin if:**
  - Age is over 75 years old

Those *without* cardiovascular disease

- **Take a high-intensity statin if:**
  - LDL-C is greater than or equal to 190 mg/dL **OR**
  - You have type 1 or 2 diabetes, age is 40-75 years old, **and** have 10-year cardiovascular risk greater than or equal to 7.5%, according to the 2013 risk calculator.

- **Take a medium-intensity statin if:**
  - LDL-C is less than 90 mg/dL, you have type 1 or 2 diabetes and age are 40-75 years old, **and** you have a 10-year cardiovascular risk less than 7.5%

- **Consider a medium- or high-intensity statin if:**
  - You don't have diabetes, age is 40-75 years old, **and** LDL-C is less than or equal to 190 mg/dL, **and** you have a 10-year cardiovascular risk greater than or equal to 7.5%

According to the 2013 guidelines, it is recommended that people start on the appropriate intensity of statin therapy as outlined above. The dose is not adjusted to meet a goal (for example, to target a certain LDL-C level). *Instead, the 2013 guidelines suggest that one take the maximum dose of moderate- or high-intensity statin that is tolerated and stick with it as tolerated.* However, the authors' mention that decreasing the statin dose may be considered when two consecutive LDL-C values are < 40 mg/dL.[6]

TO COMPLETE STEP 3: Determine what statin is right for you

Place checkmarks in any boxes that apply. Tally the number of boxes checked at the bottom of each column.

Moderate-intensity Statins		High-intensity Statins	
☐	Age > 75 years old **AND** have cardiovascular disease (including angina, previous heart attack or stroke)	☐	Age 75 years old or younger **AND** have cardiovascular disease (angina, previous heart attack or stroke)
☐	LDL-C < 90 mg/dL **AND** have type 1 or 2 diabetes **AND** age is 40-75 years old **AND** 10-year cardiovascular risk less than 7.5%	☐	LDL-C 190mg/dL or above **AND** I do **NOT** have cardiovascular disease
		☐	You do NOT have cardiovascular disease **AND** you have type 1 or 2 diabetes **AND** am between 40-75 years old **AND** 10-year cardiovascular risk is 7.5% or above according to the 2013 risk calculator

Moderate-intensity Statins	High-intensity Statins
☐ You do **NOT** have diabetes **AND** age is 40-75 years old **AND** LDL-C 190 mg/dL or above **AND** 10-year cardiovascular risk is 7.5% or above (this is not a typo, this statement should occur in both columns)	☐ You do **NOT** have diabetes **AND** age is 40-75 years old **AND** LDL-C 190 mg/dL or above **AND** 10-year cardiovascular risk is 7.5% or above (this is not a typo, this statement should occur in both columns)
Total # Checked Boxes Above:___	**Total # Checked Boxes Above:**___

If you have more checkmarks in the moderate-intensity column then a moderate-intensity statin from Table 6 is recommended. If you have more checkmarks in the high-intensity column then consider a high-intensity statin from Table 6.

Another Way to Figure Out if You Need a Statin

The ACC/AHA guidelines were developed in 2013, and in the world of healthcare 2013 was quite some time ago. As a result, *many look to the 2017 American Association of Clinical Endocrinologists/American College of Endocrinology (AACE/ACE) guidelines for added guidance*.

The 2017 AACE/ACE guidelines lay out recommendations for the treatment of dyslipidemia based on one's 10-year risk of cardiovascular disease PLUS the number of risk factors one might have.

The 2017 AACE/ACE Steps to Determining Risk and Dyslipidemia Treatment

As mentioned at the beginning of this chapter, you will have the chance to fill in some of your own data as you read this chapter and determine which group of medications may be best for you. If you'd like to record your data for the 2017 guidelines on an easy-to-use worksheet that you can take to your doctor's office, **use the worksheet in Appendix II**.

2017 AACE/ACE *Step 1*: Calculate 10-Year Risk of Cardiovascular Risk

First: According to the 2017 AACE/ACE guidelines, one should calculate their 10-year risk of cardiovascular disease using one of the following online tools.

Table 7: **Tools for Calculating 10-Year Cardiovascular Risk According to 2017 AACE/ACE Guidelines[1]***

One of the following online calculators may be used:
• **Framingham Risk Assessment Tool** (https://www.framinghamheartstudy.org/risk-functions/coronary-heart-disease/hard-10-year-risk.php) • **Multi-Ethnic Study of Atherosclerosis (MESA)** 10-year ASCVD Risk with Coronary Artery Calcification Calculator (https://www.mesa-nhlbi. org/MESACHDRisk/MesaRiskScore/RiskScore.aspx) • **Reynolds Risk Score** (http://www.reynoldsriskscore.org) • **United Kingdom Prospective Diabetes Study (UKPDS)** risk engine to calculate ASCVD risk in individuals with T2DM) (https://www.dtu.ox.ac.uk/riskengine)

*Women should use the Reynolds Risk Score or Framingham Risk Assessment Tool.

TO COMPLETE STEP 1: Determine your 10-year risk

Visit one of the following links mentioned in Table 7 to obtain your risk score.

Write your risk score in below for reference.

My CV Risk Score according to one of the tools in Table 7:	**My Score is _____ %**

2017 AACE/ACE *Step 2*: Determine Your Risk Factors

Below is a list of risk factors for cardiovascular disease as defined by the 2017 AACE/ACE guidelines. You'll notice the risk factors listed below mention something called the dyslipidemic triad. This term refers to a common pattern seen in patients at high risk for cardiovascular disease. Basically, it's low HDL-C, high TG, and small dense LDL-C (which is reflected by LDL-P and/or high Apo B). The dyslipidemic triad is a risk factor for cardiovascular disease.

Again, please refer to Appendix II for an easy, step-by-step worksheet that will help you determine how many risk factors you have.

Let's take a look at the risk factors now.

Table 8: **2017 AACE/ACE Cardiovascular Disease Risk Factors[1]***

	High, Very High, or Extreme Risk Factors
▪	Type 2 diabetes
▪	Have type 1 diabetes: -duration of more than 15 years **OR...** -with 2 or more of the following (albumin in the urine, stage 3 or 4 chronic kidney disease, initiation of intensive control of blood sugar more than 5 years after diagnosis) **OR...** -poorly controlled hemoglobin A1C **OR...** -insulin resistance with metabolic syndrome
	Major Risk Factors
▪	Age (Men 45 years and older and women 55 years and older)
▪	High LDL-C
▪	High Total cholesterol
▪	High non-HDL-C

	High, Very High, or Extreme Risk Factors
■	Family history of cardiovascular disease
■	Low HDL-C
■	High blood pressure
■	Chronic kidney disease
■	Cigarette smoking
	Additional Risk Factors
■	Obesity, abdominal obesity, overweight
■	High LDL-P
■	High Apo B
■	Presence of small, dense LDL-C (indications include: high TG with low HDL-C, insulin resistance, polycystic ovary syndrome (PCOS), high non-HDL-C, and/or high Apo B)
■	High TG
■	Dyslipidemic Triad
■	Family history of dyslipidemia (total, non-HDL-C and/ or LDL-C)
	Non-traditional Risk Factors (all not generally measured)
■	High lipoprotein (a)
■	Increased clotting factors
■	Increased inflammation markers (hsCRP, Lp-PLA2)
■	Increased homocysteine levels
■	Increased uric acid
■	Increased TG-rich remnants (RLP-TG)
_____	**Total # of risk factors checked (from the 'Major', 'Additional' and 'Non-traditional' sections.**

TO COMPLETE STEP 2: Determine your risk factors

Check the boxes in Table 8 that apply. If you checked either of the boxes in the 'High, Very High, or Extreme' risk factor sections, then move on to Step 3. Otherwise, add the number of risk factors that you checked in the 'Major', 'Additional' and 'Non-traditional' risk factor sections.

Now, if you have HDL-C > 60 mg/dL, subtract one risk factor. Record the final number of risk factors in the box below:

Number of risk factors	My Score is _____ risk factors

2017 AACE/ACE *Step 3*: Determine Your Treatment Goals

The 2013 ACC/AHA guidelines did not give much guidance on treatment goals. They are pretty clear on who should start a statin, but don't give an indication of what goal one should strive for. For example, there is no indication as to what LDL-C, non-HDL-C or Apo B one should strive to achieve.

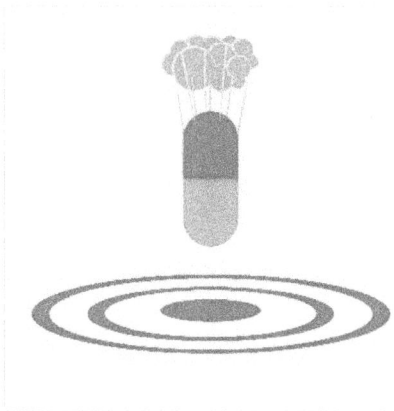

The 2017 AACE/ACE guidelines **DO** give us more guidance on treatment goals. *Based on one's 10-year risk level (calculated by using one of the online tools listed in Table 7) combined with one's risk factors, it gives an idea of what numbers one should strive to achieve.*

Table 11: **Lipid Goals Based on Risk of Cardiovascular Disease from the 2017 Guidelines**[1]

Risk Category	Risk Factors/ Calculated Risk	TC (mg/dL)	LDL-C (mg/dL)	Non-HDL-C (mg/dL)	Apo B (mg/dL)	TG (mg/dL)	HDL (mg/dL)
Low	• No risk factors	< 200	< 130	< 160	No recommendation	<150	>40 or as high as possible (>60 is best)
Mode-rate	• 2 or less risk factors and calculated 10-year risk < 10%	< 200	< 100	< 130	< 90	<150	>40 or as high as possible (>60 is best)
High	• Cardiovascular equivalent including diabetes or stage 3 or 4 chronic kidney disease with no other risk factors **OR**… • Individuals with 2 or more risk factors **and** a 10-year risk of 10% - 20%	< 200	< 100	< 130	< 90	<150	>40 or as high as possible (>60 is best)
Very High	• Established or recent hospitalization for acute coronary syndrome (ACS) **OR**… • Coronary, carotid or peripheral vascular disease, diabetes, or stage 3 or 4 CKD **with** 1 or more risk factors **OR**… • Calculated 10-year risk greater than 20% or… • Heterozygous familial hypercholester-olemia [HeFH])	< 200	< 70	< 100	< 80	<150	>40 or as high as possible (>60 is best)

Risk Category	Risk Factors/ Calculated Risk	TC (mg/dL)	LDL-C (mg/dL)	Non-HDL-C (mg/dL)	Apo B (mg/dL)	TG (mg/dL)	HDL (mg/dL)
Extreme	• Cardiovascular disease including unstable angina that persists after achieving an LDL-C <70 mg/dL **OR**… • established cardiovascular disease with diabetes, stage 3 or 4 CKD, **and/or** heterozygous familial hypercholesterolemia (HeFH) **OR**… • History of premature cardiovascular disease (<55 years of age for males or <65 years of age for females)	< 200	< 55	< 80	< 70	<150	>40 or as high as possible (>60 is best)

Note which risk category you fall into above.

TO COMPLETE STEP 3: Determine your treatment goals

Record which risk category you fall into here based on Table 10:

		My lipid goals:
■ Low Risk	LDL-C goal is < 130 mg/dL	TC = _____
■ Moderate Risk	LDL-C goal is < 100 mg/dL	*LDL-C* = _____ Non-HDL-C = _____
■ High Risk	LDL-C goal is < 100 mg/dL	Apo B = _____ TG = _____
■ Very High Risk	LDL-C goal is < 70 mg/dL	HDL = _____
■ Extreme Risk	LDL-C goal is < 55 mg/dL	

31

2017 AACE/ACE *STEP 4*: Determine How Much You Need to Lower Your Current LDL-C to Achieve Your Goal LDL-C

Ok so there's a little math involved here. You can also look to Appendix II of this book. It will take you through this process step by step.

You are going to calculate the % by which you need to lower your current LDL-C to meet your goal LDL-C. To do this, you will need to obtain your most recent LDL-C. You may need to get your most recent lab report from your doctor. Then you will need to **subtract your goal LDL-C (in Table 10) from your current LDL-C.**

Next you will **divide this number by your current LDL-C.** Finally, you will **multiply this number by 100**. This answer will equal the % by which you need to lower your current LDL-C to meet your goal LDL-C.

TO COMPLETE STEP 4: Determine how much you need to lower your current LDL-C

1. Subtract your LDL-C goal from your last LDL-C measurement

Last LDL-C - LDL-C goal	= _____
Example: 150 - 100	= 50

Divide you answer by your last LDL-C

Your answer ÷ Last LDL-C	= _____
Example: 50 ÷ 150	= 0.33

Now, multiply your answer by 100

Your answer X 100	= _____ **%**
Example: **0.33 X 100**	= **33%** **This is the % you need to reduce your current LDL-C to meet your goal LDL-C**

2017 AACE/ACE *STEP 5*: Determine which statin will give you the % reduction in LDL-C you need in order to achieve your LDL-C goal

TO COMPLETE STEP 5: Put a check in the box that matches the % decrease you just calculated. It is recommended that you choose a statin from this group.

Table 11: **Statins Grouped by % Decrease in LDL-C**

Low-intensity Statins	Moderate-intensity Statins	High-intensity Statins
▪ **Lowers LDL-C by less than 30%**	▪ **Lowers LDL-C by 30-50%**	▪ **Lowers LDL-C by more than 50%**
Simvastatin 10 mg	Atorvastatin 10-20 mg	Atorvastatin 40-80 mg
Pravastatin 10-20 mg	Rosuvastatin 5-10 mg	Rosuvastatin 20 to 40 mg
Lovastatin 20 mg	Simvastatin 20-40 mg	
Fluvastatin 20-40 mg	Pravastatin 40-80 mg	
Pitavastatin 1 mg	Lovastatin 40 mg	
	Fluvastatin XL 80 mg	
	Fluvastatin 40 mg twice daily	
	Pitavastatin 2-4 mg	

This box that you checked indicates the group of statins that you are to pick from. Discuss the choices in this group with your doctor and/or pharmacist. Drug-drug interactions and side effects of these medications should be considered.

2017 AACE/ACE *STEP 6*: Determine if other medications are needed

The 2017 guidelines recommend using other medications other than statins, if deemed necessary, to help treat dyslipidemia (for example, to help lower triglycerides or raise HDL). We will summarize them here and look at them in a little more detail in a moment.

TO COMPLETE STEP 6: Talk with your doctor to see if you may need additional medications to lower triglycerides or increase HDL-C.

Table 12: **Other Medications for the Treatment of Dyslipidemia**

Fibrates
• Gemfibrozil (Lopid®)
• Fenofibrate (Antara®, Lipofen® Lofibra®, Tricor® and Triglide®)
Fish Oil
• Prescription omega–3 fish oil
Niacin
• Niacin
Bile acid sequestrants
• Cholestyramine (Questran®, Prevalite®)
• Colestipol (Colestid®)
• Colesevelam (Welchol®)
Cholesterol absorption inhibitors
• Ezetimibe (Zetia®)
PCSK9 Inhibitors
• Alirocumab (Praluent®)
• Evolocumab (Repatha®)
MTP Inhibitors
• Lomitapide (Juxtapid®)
Antisense Apolipoprotein B Oligonucleotide
• Mipomersen (Kynamro®)

What Do I Do with This Information?

So what were the results of your assessments? Did both sets (2013 and 2017) of guidelines recommend the same group of statins for you? You are encouraged to take this information with you to your doctor to discuss the results.

Key to Success

Consider using information from these risk assessments combined with items such as your LDL-P, non-HDL-C, Apo B level, cardiovascular health, weight, and family history to determine if a statin or other cholesterol medication is for you. Information from this assessment should be discussed with your doctor so that a customized plan of treatment can be outlined for you. Remember that statins and other cholesterol medications carry the risk of certain side effects.

The medications listed above should be used in conjunction with lifestyle modifications like eating healthy, increasing physical activity, and quitting tobacco products.

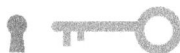

Now that we've looked at each set of guidelines, let's take a closer look at the medications available to treat dyslipidemia.

Medications

The 2013 ACC/AHA guidelines recommend focusing on statins to reduce LDL-C. They assert that using the highest dose tolerated of a medium-intensity or high-intensity statin is necessary to see results. They believe that trying to change the dose to achieve a goal LDL-C could result in under-treatment. They also emphasize that statins should be used in conjunction with lifestyle modifications such as eating a healthy diet and increasing physical activity. The

2013 guidelines emphasize that lifestyle modifications and statin adherence should be emphasized before non-statin drugs are added to therapy.[6]

The 2017 AACE/ACE guidelines also recommend a combination of medications and lifestyle modifications, but they state that this should be to achieve certain cholesterol goals (see Table 9). Also in contrast to the 2013 guidelines, the 2017 guidelines say that it's ok to use non-statin drugs, if needed.

When beginning any of the therapies below, seek emergency medical attention immediately if you have any of the following symptoms:

- Hives
- Difficulty breathing
- Swelling of the face, lips, tongue, or throat

Here is a rundown of cholesterol medications.

Statins

As mentioned earlier, examples of statins include atorvastatin (Lipitor®), fluvastatin (Lescol®), lovastatin (Mevacor®, Altocor®), pitavastatin (Livalo®), pravastatin (Pravachol®), simvastatin (Zocor®), and rosuvastatin (Crestor®).

Statins are a class of medications (also called HMG-CoA reductase Inhibitors). Statin drugs are recommended by the 2013 ACC/AHA and 2017 AACE/ACE guidelines as the primary medications that should be used to treat dyslipidemia.[1, 6] They can lower LDL-C by 21 to 55%. They can decrease triglycerides by anywhere from 6 to 30%. They also may increase HDL-C by 2 to 10%.[1]

According to the 2017 guidelines, those in the high risk and very high-risk categories may consider lowering their LDL-C below the targets mentioned in Table 9 as some studies have shown this to further decrease the risk of cardiovascular events (like heart attack and stroke). [1]

Side Effects

- Liver problems, nerve problems, and muscle pain.
    - o It is a good idea to get a baseline measurement of your liver enzymes so that your liver function can be monitored if you begin having symptoms of liver toxicity (tiredness, weakness, loss of appetite, dark-colored urine, yellowing of the skin or eyes).[6]
- Raised blood sugar levels and type 2 diabetes
    - o Although they appear to be less frequent with pravastatin or pitavastatin.[1]
    - o The risk of developing increased blood sugar and type 2 diabetes by using statins does not outweigh the benefits of using a statin according to the guidelines. [1]
    - o People taking statins should be screened for new-onset diabetes according to the newest diabetes guidelines. If diabetes develops, they encourage one to continue to statin therapy and focus on adhering to a heart healthy diet and increase physical activity. One is also encouraged to maintain a healthy body weight and avoid tobacco.[6]
- Rhabdomyolysis
    - o A rare, serious condition called rhabdomyolysis can occur. This is where muscle fibers break down, releasing proteins into the blood that can damage the kidneys.
    - o Report any muscle pain to your doctor while you are taking a statin.
    - o Your doctor may want to measure your creatine kinase (CK) level.[6] This can tell him/her if the pain might be due to rhabdomyolysis.

o The 2013 authors also advise stopping the statin following symptoms of rhabdomyolysis such as extreme fatigue or muscle pain.[6]
- Finally, if confusion or memory loss develops while taking a statin, the you should be evaluated by your doctor for a variety of causes, including statin use.[6]

If a statin is started in someone > 75 years old, caution is advised especially, if they are taking medications that interact with the statin which can potentially increase the risk of side effects.[20]

Fibrates

Examples of fibrates include gemfibrozil (Lopid®), fenofibrate (Antara®, Lipofen® Lofibra®, Tricor® and Triglide®). According to the 2017 AACE/ACE guidelines, fibrates should be used to lower triglycerides when they are > 500 mg/dL. They should also be considered when triglycerides are 200 mg/dL or more.[1]

Fibrates can lower triglycerides by 20 to 35%. They can also increase HDL-C by 6 to 18%. However, fibrates may cause an actual net increase in LDL-C by 10 to 15% which may seem bad at first, but it is thought that the lipid profile is transformed so that it contains larger, less harmful LDL-C particles.[1]

Side Effects

Possible side effects include:
- Upset stomach, nausea, diarrhea, gall bladder stones, and muscle disorders.
- Possible kidney dysfunction
  - o Kidney function should be measured before starting fenofibrate therapy, 3 months after starting, and every 6 months thereafter.
  - o Fenofibrate should not be used if one's glomerular filtration rate (GFR, a measure of kidney function) is < 30 mL/min.

- o If the GFR is 30 to 59 mL/min, the dose should be reduced.[6]
- Rhabdomyolysis
  - o Gemfibrozil should not be started in people taking statin therapy because of an increased risk for rhabdomyolysis.
  - o Fenofibrate may be considered in people taking low to moderate intensity statins when triglycerides are > 500 mg/dL if the patient and physician decide the benefits of therapy outweigh the potential for side effects. [6]
- Gemfibrozil may actually help improve diabetic retinopathy (a condition in diabetes where the retina in the eye is damaged leading to vision problems).[1]

Omega–3 Fish Oil

Prescription (2 to 4 grams per day) omega–3 fish oil is recommended when triglycerides are > 500 mg/dL.[1] Over-the-counter fish oil is NOT recommended in the guidelines because, by law, over-the-counter drugs cannot make claims to treat or cure disease. Thus they stick with the recommendation to use prescription fish oil instead.

Omega–3 fish oil can lower triglycerides by 27 to 45 %, total cholesterol by 7 to 10%, VLDL-C by 20 to 42%, and Apo B by 4%. The guidelines recommend that LDL-C be monitored closely while taking fish oil because omega–3 fatty acids can actually increase LDL-C by as much as 45%.[1] It is thought that even though fish oil can increase LDL-C, it may transform it into the larger, less clot-provoking kind that doesn't increase one's risk of cardiovascular disease.

Side Effects

- Prolonged bleeding time
  - o Omega–3 fish oil can prolong bleeding time and should be used with caution with patient's using

blood thinners or a history of bleeding (like brain or stomach bleeds).
- o If you notice signs of bleeding (like a nosebleed or dark, tarry stools), let your doctor know right away.
- Allergic reactions
  - o People who have allergies to fish or shellfish should use fish oil cautiously.
- Aggravation of atrial fibrillation
  - o Omega–3 fish oil can aggravate atrial fibrillation (a. fib.) in people who have a. fib.
- Other common side effects include joint pain, belching, heartburn, indigestion, nausea, loose stools, taste changes, constipation, vomiting, rash, and itching.

Niacin

Niacin is recommended as an adjunct (in addition to) fibrates and fish oil to help lower triglycerides. The guidelines say that niacin should NOT be used in people aggressively treated with a statin because studies failed to show added benefit of adding niacin to a statin.[1]

Niacin should be started at a low dose then slowly increased over a period of weeks. It should be taken with food.

It can decrease LDL-C by 10 to 25%. It is thought to transform LDL-C particles to the less damaging, larger size. It is also thought to decrease LDL particle concentration. It may also decrease triglycerides by 20 to 30 % and increase HDL-C by 10 to 35%.[1]

Side Effects

- Skin flushing.
  - o Ask your doctor if taking aspirin 325mg before your niacin dose to prevent skin flushing symptoms is ok.[6]

> o Discontinue niacin if severe skin symptoms occur[6]

- Itching
- Nausea, peptic ulcer, abdominal discomfort
- Atrial fibrillation
  - o Discontinue niacin if new atrial fibrillation occurs[6]
- Increased uric acid levels that can lead to gout.
  - o Uric acid should be measured prior to starting niacin
- Liver dysfunction
  - o It is recommended that your doctor obtain baseline liver function tests prior to therapy and during therapy
  - o Niacin should not be used if liver function tests are 2 to 3 times the upper normal limit
- Increased blood sugar
  - o Fasting blood glucose or hemoglobin A1C (to measure blood sugar control) should be measured before starting niacin. These should also be checked every 6 months after starting niacin.[6]
- Discontinue niacin if persistent high blood sugar occurs[6]

Bile Acid Sequestrants

Examples of bile acid sequestrants include cholestyramine (Questran®, Prevalite®), colestipol (Colestid®), and colesevelam (Welchol®). These drugs can be considered when help decreasing LDL-C and Apo B are desired. They may also increase HDL-C. On the down side, they may increase triglycerides.[1]

These medications can lower LDL-C by 15 to 25%. Colesevelam may actually decrease blood sugar levels and improve hemoglobin A1C by 0.5%; therefore, it is also FDA approved to treat type 2 diabetes.[1]

Side Effects

Since they stay in the gut and are not absorbed, they do not cause many side effects.

- Increased triglycerides
    - Bile acid sequestrants should not be used in people with triglyceride levels 300 mg/dL or greater.
    - A fasting lipid panel should be obtained before starting therapy and then every 6 to 12 months thereafter.
    - If baseline triglycerides are 250 to 299 mg/dL, another fasting lipid panel should be obtained 4 to 6 weeks after starting treatment. [6]
- Constipation, bloating, flatulence, and diarrhea are potential side effects.
- They may also reduce the absorption of folic acid and fat-soluble vitamins like vitamin A, D and K.

Cholesterol Absorption Inhibitors

Ezetimibe (Zetia®) may be used alone or in combination with a statin to reduce LDL-C and Apo- B[1]. It may be a good choice for people who cannot tolerate statins.

Ezetimibe can lower LDL-C by 10 to 18%. It can decrease Apo B 11 to 16%. In combination with statins or fenofibrate, LDL-C can be lowered even more.[1]

Side Effects

- Muscle pain and rhabdomyolysis
    - These are rare with this drug, but when given with a statin, the risk of these side effects goes up.

- Numbness, tingling
- Stomach pain, diarrhea
- Fatigue, headache, dizziness
- Depression, cold symptoms, and joint and/or back pain.
- Liver dysfunction
    - Your doctor may want to obtain baseline liver function tests before starting ezetimibe therapy, especially if a statin is also being prescribed. Ezetimibe should be stopped if ALT (one of the liver enzymes) increases to over 3 times the upper normal limit.[6]

PCSK9 Inhibitors

These are newer lipid-lowering drugs. Examples of these drugs include alirocumab (Praluent®) and evolocumab (Repatha®). They are typically used when statins don't work. These drugs appear to affect the immune system.

PCSK9 Inhibitors can lower LDL-C by 48 to 71% and lower on-HDL-C by 49 to 58%. They can also lower total cholesterol by 36 to 42% and decrease Apo B by 42 to 55%.[1]

One downfall is these drugs require subcutaneous self-injection. They usually need to be refrigerated. They may also be expensive.

Side Effects

- Joint pain, muscle pain, injection site reactions
- Headache
- Fatigue
- Trouble swallowing
- Reddening of the skin
- Fever, Influenza, bronchitis, and urinary tract infections.
- Diarrhea

MTP Inhibitors

Lomitapide (Juxtapid®) is approved as an additional lipid-lowering agent in people with genetically high lipid levels (homozygous familial hypercholesterolemia (HoFH)). It can decrease LDL-C up to 40%, decrease total cholesterol by 36%, decrease Apo B by 39%, decrease non-HDL-C by 40%, and decrease triglycerides by 45%.[1]

Side Effects

- Liver dysfunction
    - The FDA requires that liver enzymes be reported by your prescriber through a special reporting program while you are prescribed the medication.
    - Lomitapide can cause a condition called 'fatty liver' where excess fat is stored in the liver.
- It can also cause fatty deposits in the small intestine which can cause abdominal pain, vomiting, gas, diarrhea, constipation, weight loss, and fatty stools.
- Lomitapide can also cause fat-soluble vitamin deficiency, so taking vitamin supplements while on this medication is recommended. [1]
- Stop using lomitapide and call your doctor immediately if you have any of the following symptoms of liver dysfunction:
    - Nausea
    - Fatigue
    - Dark urine
    - Clay-colored stools
    - Yellowing of the skin or eyes

Antisense Apolipoprotein B Oligonucleotide

That's a mouthful! Mipomersen (Kynamro®) is also used to treat homozygous familial hypercholesterolemia (HoFH). This is an inherited condition that leads to dyslipidemia. It is given by subcutaneous injection.

Mipomersen can decrease LDL-C by 21%, decrease total cholesterol by 19%, decrease non-HDL-C by 22% and decrease Apo B by 24%.[1]

Side Effects

- Liver dysfunction, fatty liver
  - Like with lomitapide, prescribers must enroll in a special program that requires them to report your liver enzymes while they are prescribed the medication because there is such a high risk of liver damage. [1]
- Nausea, headache, and fatigue. [1]
- Stop mipomersen and call your doctor if you experience any of the following symptoms:
  - Flu symptoms
  - Joint pain
  - Pain, swelling, bruising where the injection was given
  - Symptoms of liver dysfunction:
  - Nausea
  - Fatigue
  - Dark urine
  - Clay-colored stools
  - Yellowing of the skin or eyes

Diet and Exercise: The Best Medicine

Both the 2013 and 2017 guidelines agree that lifestyle modifications such as avoiding tobacco products, maintaining a healthy weight, and healthy amounts of physical activity are critical to reducing the risk of cardiovascular disease.[1, 6] The 2017 AACE/ACE Guidelines tell us that a healthy approach to lipid management should include lifestyle modifications, such as eating a healthy diet and getting plenty of physical activity. They go on to recommend at least 30 minutes of moderate-intensity physical activity, 4 to 6 times a week. They define moderate-intensity activities as those that burn at least 200 calories (or about 4-7 calories per minute).[1]

The physical activity mentioned above can be accomplished in one 30-minute session or broken up into several 10 minutes sessions throughout the day.[1] Physical activity doesn't have be to be boring-old exercise, although exercise (like going to the gym) is fine if you prefer it. Moderate-intensity activities include walking at a fast pace, riding a bike, scrubbing the bathtub, mowing the lawn, or playing sports. These are activities that raise your heart rate but can be sustained for a period of time.

In addition to the physical activity described above, strength training at least 2 days a week is recommended.[1] Strength training uses resistance to build muscle and increase strength. This resistance can be accomplished several different ways. Examples include lifting weights, using your own weight as resistance (like with pushups), or using exercise bands.

It is recommended that adults partake in a reduced-calorie diet rich in fruits and vegetables (at least 5 servings per day), whole grains, fish, and lean meat. Adults should limit saturated fats, trans fats, and cholesterol. Plant stanols/sterols (about 2 grams per day) are encouraged. Foods that contain plant sterols include cereals, legumes, nuts, seeds, fruits, and vegetables. They also recommend 10-25 grams of soluble fiber per day.

The Best Bang for Your Buck

So which options are the most cost-effective? In other words, where can you get the best bang for your buck? Well measures like changing one's diet and increasing physical activity are the cheapest options if protection against cardiovascular events is the goal. When these options aren't enough, lipid-lowering medications are recommended.

Both the 2013 and 2017 guidelines agree that statins appear to be the most cost-effective medications for those seeking to decrease their risk of cardiovascular events. This goes for people who have or have not already had a cardiovascular event.[1, 6]

If lowering triglycerides and raising HDL-C is the goal, fibrates are cost-effective options according to the 2017 guidelines. They can be used alone or in combination with other lipid-lowering agents. However, even though they lower triglycerides and raise HDL-C, they do not actually reduce the number of heart attacks or strokes unless one's triglycerides is > 200 mg/dL and HDL-C is < 40 mg/dL.[1]

The 2013 guidelines do not recommend routinely using other medications in addition to statins because they believe there is insufficient evidence to show they add any additional decrease in cardiovascular events.[6]

Studies in Canada and the United Kingdom have shown the combination of ezetimibe with a statin to be cost-effective in lowering LDL-C and reducing the number of cardiovascular events according to the 2017 guidelines.[1]

Despite the lower cost of generic medications, bile acids sequestrants are not considered by the 2017 guidelines to be cost-effective LDL-C lowering agents when compared to statins.[1]

How Often Should One Be Screened for Cardiovascular Disease?

The 2013 ACC/AHA and 2017 AACE/ACE guidelines give us some direction on how often we should be screened for cardiovascular risk. They have this to say about how people should be screened:

1. Young adults in their 20's[1]

- Should be evaluated every 5 years (or more frequently if there is a family history of heart attack or sudden death before age 55 in first-degree male relative).

- More frequent assessments may be necessary if risk factors for cardiovascular disease are present.

- Young adults with diabetes should get a lipid screening and lipid panel done at the time of diabetes diagnosis. If the LDL-C is < 100 mg/dL, then it's reasonable to repeat the lipid panel every 3 to 5 years.

2. Middle-aged adults (men 45-64 years old and women 55-64 years old) [1,6]

- Middle-aged individuals should be screened every 1 to 2 years.

- More frequent screening is recommended when multiple risk factors are present.

- Middle-aged adults with diabetes should get a lipid screening and lipid panel performed at the time of diabetes diagnosis, and then yearly thereafter.

3. Men and women over 65 years old

- It is recommended that all adults 65 to 75 years old with 0 to 1 cardiovascular risk factors should be screened annually for dyslipidemia.

4. People should be screened to see if dyslipidemia is in their family (familial hypercholesterolemia (FH)) when there is a family history of:

- Premature cardiovascular disease (history of a heart attack or sudden death before age 55 years in father or other male first-degree relative, or before age 65 years in mother or other female first-degree relative), or

- Dyslipidemia (total, non-HDL-C and/ or LDL-C) consistent with FH

How Often Should One Follow-up with the Doctor After Starting Treatment?

Here is what the 2017 guidelines have to say about follow up and monitoring of lipid therapy: [1]

1. One should generally be reassessed 6 weeks after starting therapy and at 6-week intervals until the treatment goal is achieved.

2. Once stable, one should be tested every 6 to 12 months. More frequent lipid testing should be considered in situations where changes that may affect lipid control occur such as a change in medications or change in weight or health condition.

3. If taking niacin or fibric acid, liver function should be checked within 3 months of starting treatment and then periodically thereafter.

4. If taking a statin, creatine kinase should be measured if muscle pain is experienced.

What Does It All Mean?

Well it is disturbing that lipid-lowering interventions are aimed at the population (older adults) that, according to some data, could be negatively affected. As discussed above, some data shows *decreased LDL-C levels* in those over 50 years old may be associated with an *increased* risk of death. Should those over 50 years old continue to take their lipid-lowering agent (most likely a statin drug)?

As discussed, when it comes to one's risk of heart attack or stroke, there may be more going on in one's body then just high LDL-C. Other tests such as LDL-P, non-HDL-C, and Apo B can be helpful in determining what's going on and if you are truly at risk for cardiovascular disease. Recall the information from Table 3 that suggests those with high LDL-C and low LDL-P appear to be at low risk. Those with low LDL-C and high LDL-P appear to be at high risk.[7] Also, other factors like family history, the presence of diabetes, and maintaining a healthy weight also come into play.

Whatever you do, do not stop taking your statin or other lipid-lowering medication without speaking with your doctor. It is recommended that you and your doctor consider all of the data and come up with a treatment plan together that not only involves monitoring your LDL-C, but perhaps also your Apo B, non-HDL-C, triglycerides, and other tests. The 2013 and 2017 guideline criteria for determining risk of cardiovascular disease is a good starting point. When interpreting your risk level from these guidelines, also consider other lab tests discussed above. Everyone is different and the point of the guidelines is not to be a 'one size fits all' standard. The intention is to look at the whole picture, including your

The Bottom Line

Refer to Appendix I and II for step-by-step worksheets that will help you determine which cholesterol therapies may be right for you.

When learning about high cholesterol, you may hear a term called 'hyperlipidemia' used. Hyperlipidemia is just a fancy word for high cholesterol. '*Hyper*' literally means *high*, '*lipid*' means *fat* and '*emia*' means in the *blood*. So '**hyperlipidemia**' means 'a **high amount of fats in the blood**'.

'*Dyslipidemia*' is an even better description because it has now been learned that some of the people who may be at high risk for heart attack and stroke don't have high cholesterol (high LDL-C); they may actually have low cholesterol.[7] '*Dys*' means *abnormal*. So '**dyslipidemia**' means '**abnormal fats in the blood**'.

'Arteriosclerotic cardiovascular disease (ASCVD)' or just **'cardiovascular disease'** refer to the clogging of the arteries throughout the body, particularly in the heart and brain. When the cells of the heart are deprived of oxygen long enough, fatal arrhythmias (deadly irregular heart beat or rhythms) can happen. When the cells of the brain are deprived of oxygen, a stroke can happen.

'Cardiovascular events' or **'arteriosclerotic cardiovascular disease (ASCVD')** refer to a group of events that are known to be caused by the blockage of blood flow to various areas of the body (namely heart attack, angina, stroke, transient ischemic attack (TIA), and peripheral arterial disease).

In order for your doctor to determine if you are at risk for heart attack or stroke, he/she may order a blood lipid panel for you to have done at a lab. This will involve drawing some blood. You will need to fast (eat or drink nothing except for water) approximately 8 to 12 hours prior to the test.

Commonly Ordered types of blood lipid tests that may be drawn at a lab

- **Total cholesterol**-The total cholesterol, including 'good' and 'bad' cholesterol, in your blood stream.

- **LDL-C AKA 'bad' cholesterol**-This type of cholesterol is believed to play a big role in the formation of blockages in the arteries; however, it's now recognized that LDL-C alone may not be the best measure of one's risk for heart attack or stroke.

- **HDL-C AKA 'good' cholesterol**-This type of cholesterol helps keep blockages from forming in the arteries. You want this number to be at least 40 mg/dL or as high as possible (> 60 mg/dL is best). Things that can make this number go up include increased physical activity, weight loss, quitting tobacco, and statin drugs.

- **VLDL-C**-There is no easy way to measure VLDL-C so it is usually estimated as a percentage of your triglycerides. High VLDL-C has been implicated in the production of artery-clogging plaques. You can help lower VLDL-C by lowering triglycerides.

- **<u>Triglycerides (TG)</u>**-Your body converts calories you don't eat into triglycerides a type of fat in the blood. Eating more calories than your body can use on a regular basis can lead to high triglycerides. High triglycerides indicate a higher risk of cardiovascular disease. High triglycerides are commonly found in those with metabolic syndrome and diabetes. Metabolic syndrome is a group of conditions found in one person that include abdominal obesity, high blood pressure, dyslipidemia, and increased blood clotting. Metabolic syndrome appears to be a product of insulin-resistance and is a precursor to type 2 diabetes.

- **<u>Apo B</u>**-Apo B represents the number of blockage-forming particles in the blood, similar to LDL-P.

- **<u>LDL-P</u>**-LDL-P represents the number of blockage-forming particles in the blood, similar to Apo B.

- **<u>Non-HDL-C</u>**--*Equal to Total cholesterol minus HDL-C.* This represents the number of ALL blockage-forming particles in the blood. This is nice because it does not require another test outside of a basic lipid panel.

Until recently, it was believed that LDL-C was the best marker to indicate who may be at risk for cardiovascular disease and death. However, we are now finding that **LDL-C alone may not be the best marker to evaluate one's risk of cardiovascular disease.**[7]

It has been proposed that the cholesterol particles in our blood are much like cars driving down a narrow road. LDL-C measures the amount of cholesterol contained in the LDL particles. So LDL-C measures the 'number of passengers in the cars'. LDL-P (number of LDL particles) measures the 'number of cars' on the road. **Studies show that it is the number of cars on the road (LDL-P), not the number of passengers in the cars (LDL-C), that may better predict one's risk of developing cardiovascular disease.**[7] Logic says that the more cars on the road, the more likely some of them will crash into the walls (of the arteries). Once LDL particles start 'sticking' to the sides of the arteries, blockages can form. As mentioned above, blockages can cut off the oxygen-rich blood supply, causing a heart attack or a stroke.

With all of this in mind, when a person gets their LDL-C measured and their LDL-C is low, they may believe that they are at low risk for cardiovascular disease. However, this may not be the case. Measuring LDL-P or Apo B could help more accurately determine if one is at high risk. *People with low LDL-C and high LDL-P appear to be at very high risk for cardiovascular disease* because their LDL-P is elevated even though their LDL-C is low.[7]

People with high LDL-C but low LDL-P appear to be at a low risk of cardiovascular disease.[7] Unfortunately, these people are very likely to be prescribed a statin because of their high LDL-C. Statins are not without side effects. Liver dysfunction, nerves problems, and serious muscle conditions are potential side effects of statins.

Summary of Blood Lipid Findings

Cholesterol		Potential Risk
LDL-C↑	LDL-P↓	Low risk
LDL-C↓	LDL-P↓	Low risk
LDL-C↑	LDL-P↑	High risk
LDL-C↓	LDL-P ↑	High risk

Measuring Apo B has been proposed to help determine one's risk of cardiovascular disease. Each of these clot-containing particles carries only one Apo B molecule; so the total Apo B level reflects the total number of circulating clot-causing particles.

Apo B basically tells us how many LDL particles (LDL-P) there are. Fasting is not required for Apo B testing.

There are 2 main sets of guidelines that health providers look to when diagnosing and treating dyslipidemia. These are the *2013 American College of Cardiology/American Heart Association (ACC/AHA) guidelines* and the *2017 American Association of Clinical Endocrinologists/American College of Endocrinology (AACE/ACE) guidelines*.

Again, refer to Appendix I and II for step-by-step worksheets that will help you determine which cholesterol therapies may be right for you.

The 2013 ACC/AHA Lipid Guidelines

The 2013 ACC/AHA Lipid Guidelines Note There are 4 Groups of People Who Should Take a Statin Drug: [6]

1. Anyone with cardiovascular disease, including angina, previous heart attack, or stroke.

2. Anyone with very high LDL-C (190 mg/dL or above)

3. Anyone with type 2 diabetes between 40 and 75 years old with LDL-C 70-189 mg/dL and without cardiovascular disease

4. Anyone without cardiovascular disease or diabetes, between 40 to 75 years old with a 10-year risk of heart attack or stroke greater than 7.5% (according to the 2013 risk calculator).

These 4 groups are meant to include people who have not had a heart attack or stroke, but who may be at risk for one. These groups also include people who have had a heart attack or stroke who ***do not have heart failure and are not receiving hemodialysis***.

The 2013 ACC/AHA Lipid guidelines attempt to figure out how intense statin therapy should be based on your risk score (obtained by visiting www.cvriskcalculator.com) and answers to some questions about other health conditions.

Here is a breakdown of who should take medium intensity and who should take high intensity statins (from the 2013 guidelines). [6]

Those *with* cardiovascular disease

- Take a high-intensity statin if age is less than or equal to 75 years old.

- Take a medium-intensity statin if age is over 75 years old

Those *without* cardiovascular disease

Take a high-intensity statin if:

- LDL-C is greater than or equal to 190 mg/dL
- You have type 1 or 2 diabetes, age is 40-75 years old and have 10-year cardiovascular risk greater than or equal to 7.5% according to the 2013 risk calculator.

Take a medium-intensity statin if:

- LDL-C is less than 90 mg/dL, you have type 1 or 2 diabetes and age is 40-75 years old and 10-year cardiovascular risk less than 7.5%

Consider a medium- or high-intensity statin if:

- You don't have diabetes, age is 40-75 years old <u>and</u> LDL-C is less than or equal to 190 mg/dL <u>and</u> 10-year cardiovascular risk is greater than or equal to 7.5%

Breakdown of Moderate and High-intensity Statins

Moderate-intensity Statins	High-intensity Statins
Lowers LDL-C by 30-50%	Lowers LDL-C by more than 50%
Atorvastatin 10-20 mg	Atorvastatin 40-80 mg
Rosuvastatin 5-10 mg	Rosuvastatin 20-40 mg
Simvastatin 20-40 mg	
Pravastatin 40-80 mg	
Lovastatin 40 mg	
Fluvastatin XL 80 mg	
Fluvastatin 40 mg twice daily	
Pitavastatin 2-4 mg	

The 2013 guidelines note that the addition of other therapies (like niacin) to statins can help lower LDL–C, but they did not further reduce cardiovascular events in studies. Therefore, other medications besides statins are not generally recommended in the 2013 guidelines because it is believed that the benefit of using them does not outweigh the potential for side effects.

The 2017 AACE/ACE Guidelines

The 2017 AACE/ACE guidelines help you determine which cholesterol medications may be right for you based on your cardiovascular risk score and your risk factors. First, they have you calculate your 10-Year Cardiovascular Risk using one of the online tools listed below[1]*

Online Risk Calculators Preferred by the 2017 AACE/ACE Guidelines

- **Framingham Risk Assessment Tool** (https://www.framinghamheartstudy.org/risk-functions/coronary-heart-disease/hard-10-year-risk.php)
- **Multi-Ethnic Study of Atherosclerosis (MESA)** 10-year ASCVD Risk with Coronary Artery Calcification Calculator (https://www.mesa-nhlbi. org/MESACHDRisk/MesaRiskScore/RiskScore.aspx)
- **Reynolds Risk Score** (http://www.reynoldsriskscore.org)
- **United Kingdom Prospective Diabetes Study (UKPDS)** risk engine to calculate ASCVD risk in individuals with T2DM) (https://www.dtu.ox.ac.uk/riskengine)

*Women should use the Reynolds Risk Score or Framingham Risk Assessment.

The 2017 AACE/ACE guidelines then have you look at how many risk factors you have.

2017 AACE/ACE Guidelines Risk Factors

High, Very High, or Extreme Risk Factors
Type 2 diabetes

Have type 1 diabetes:
 -duration of more than 15 years **OR...**
     -with 2 or more of the following (albumin in the urine, stage 3 or 4 chronic kidney disease, initiation of intensive control of blood sugar more than 5 years after diagnosis) **OR...**
     -poorly controlled hemoglobin A1C **OR...**
     -insulin resistance with metabolic syndrome

Major Risk Factors
Age (Men 45 years and older and women 55 years and older)
High LDL-C
High total cholesterol
High non-HDL-C
Family history of cardiovascular disease
Low HDL-C
Diabetes
High blood pressure
Chronic kidney disease
Cigarette smoking
Additional Risk Factors
Obesity, abdominal obesity, overweight
High LDL-P
High Apo B
Presence of small, dense LDL-C (indications include: high TG with low HDL-C, insulin resistance, polycystic ovary syndrome (PCOS), high non-HDL-C, and/or high Apo B)
High TG
Dyslipidemic Triad
Family history of dyslipidemia (total, non-HDL-C and/ or LDL-C)
Non-traditional Risk Factors (all not generally measured)
High lipoprotein (a)
Increased clotting factors
Increased inflammation markers (hsCRP, Lp-PLA2)
Increased homocysteine levels
Increased uric acid
Increased TG-rich remnants (RLP-TG)

The 2017 AACE/ACE guidelines then have you see what risk category you fall into.

2017 AACE/ACE Guidelines Risk Categories	
Risk Category	**Risk Factors/ Calculated Risk**
Low	• No risk factors
Moderate	• 2 or less risk factors <u>and</u> calculated 10-year risk < 10%
High	• Cardiovascular equivalent including diabetes or stage 3 or 4 chronic kidney disease with no other risk factors **OR**… • Individuals with 2 or more risk factors **and** a 10-year risk of 10% - 20%
Very High	• Established or recent hospitalization for acute coronary syndrome (ACS) **OR**… • Coronary, carotid or peripheral vascular disease, diabetes, or stage 3 or 4 CKD **with** 1 or more risk factors **OR**… • Calculated 10-year risk greater than 20% or… • Heterozygous familial hypercholesterolemia [HeFH])
Extreme	• Cardiovascular disease including unstable angina that persists after achieving an LDL-C <70 mg/dL **OR**… • established cardiovascular disease with diabetes, stage 3 or 4 CKD, **and/or** heterozygous familial hypercholesterolemia (HeFH) **OR**… • History of premature cardiovascular disease (<55 years of age for males or <65 years of age for females)

The **2017 AACE/ACE guidelines** then breaks down your LDL-C goal based on what risk category you are in.

2017 AACE/ACE Guidelines Risk Categories and LDL-C Goals

▣	**Low Risk**	**LDL-C goal is < 130 mg/dL**
▣	**Moderate Risk**	**LDL-C goal is < 100 mg/dL**
▣	**High Risk**	**LDL-C goal is < 100 mg/dL**
▣	**Very High Risk**	**LDL-C goal is < 70 mg/dL**
▣	**Extreme Risk**	**LDL-C goal is < 55 mg/dL**

The **2017 AACE/ACE guidelines** indicate that you should choose a statin drug based on how much you need to lower your current LDL-C to meet your LDL-C goal.

Low, Moderate, and High-intensity Statin Drugs[6]

Low-intensity Statins	Moderate-intensity Statins	High-intensity Statins
Lowers LDL-C by less than 30%	Lowers LDL-C by 30-50%	Lowers LDL-C by more than 50%
Simvastatin 10 mg	Atorvastatin 10-20 mg	Atorvastatin 40-80 mg
Pravastatin 10-20 mg	Rosuvastatin 5-10 mg	Rosuvastatin 20-40 mg
Lovastatin 20 mg	Simvastatin 20-40 mg	
Fluvastatin 20-40 mg	Pravastatin 40-80 mg	
Pitavastatin 1 mg	Lovastatin 40 mg	
	Fluvastatin XL 80 mg	
	Fluvastatin 40 mg twice daily	
	Pitavastatin 2-4 mg	

Unlike the 2013 guidelines, the 2017 guidelines note that other medications may be added to statin therapy, if needed. Here is a breakdown of other medications used for dyslipidemia:

Other Medications for the Treatment of Dyslipidemia

Fibrates
• Gemfibrozil (Lopid®)
• Fenofibrate (Antara®, Lipofen® Lofibra®, Tricor® and Triglide®)
Fish Oil
• Prescription omega–3 fish oil
Niacin
• Niacin

Bile acid sequestrants
• Cholestyramine (Questran®, Prevalite®)
• Colestipol (Colestid®)
• Colesevelam (Welchol®)
Cholesterol absorption inhibitors
• Ezetimibe (Zetia®)
PCSK9 Inhibitors
• Alirocumab (Praluent®)
• Evolocumab (Repatha®)
MTP Inhibitors
• Lomitapide (Juxtapid®)
Antisense Apolipoprotein B Oligonucleotide
• Mipomersen (Kynamro®)

What Do I Do with This Information?

So what were the results of your assessments? Did both sets of guidelines recommend the same group of statins for you? You are encouraged to take this information with you to your doctor to discuss the results.

Remember:

__Adverse effects, drug-drug interactions, and patient preferences should be considered before taking a statin.__

You and your doctor might also want to think about other factors as well. *__Consider using information from the risk assessment combined with items such as your LDL-P, non-HDL-C, Apo B level, cardiovascular health, weight, and family history to determine if a moderate to high dose statin is for you. Also, remember that statins carry the risk of certain side effects.__*

At the end of the day, the guidelines we just reviewed in this chapter are just that – guidelines. They are meant to supply you with valuable insights into your lipid health and give you information that can help you determine if you should consider a lipid-lowering medication and which ones you might want to consider.

REFERENCES

1. Jellinger PS, Handelsman Y, Rosenblit PD, et al. American Association of Clinical Endocrinologists and American College of Endocrinology guidelines for the management of dyslipidemia and prevention of cardiovascular disease. *Endocr Pract* 2017; 23:1-87

2. Anderson KM, Castelli WP, Levy D. Cholesterol and mortality. 30 years of follow-up from the Framingham study. JAMA 1987 Apr 24; 257 (16): 2176-80.

3. Robert DuBroff and Michel de Lorgeril. Cholesterol confusion and statin controversy. World J Cardiol. 2015. Jul 26; 7(7): 404-409.

4. Al-Mallah, MH, Hatahet H, Cavalcante JL, Khanal S. Low admission LDL-cholesterol is associated with increased 3-yearm all-cause mortality in patients with non STmsegment elevation myocardial infarction. Cardiol J 2009;16:227-33.

5. Krumholz HM et al. Lack of association between cholesterol and coronary heart disease mortality and morbidity and all-cause mortality in persons older than 70 years. JAMA.272, 1335-40, 1994.

6. Stone NJ, Robinson JG, Lichtenstein AH, Bairey Merz CN, Blum CB, Eckel RH, Goldberg AC, Gordon D, Levy D, Lloyd-Jones DM, et al. 2013 ACC/AHA guideline on the treatment of blood cholesterol to reduce atherosclerotic cardiovascular risk in adults: a report of the American College of Cardiology/American Heart Association Task Force on Practice Guidelines. J Am Coll Cardiol. 2014; 63:2889–2934.

7. Cromwell WC, Otvos JD, Keyes MJ, et al. LDL particle number and risk of future cardiovascular disease in the framingham offspring study - implications for LDL management. *J clin lipidol.* 2007;1(6):583-592. Accessed 20110204. doi:10.1016/j.jacl.2007.10.001.

8. The effects of lowering LDL cholesterol with statin therapy in people at low risk of vascular disease: meta-analysis of individual data from 27 randomized trials.

Cholesterol Treatment Trialists' (CTT) Collaborators., Mihaylova B, Emberson J, Blackwell L, Keech A, Simes J, Barnes EH, Voysey M, Gray A, Collins R, Baigent C Lancet. 2012 Aug 11; 380(9841):581-90.

9. Efficacy and safety of more intensive lowering of LDL cholesterol: a meta-analysis of data from 170,000 participants in 26 randomised trials.

Cholesterol Treatment Trialists' (CTT) Collaboration., Baigent C, Blackwell L, Emberson J, Holland LE, Reith C, Bhala N, Peto R, Barnes EH, Keech A, Simes J, Collins R Lancet. 2010 Nov 13; 376(9753):1670-81.

10. Review Statins for the primary prevention of cardiovascular disease.

Taylor F, Huffman MD, Macedo AF, Moore TH, Burke M, Davey Smith G, Ward K, Ebrahim S Cochrane Database Syst Rev. 2013 Jan 31; (1):CD004816.

11. Downs JR, Clearfield M, Weis S, et al. Primary prevention of acute coronary events with lovastatin in men and women with average cholesterol levels: results of AFCAPS/TexCAPS. Air Force/Texas Coronary Atherosclerosis Prevention Study. JAMA. 1998;279:1615–1622.

12. ALLHAT Officers and Coordinators for the ALLHAT Collaborative Research Group Major outcomes in moderately hypercholesterolemic, hypertensive patients randomized to pravastatin vs. usual care: the Antihypertensive and Lipid Lowering Treatment to Prevent Heart Attack Trial (ALLHAT-LLT) JAMA. 2002;288:2998–3007.

13. Sever PS, Dahlöf B, Poulter NR, et al. Prevention of coronary and stroke events with atorvastatin in hypertensive patients who have average or lower-than-average cholesterol concentrations, in the Anglo-Scandinavian Cardiac Outcomes Trial-Lipid Lowering

Arm (ASCOT-LLA): a multicentre randomised controlled trial. Lancet. 2003;361:1149–1158.

14. Neil HA, DeMicco DA, Luo D, et al. Analysis of efficacy and safety in patients aged 65-75 years at randomization: Collaborative Atorvastatin Diabetes Study (CARDS) Diabetes Care. 2006;29:2378–2384.

15. Nakaya N, Mizuno K, Ohashi Y, et al. Low-dose pravastatin and age-related differences in risk factors for cardiovascular disease in hypercholesterolaemic Japanese: analysis of the management of elevated cholesterol in the primary prevention group of adult Japanese (MEGA study) Drugs Aging. 2011;28:681–692.

16. Lemaitre RN, Psaty BM, Heckbert SR, et al. Therapy with hydroxymethylglutaryl coenzyme a reductase inhibitors (statins) and associated risk of incident cardiovascular events in older adults: evidence from the Cardiovascular Health Study. Arch Intern Med. 2002;162:1395–1400.

17. Shepherd J, Blauw GJ, Murphy MB, et al. Pravastatin in elderly individuals at risk of vascular disease (PROSPER): a randomised controlled trial. Lancet. 2002;360:1623–1630.

18. Glynn RJ, Koenig W, Nordestgaard BG, et al. Rosuvastatin for primary prevention in older persons with elevated C-reactive protein and low to average low-density lipoprotein cholesterol levels: exploratory analysis of a randomized trial. Ann Intern Med. 2010;152:488–496.

CHAPTER 2

HIGH BLOOD PRESSURE

The Empowered Medicine Guide to High Blood Pressure

How to Use This Chapter

This chapter is arranged in a step-by-step fashion. First, we will go over the basics of high blood pressure such as what it is, how to tell what stage of high blood pressure you may have, and why treating it is important. Then we will follow a step-by-step process for figuring out what your blood pressure goals should be. Feel free to write your own information in the blanks provided to aid in your calculations. Finally, we will look at the different medications recommended (and NOT recommended) for treating high blood pressure.

If you wish, use Appendix III in the back to log your own information for easy calculations and sharing with your doctor. Also, at the end of this chapter you will find a section called 'The Bottom Line'. This box sums up the main points of the chapter.

High Blood Pressure: The Basics

The heart is an organ that pumps blood into the arteries. The arteries are a type of blood vessel that carries blood rich in oxygen from the heart to the rest of the body. The body needs oxygen to function properly.

'Blood pressure' refers to the pressure the blood exerts against the artery walls. It tells us how hard the heart is working to pump blood. When your heart has to work too hard (like when your blood pressure is too high), it puts strain on the heart. The heart can deal with this extra work for a while, but long term this strain can weaken the heart and cause health problems.

High blood pressure is also called **hypertension.** When blood pressure is high, this can mean that the arteries are constricting or narrowing. Sometimes this narrowing of the arteries is caused by the build-up of plaques along the inside of the artery walls. This buildup of plaque is called ***atherosclerosis or cardiovascular disease (CVD).***

Over time, atherosclerosis causes the arteries to become narrow and stiff, causing high blood pressure. This narrowing of the arteries decreases the amount of blood that can reach vital organs like the kidneys, eyes, heart, and brain.

ATHEROSCLEROSIS

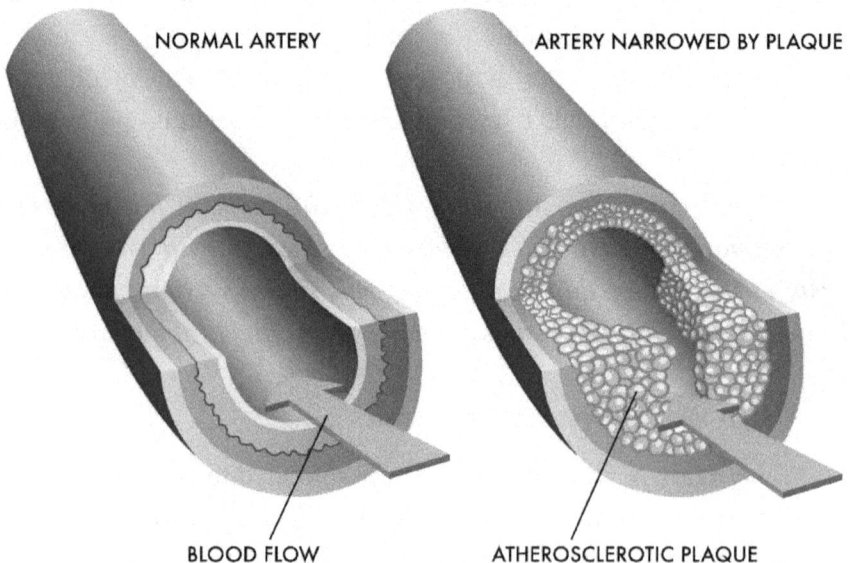

NORMAL ARTERY   ARTERY NARROWED BY PLAQUE

BLOOD FLOW   ATHEROSCLEROTIC PLAQUE

If left unchecked, high blood pressure can increase your risk of developing other devastating health conditions. ***For example, high*** *blood pressure can damage the blood vessels in the brain, causing dementia or even a stroke. Damaged blood vessels in the heart can lead to a decrease in oxygen to the heart. This can cause heart failure or a heart attack. Lack of blood flow can affect other organs in the body as well, potentially causing blindness and/or kidney failure.*

Hypertension

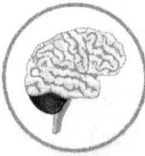

Stroke

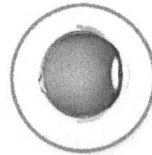

Blindness

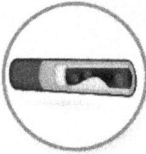

Arteriosclerosis (blood vessel damage)

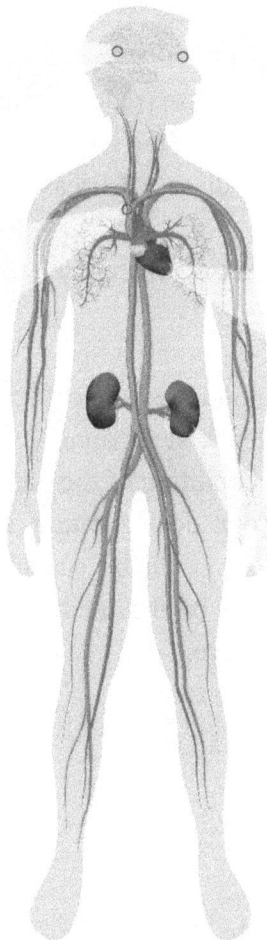

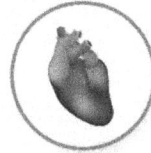

Heart attack and heart failure

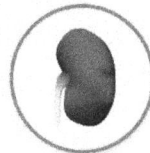

Kidney failure

High blood pressure can be caused by lifestyle factors such as smoking, being overweight, lack of physical activity, stress, or too much salt or alcohol. Other causes of high blood pressure include health issues like chronic kidney disease, adrenal gland disorders, or thyroid disorders. High blood pressure can also run in one's family.

Screening for 'other causes' of high blood mentioned above should take place, especially if any of the following apply to you:[4]

1. High blood pressure requiring 3 or more medications
2. Diagnosis of high blood pressure before 30 years old
3. Organ damage from high blood pressure
a. Heart failure
b. Kidney dysfunction
c. Peripheral artery disease (reduced blood flow in the limbs)
d. Retinopathy (disease of the retina in the eye)
e. Cerebral vascular disease (disease of the blood vessels in the brain)
4. High blood pressure in older adults with low serum potassium

Screening for high blood pressure causes might include tests for kidney disease, eye problems, sleep apnea, thyroid dysfunction, and primary aldosteronism (a condition of the adrenal glands that leads to high blood pressure). Your doctor might also see if any of the medications you are taking could be causing high blood pressure. The table below lists some of the medications that may cause or exacerbate high blood pressure.

Table 1. **Medications That Can Cause High Blood Pressure or Make it Worse**[4]

1. Nonsteroidal anti-inflammatory Drugs (NSAIDs)
a. ibuprofen
b. naproxen
c. celecoxib
d. indomethacin
e. ketoprofen
f. piroxicam
g. salsalate
2. Corticosteroids
a. prednisone
b. methylprednisolone
c. betamethasone
d. triamcinolone
e. hydrocortisone
f. cortisone
g. prednisolone
h. triamcinolone
i. dexamethasone
3. Decongestants
a. pseudoephedrine
b. oxymetazoline
c. phenylephrine
4. Caffeine
5. Monoamine oxidase inhibitors (MAOI)
a. rasagiline
b. selegiline
c. isocarboxazid
d. phenelzine
e. tranylcypromine
6. Other antidepressants
a. venlafaxine
b. bupropion
c. desipramine
7. Cyclosporine

8. Estrogens
a. estradiol
b. conjugated estrogens
c. estropipate
9. Testosterones
10. Nicotine

How Big is the High Blood Pressure Problem?

High blood pressure is a serious problem in the United States. As discussed above, having high blood pressure puts you at a much higher risk for heart attack, stroke, kidney failure, and blindness. [1] Here are a few facts about high blood pressure in the United States:

Table 2. **High Blood Pressure Facts**

1 in 3 American adults have high blood pressure (about 75 million people). [2]
Only 54% of people with high blood pressure have their blood pressure under control.[2]
About 8 out of 10 people who have a first stroke have high blood pressure.[3]
7 out of 10 people who have their first heart attack have high blood pressure.[3]
7 out of 10 people who have chronic heart failure have high blood pressure.[3]
Each 20 mm Hg higher SBP and/or 10 mm Hg higher DBP are each associated with a **doubling** in the risk of death from stroke, heart disease, or other diseases of the blood vessels.[4]

Now that we understand the importance of maintaining a healthy blood pressure, let's take a look at the recommended way to take your blood pressure. It's important to get an accurate reading so that you and your doctor can determine the best possible treatment.

Do It Right

Your blood pressure reading is expressed as two numbers. For example, your blood pressure may be 138/78 mmHg. The top number is called the **systolic blood pressure (SBP)**; the bottom number is called the **diastolic blood pressure (DBP)**. The systolic blood pressure number (the top number) reflects the highest pressure in the arteries. This is the pressure produced while the heart is contracting, pushing blood into the arteries. The diastolic blood pressure (the bottom number) reflects the pressure in the arteries when the heart is resting between beats.

Proper technique is important when measuring blood pressure. Make sure when you get your blood pressure checked that it is done properly. For the most accurate readings, the patient should be seated quietly for at least five minutes prior to the reading. Ideally, feet should be planted on the floor. For best results, the arm on which the reading is taken should be supported at heart level. A blood pressure cuff of appropriate size should be used. The bladder of the cuff (the part that fills with air) should be able to wrap at least 80% of the way around the patient's upper arm. The most accurate readings are done over a bear arm and not over a sleeve of a shirt. An accurate blood pressure reading relies on the ability of the clinician and/or the machine to detect sounds within the blood vessels. If the person or device that listens to the blood vessels is trying to listen through clothing, the reading may be less accurate.

Blood pressure can vary throughout the day. It is important to take an average blood pressure based on more than 2 readings obtained on more than 2 occasions to estimate your blood pressure.[4] Try taking two or three blood pressure readings at least twice a day to get a more accurate measure of your blood pressure.

It is recognized that some people will have higher blood pressure readings at the doctor's office than at home. This is due to a phenomenon called *white coat syndrome*. White coat syndrome is thought to be caused by the fact that many people are nervous when they visit the doctor. When you are nervous, your blood pressure can go up. People with this condition will have higher blood pressure readings in the doctor's office than at home.

For these people, there are alternative methods for getting accurate blood pressure readings. One could purchase an automated blood pressure device from the store and take several blood pressure readings at home. These types of devices are fully automated and are usually battery operated. One only has to put the cuff around their arm and push a button.

There are more sophisticated monitoring devices available as well. For example, ambulatory blood pressure monitoring (ABPM) can monitor blood pressure while one goes about their daily business and at night during sleep. This type of blood pressure monitoring is typically done in coordination with your doctor's office. If you suspect that your readings in the doctor's office are artificially high because of white coat syndrome, ask your doctor if one of these methods of measurement is right for you.

Key to Success

Unfortunately, about **1 out of 5 U.S. adults** with high blood pressure do not know that they have it.[3] Know your numbers and decrease your risk of heart attack, heart failure, kidney failure, and stroke today.

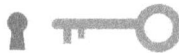

What Should My Blood Pressure Be?

So who decides what our blood pressure goals should be? The following represent some of the most used blood pressure guidelines that health professionals look at today:

1. 2014 Eighth Joint National Committee (JNC 8) of the National Heart, Lung, and Blood Institute (NHLBI) guidelines

2. 2017 American College of Cardiology and The American Heart Association Task Force on Clinical Practice Guidelines (ACC/AHA) guidelines

3. The American Society of Hypertension (ASH) guidelines

4. 2017 American Academy of Family Physicians and American College of Physicians (AAFP/ACP) guidelines for high blood pressure in adults over 60 years old.

When it comes to high blood pressure, guidelines from the JNC 8 and ACC/AHA are the most commonly referred to guidelines in health care. These will be the main guidelines we will focus on in this chapter. However, the ASH and 2017 ACP/AAFP guidelines may be mentioned from time to time.

Regardless of which guidelines you are looking at, each of these panels have scoured data from scientific research trials, and then provided recommendations on high blood pressure goals and medication choices based on the data from these trials. *This method of utilizing scientific evidence to help create sound health recommendations is called 'evidence-based medicine'*. It is the gold standard. This is how health care providers are encouraged to practice medicine today.

The professionals of the organizations mentioned above recognize that the higher your blood pressure is above optimal readings, the higher your risk of heart attack, stroke, and other complications. Although as we will see in a moment, there seems to be some disagreement, however, as to what those optimal readings should be.

The 2017 ACC/AHA guidelines break down high blood pressure into the following stages in Table 3.

STEP 1: Determine What Stage of High Blood Pressure You May Have

Check which box in the table below applies to your blood pressure

Table 3. **High Blood Pressure Stages*[4]**

*BP = blood pressure, SBP = systolic blood pressure, DBP = diastolic blood pressure

Check Which Applies to You	Stage	Blood Pressure Reading	
▪	Normal	SBP < 120	DBP < 80
▪	Elevated	SBP 120 - 129	BBP < 80
▪	Stage 1 high blood pressure	SBP 120 - 139	DBP 80 - 89
▪	Stage 2 high blood pressure	SBP > or = to 140	DBP > or = to 90

Figuring Out Your Blood Pressure Goal

Once you find out which stage of high blood pressure you have, it's time to figure out your blood pressure goal. In order to determine your blood pressure goal, you will first need to figure out your 10-year cardiovascular disease (CVD) risk (don't worry, calculating this is easy). This is a calculation of the likelihood of getting CVD in the next 10 years. Remember, CVD is typically caused by plaques that form in the arteries. These plaques limit blood flow and puts one at a higher risk of heart attack, stroke, kidney disease, and blindness.

High blood pressure and cardiovascular disease are connected. Where there is one, you are likely to find the other. Your 10-year CVD score can be calculated by using any of the following online tools.

Table 4. **Calculators to Calculate Your 10 Year CVD Risk**

One of the following online calculators may be used:
• **Framingham Risk Assessment Tool** (https:// www.framinghamheartstudy.org/risk-functions/coronary-heart-disease/hard-10-year-risk.php) • **Multi-Ethnic Study of Atherosclerosis (MESA)** 10-year ASCVD Risk with Coronary Artery Calcification Calculator (https://www.mesa-nhlbi. org/MESACHDRisk/MesaRiskScore/RiskScore.aspx) • **Reynolds Risk Score** (http://www.reynoldsriskscore.org) • **United Kingdom Prospective Diabetes Study (UKPDS)** risk engine to calculate ASCVD risk in individuals with T2DM) (https://www.dtu.ox.ac.uk/riskengine) • **ACC ASCVD Risk Estimator Plus** tool created by the American College of Cardiology (considered by some to be sub-par by some standards as it was not validated prior to putting into practice) (http://tools.acc.org/ASCVD-Risk-Estimator/)

After using one of the online tools above, you will receive a score which will be a percentage. ***This is the percent risk you have of developing CVD in the next 10 years.*** This information will be used below to help figure out what your blood pressure treatment goals should be.

If you have already been diagnosed with cardiovascular disease, then you can skip to Step 3

If you have NOT been diagnosed with cardiovascular disease, please continue on to Step 2.

STEP 2: Calculate Your 10 Year Risk of Cardiovascular Disease

Write your 10-year risk score in below for reference.

My CVD Risk Score according to the Calculator (based on one of the online tools in Table 4)	My Score is _____ %

Now it's time to calculate your blood pressure goal. Each guideline tells us at what blood pressure reading that it is recommended that one start high blood pressure treatment. We'll also look at the recommended blood pressure goals once one starts treatment. Note: not all categories below are covered by each guideline. This is because each guideline may break down the categories a bit differently.

Check all that apply:

Table 5. **When to Treat and Treatment Goals**[*][1,4]

*BP = blood pressure, SBP = systolic blood pressure, DBP = diastolic blood pressure

Check all that apply	**Criteria**	**JNC 8**	**ACC/AHA**	**ACC/AAFP**	**ASH**
■	Age > 60 years old (without diabetes or chronic kidney disease)	**Treat when:** BP > 150/90		**Treat when:** SBP > 150	**Treat when:** BP > 140/90 unless age is > 80 years old, then consider treating when BP > 150/90
		Goal: BP < 150/90		**Goal:** SBP < 150	**Goal:** BP < 140/90 unless age > 80 years old, then consider goal BP < 150/90

Check all that apply	Criteria	JNC 8	ACC/AHA	ACC/AAFP	ASH
☐	Age 18 to 59 years old (without diabetes or chronic kidney disease)	**Treat when:** BP > 140/90			
		Goal: BP < 140/90			
☐	Age 18 or older with no clinical CVD and 10-year ASCVD risk < 10%		**Treat when:** BP > 140/90		
			Goal: BP < 130/80		
☐	CVD or 10-year ASCVD risk > or = to 10%		**Treat when:** BP > 130/80		
			Goal: BP < 130/80		
☐	Diabetes mellitus	**Treat when:** BP > 140/90	**Treat when:** BP > 130/80		
		Goal: BP < 140/90	**Goal:** BP < 130/80		

Check all that apply	Criteria	JNC 8	ACC/AHA	ACC/AAFP	ASH
◼	Chronic kidney disease (includes those with transplant)	**Treat when:** BP > 140/90	**Treat when:** BP > 130/80		
		Goal: BP < 140/90	**Goal:** BP < 130/80		
◼	Age 18 years or older with chronic kidney disease or diabetes	**Treat when:** BP > 140/90			
		Goal: BP < 140/90			**Goal:** Consider BP < 130/80 if there is albumin in the urine
◼	Age > or = to 65 years old, not in assisted living		**Treat when:** BP > 130/80		
			Goal: BP < 130/80		
◼	Heart Failure		**Treat when:** BP > 130/80		
			Goal: BP < 130/80		

Check all that apply	Criteria	JNC 8	ACC/AHA	ACC/AAFP	ASH
▪	History of stroke		**Treat when:** BP > 140/90 OR BP > 130/80 if lacunar stroke		
			Goal: BP < 130/80		
▪	Peripheral arterial disease		**Treat when:** BP > 130/80		
			Goal: BP < 130/80		

STEP 3: Discover Your Blood Pressure Goals and When to Treat High Blood Pressure

Note which boxes you checked above. In the box below write in any 'when to treat' and any 'goal blood pressures' that were recommended for you in the table above.

List any blood pressure reading(s) that were recommended as 'when to treat'	_____ , _____ , _____
List any 'Blood Pressure Goal(s)' that were recommended	_____ , _____ , _____

Not Everyone Agrees…

Some of you may have several different recommendations for blood pressure goals using the steps above. This is because each of the guideline committees do not agree with each other on all of these numbers. If you have several different blood pressure goals that conflict with each other (i.e. 140/90 and 150/80) *it is recommended that you bring these numbers to your doctor to discuss which blood pressure goal may be right for you*.

For example, the JNC 8 recommendations have been quite controversial. The JNC 8 panel attempted to relax the old stringent guidelines a little bit by replacing blood pressure goals with higher, easier to achieve goals. The result was a simplified document that is easier to follow, with slightly higher blood pressure goals. However, organizations like the ASH, AHA and ACC have raised concerns.

American Heart Association Past President Mariell Jessup, M.D. has this to say about the JNC 8 guidelines raising the systolic blood pressure goal for adults older than 60 from 140 to 150: "We believe there's just not enough evidence at this point to justify such a major change in how we treat people with high blood pressure."

Dr. Jessup was also quoted on the AHA's website as saying, "Much of our great success in reducing deaths from stroke has been attributed to better blood pressure control. However, even with the current target of less than 140, many individuals have high blood pressure that is out of control, and they continue to be at serious risk, especially for heart failure and for stroke. If the target is raised, almost certainly blood pressure in many people will be even higher."

Evidence from studies shows that the incidence of stroke and heart attack are significantly higher in individuals with SBP>140 than among those with SBP<140. Raising the SBP threshold from 140 to 150 as a new target for hypertension treatment in older individuals could have a detrimental effect on stroke risk reduction.[12]

On the other side of the spectrum, the 2017 ACC/AHA guidelines recommend much more strict blood pressure control. The

ACC/AHA guidelines recommend a goal of 130/80 for adults > 18 years old (including those > 60 years old). This is in stark contrast to the goal of 150/90 for adults > 60 years old recommended by JNC 8.

Picking Sides

The ACP/AAFP has chosen to continue to endorse the 2014 JNC 8 guidelines and has taken the position to **not** endorse the new 2017 ACC/AHA guidelines for several reasons:

1. They do not agree with the new ACC/AHA recommendation to treat anyone with blood pressure > 130/80 (instead of 140/90 mmHg) because this would translate into 46% of the U.S. adult population being started on treatment (as opposed to 32% with the 140/90 threshold).

2. They do not believe the bulk of the guidelines were based on systematic evidence review. For example, it refers to using the ACC/AHA cardiovascular disease risk tool which it says is unvalidated (meaning it hasn't been tested to be accurate before being put into use)

3. They claim the harm of treating a patient to the lower blood pressure goal of 130/80 was not evaluated.

4. Both the ACP/AAFP and ACC/AHA agree that there might be a small benefit of lower treatment targets (such as 130/80) in decreasing the number of cardiovascular events, but this did not translate to a decrease in mortality (death) from cardiovascular events in the studies (instead some studies showed a decrease in mortality from any cause). So the AAFP recommends considering the lower target of 130/80 only in certain people as deemed appropriate by their doctor.

5. The ACP/AAFP believe there was a conflict of interest within the ACC/AHA committee that may have skewed the final recommendations (i.e. committee members that had possible ties to drug companies that supply medications for the treatment of high blood pressure).

So as you can see, there is some disagreement between these organizations with regard to blood pressure goals. The thing is, the guidelines are just that guidelines. They are not hard and fast rules. They are meant to be used as a tool. It is suggested that you and your doctor consider the recommendations from each set of guidelines and make a treatment plan tailored for your unique situation.

Key to Success

If there was more than one goal blood pressure recommended for you when following the steps above, you will want to discuss with your doctor which blood pressure goal you should go with.

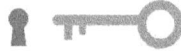

High Blood Pressure Treatment

Non-medication Treatment

In addition to medical treatment, patients should make an effort to make lifestyle changes like eating healthier and exercising. These types of changes help lower blood pressure naturally. A sensible plan should include a heart-healthy diet that includes sodium restriction, alcohol restriction, and possibly potassium supplements.

Research shows that a Mediterranean diet based on typical foods and recipes found in Mediterranean-style cooking lowers one's risk of heart disease. This type of diet generally consists primarily of fresh fruits and vegetables, and heart-healthy monounsaturated fats like those found in fish, nuts, seeds, and olive oil. Limiting one's intake of unhealthy saturated fats (found in butter and red meat) and trans fats (found in margarine and hydrogenated oils) is also key. This type of eating also incorporates some whole grains.

The Mediterranean-style diet also incorporates red wine, in moderation. However, the ACC/AHA guidelines assert that men should limit themselves to no more than 2 drinks per day and women to no more than 1 drink per day.[4] If you have trouble limiting your alcohol consumption, have a family history of alcohol abuse or have liver problems, it may be best if you avoid wine and other forms of alcohol.

Weight loss for overweight patients is also recommended as part of one's high blood pressure treatment plan. Increased physical activity is highly recommended. The 2015-2020 Physical Activity Guidelines for Americans released by the U.S. Department of Health and Human Services recommends at least 150 minutes a week of moderate-intensity physical activity and strength training on two or more days of each week. They also recommend that children ages 6 to 17 years old get 60 minutes of physical activity (which could include aerobic, strength training, etc.) per day.

Physical activity is key to improving not only one's blood pressure but also their overall health in general. The 2018 Physical Activity Guidelines Advisory Committee Scientific Report tells us that physically active adults sleep, feel, and function better. Physical activity also improves blood pressure, improves insulin sensitivity (how your body processes sugar), reduces anxiety, reduces the risk of falls, reduces the risk of dementia, and improves cognition (how you think and understand). There is even evidence to support the notion that regular, moderate-intensity physical activity reduces the risk of cancers of the breast, colon, bladder, endometrium, esophagus, kidney, lung, and stomach.

Typically, lifestyle changes can be expected to lower one's SBP blood pressure by 4-5 mm Hg and DBP by 2-4 mmHg. However according to guidelines, a diet full of fruits, vegetables, and healthy grains that is low in saturated fat may lower SBP by as much as 11 mm Hg.[4]

Making lifestyle changes like these can be challenging, but in the long run can reduce your risk for heart attack, stroke, blindness, and kidney failure. They can also increase your overall health and help you feel better.

Medications

There are dozens of high blood pressure medications on the market today. Not all of these medications have been shown to perform equally when it comes to how they work, their cost, and their side effect profiles. With so much at stake, it's important to choose wisely. Thankfully for health care providers and their patients, the guidelines are available to help them evaluate how each medication stacks up based on how they performed in clinical trials. These guidelines can help you and your doctor decide which high blood pressure medication may work best for you and your unique situation.

Empowered U

True or False:

Men should limit their alcohol to 3 drinks per day.

Answer: False (men should limit themselves to 2 drinks per day)

We'll review the panels' medication recommendations in just a moment. First let's look at each of the groups of medications generally used for the treatment of high blood pressure. There are 4 major groups of medications that the JNC 8 panel and the 2017 ACC/AHA panel consider to be key in treating high blood pressure: ***thiazide diuretics, calcium channel blockers (CCB), angiotensin*** *converting enzyme inhibitors (ACEI), and angiotensin receptor blockers (ARB).* These names are quite a mouthful so *it may be easier to just remember them as: thiazides, CCBs, ACEIs, and ARBs.*

Below you'll find a table that summarizes these 4 groups and one that summarizes medications less commonly used for high blood pressure.

Table 6. **Four Main Drug Classes Recommended for the Initial Treatment of Blood Pressure**

Class of Medications	Examples Recommended by Panel
Thiazide diuretics	Chlorthalidone (Thalitone®), Hydrochlorothiazide (Microzide®, Hydrodiuril®), Indapamide (Lozol®)
ACEI (angiotensin converting enzyme inhibitors)	Captopril (Capoten®), Enalapril (Vasotec®), Lisinopril (Prinivil®, Zestril®, Qbrelis®)
ARB (angiotensin receptor blocker)	Eprosartan (Teveten®), Candesartan (Atacad®), Losartan (Cozaar®), Valsartan (Diovan®), Irbesartan (Avapro®)
CCB (calcium channel blocker)	Amlodipine (Norvasc®), Diltiazem extended release, Verapamil

Remember, these 4 classes of drugs are those recommended for the *initial* treatment of high blood pressure. In other words, when one is first diagnosed with high blood pressure, it is recommended the doctor prescribe a drug from one of these categories. However, many people may require a combination of drugs from these 4 groups, or even the addition of drugs outside of these 4 groups, to control their high blood pressure.

Table 7. **Other Medications that are Less Commonly Used for High Blood Pressure**

Class of Medications	Examples
Loop Diuretics	Bumetanide (Bumex®), Furosemide (Lasix®) and Torsemide (Demadex®).
Potassium-sparing diuretics	Amiloride (Midamor®) and Triamterene. Eplerenone (Inspra®) and Spironolactone (Aldactone®)
β-blockers (or 'beta blockers')	• Atenolol (Tenormin®) Betaxolol (Kerlone®) • Bisoprolol (Zebeta®) • Metoprolol (Lopressor®, Toprol-XL®) • Nebivolol (Bystolic®) • Nadolol (Corgard®) • Propranolol (Inderal®) • Acebutolol (Sectral®) • Penbutolol (Levatol®) • Pindolol (Visken®) • Carvedilol (Coreg®) • Labetalol (Normodyne®, Trandate®)
Alpha Blockers	Doxazosin (Cardura®), Prazosin (Minipress®), Terazosin (Hytrin®)
Centrally-acting Drugs	Clonidine (Catapress®), Methyldopa (Aldomet®), Guanfacine (Tenex®)
Vasodilators	Hydralazine (Apresoline®), Minoxidil (Loniten®)
Renin Inhibitors	Aliskiren (Tekturna® and Rasilez®)

The medications listed in Table 7 are **not** generally recommended for the initial treatment of high blood pressure by the panel. These medications were not necessarily omitted because they are harmful. In some cases, there just may have not been enough evidence to support recommending them for the initial treatment of high blood pressure.

Let's now review the medications used for treating high blood pressure.

Diuretics

Diuretics are often called 'water pills'. They work by causing the body to lose extra water. Getting rid of extra fluid in the body can lower blood pressure and decrease the work on the heart. There are different classes of diuretics. Let's break them down:

Thiazide Diuretics

Examples of thiazide diuretics include hydrochlorothiazide (Microzide®, Hydrodiuril®), chlorthalidone (Thalitone®), and indapamide (Lozol®).

Thiazide diuretics are one of the groups of drugs recommended as a first drug of choice for the treatment of high blood pressure in black and non-black people[1]. The term 'black people' in the context of these guidelines is used by the authors of the guidelines to describe people primarily of sub-Saharan African descent.

Notice that 'thiazide' diuretics are the only diuretics recommended for the initial treatment of high blood pressure. The other classes of diuretics are NOT usually recommended as a first choice. *Thiazide diuretics may also be considered a drug of first choice for treating high blood pressure in patients with heart failure.[1] However, the ACC/AHA consider loop diuretics to be a drug of choice for heart failure patients as well.[4]*

Thiazide diuretics can cause low levels of sodium and potassium in the blood. Your doctor may need to monitor your sodium and potassium levels and may advise you to eat more potassium-rich foods like bananas, sweet potatoes, spinach, and lentils. He or she may also advise you to take potassium supplements.

Maintaining proper potassium balance is critical because having a potassium level that is too high or too low can cause serious or even deadly heart problems like an abnormal heart rate and/or rhythm. Maintaining proper sodium levels is important for brain and nerve function. Sodium that is too low can cause nausea, vomiting, headache, loss of consciousness, and even death. It's important to work with your doctor when managing your sodium and potassium levels. Do not take sodium or potassium supplements without first consulting your doctor.

Thiazide diuretics have also been shown in trials to increase the risk of developing diabetes.[5] Increased blood cholesterol is another possible side effect of thiazide diuretics. Despite these potential effects, studies have shown that thiazide diuretics decrease the risk of cardiovascular-related health issues and cardiovascular-related death.[6,7] For these reasons, the JNC 8 panel feels that the benefits outweigh the risks of using these medications.[1]

Thiazide diuretics should be used with caution in people with gout, unless that person is on uric-acid lowering medication because thiazides can increase uric acid levels and exacerbate gout.[4]

People who are allergic to sulfonamides (AKA 'sulfa drugs') should not take thiazides due to an increased risk of having an allergic reaction.

Loop Diuretics

Examples of loop diuretics include bumetanide (Bumex®), furosemide (Lasix®) and torsemide (Demadex®).

Loop diuretics are often used to lower blood pressure in emergency situations or for the treatment of high blood pressure in combination with other drugs. During the JNC 8 panel's review, there were no trials of fair quality comparing loop diuretics to the 4 recommended classes of high blood pressure medications; therefore, *they are NOT recommended by the JNC 8 as first line medications to treat high blood pressure.[1] However, they are recommended by the 2017 ACC/AHA guidelines as a preferred choice for people with heart failure.*

Loop diuretics work by increasing the amount of salt that leaves the body in the urine. Salt can cause the body to retain water and can raise one's blood pressure.

In addition to increasing the amount of salt we lose, these types of diuretics also cause us to lose potassium. For this reason, many people need to increase the amount of potassium-rich food in their diets while taking these drugs. As with thiazide diuretics, your doctor may ask that you take potassium supplements while taking these drugs as well. As mentioned before, do not take potassium supplements without talking to your doctor first.

Increased blood sugar, increased blood lipids, and hypocalcemia (low calcium levels in the blood) are possible side effects of loop diuretics. Also, if you've been diagnosed with gout (a condition where uric acid crystals form in the joints causing arthritis), loop diuretics may make your symptoms worse.

A somewhat unique side effect of loop diuretics is the potential for hearing loss. This loss might be temporary or permanent. Finally, although very uncommon, one may be at a higher risk of developing kidney stones while taking loop diuretics.

As with thiazides, people who are allergic to sulfonamides should not take loop diuretics.

Potassium-sparing diuretics

Examples of potassium-sparing diuretics include amiloride (Midamor®) and triamterene. Eplerenone (Inspra®) and spironolactone (Aldactone®) are specific types of potassium-sparing diuretics called aldosterone antagonists. All 4 of these potassium-sparing diuretics help get rid of extra fluid in the body without getting rid of extra potassium.

The JNC 8 and ACC/AHA panels consider potassium-sparing diuretics to be minimally effective for the treatment of high blood pressure. For this reason, the panels do **NOT** recommend potassium-sparing diuretics as a first choice for the treatment of high blood pressure. They do go onto note that *potassium-sparing diuretics may be useful in people with resistant high blood pressure.[4] Also, potassium-sparing diuretics are often prescribed to help offset potassium lost from other diuretics or may be prescribed for patients with heart failure.[1]*

Potential side effects of potassium-sparing diuretics include high potassium levels and/or low sodium levels. The elderly, patients with chronic kidney disease, and those who take ACEIs, ARBs and/or NSAIDS are at particular risk for high potassium levels. In fact, potassium-sparing diuretics should be avoided in people with kidney disease, those taking other potassium-sparing diuretics, and with those taking potassium supplements.[4]

Finally, aldosterone antagonists like spironolactone can cause hormone disturbances resulting in gynecomastia (enlarged breasts in men). In women, aldosterone antagonists can contribute to menstrual irregularities.

More on Diuretic Side Effects

One potential side effect of diuretics in general is orthostatic hypotension (low blood pressure when standing up). This can cause you to feel dizzy when getting up from the seated or lying position. To avoid this, rise slowly when getting up out of a chair or out of bed.

Generally, low blood pressure, dizziness, headache, muscle cramps, and thirst are also potential side effects. Diuretics can cause dehydration. Dizziness, headache, low blood pressure, and excessive thirst can all be signs of dehydration. If you experience a very dry mouth despite drinking more fluids or if your urine is very dark-yellow colored, talk to your doctor. It is possible your diuretic dose may need to be adjusted.

Persistent headaches, muscle cramps, and dizziness can be signs of abnormal levels of potassium, sodium, or other electrolytes in the blood. All classes of the diuretics are capable of throwing one's electrolytes off balance. It's worth mentioning again that abnormal amounts of certain electrolytes in the blood can cause serious problems like irregular heart rates and/or rhythms (in the case of potassium), and/or even slipping into a coma (in the case of sodium). If you experience any of these symptoms, let your doctor know right away.

Finally keep in mind that diuretics will also likely increase the amount and number of times you need to urinate each day since your body will be trying to rid itself of extra fluid. For this reason, you may want to take them earlier in the day so you are not up all night using the bathroom. For example, if you take your diuretic once a day, you may want to take it at 6:00 a.m. If you take it twice daily, you may consider taking it at 6:00 a.m. and 4:00 p.m.

Diuretics can be very useful medications. However, they are capable of a variety of side effects. Just because something is listed as a side effect doesn't mean one will experience it. It simply means that some people may experience it while taking the drug. Here is a summary of some of the more common side effects possible with diuretics.

Table 8. **Common Side Effects of Diuretics**

- Dehydration
- Low potassium in the blood (thiazides, loop diuretics)
- High potassium in the blood (potassium-sparing diuretics)
- Low sodium in the blood (thiazides, loop diuretics)
- High calcium in the blood (thiazides)
- Low calcium in the blood (loop diuretics)
- Low magnesium in the blood (thiazides, loop diuretics)
- Headache (all diuretics)

- Light headedness (all diuretics)
- Irregular heart rate and/or rhythm (all diuretics)
- Vomiting (all diuretics)
- Muscle cramps and/or weakness (all diuretics)
- Constipation (all diuretics)
- Loss of consciousness (all diuretics)
- Increased risk of diabetes/increased blood sugar (thiazides, loop diuretics)
- Increased risk of high cholesterol (thiazides, loop diuretics)
- Increase uric acid levels/make gout worse (thiazides, loop diuretics)
- Possible allergy if allergic to sulfa drugs (thiazides, loop diuretics)
- Hearing loss (loop diuretics)
- Kidney stones (loop diuretics)
- Enlarged breasts in men (Eplerenone, Spironolactone)
- Menstrual irregularities (Eplerenone, Spironolactone)

ACE Inhibitors (ACEI)

Angiotensin converting enzyme inhibitors (ACEI) work by blocking the action of an enzyme in the body that constricts the blood vessels. When blood vessels are constricted, the heart has a tougher time pumping blood. So by helping to relax blood vessels, ACEIs make the heart's job easier.

ACEIs also increase the amount of sodium and water the body gets rid of. This also helps make the heart's job easier and lowers blood pressure. Examples of these medications include the following:

- Captopril (Capoten®)
- Enalapril (Vasotec®)
- Lisinopril (Prinivil®, Zestril®)
- Benazepril (Lotensin®)
- Fosinopril (Monopril®)

• Ramipril (Altace®)
• Quinapril (Accupril®)
• Perindopril (Aceon®)
• Trandolapril (Mavik®)
• Moexipril (Univasc®)

ACEIs are one of the 4 classes of drugs recommended as a first choice for the treatment of high blood pressure in the general non-black population (including those with diabetes). They are also recommended as initial (or add-on) therapy in people 18 years or older with chronic kidney disease (regardless of race or diabetes status).[1] However potassium levels should be monitored closely in these people.

ACEI are not recommended as a first choice in the black population (*unless the patient has chronic kidney disease*) because in one study there was a 51% higher rate of stroke in black persons where an ACEI was used as initial therapy (compared to CCBs).[1] ACEI were also less effective at lowering blood pressure in the black population in this study.[1] *Therefore CCB or thiazides are recommended to try first in the black population.*[1]

ACEIs can cause high levels of potassium in the blood. People with acute or severe kidney disease, those taking potassium supplements, and those on other drugs that increase potassium should consult their doctor if they are taking an ACEI. ACEI have been shown in studies to have a kidney-protective effect. However, depending on your situation, your doctor may ask you to discontinue your ACEI if you have acute or severe kidney disease because kidney disease in itself can increase potassium levels. As mentioned in the 'Diuretics' section, abnormal potassium levels can to lead to abnormal heart rates/rhythms. Speak with your doctor if you experience any persistent dizziness, palpitations, or weakness while taking ACEIs.

ACEIs are sometimes not tolerated well because of a troublesome side effect – a cough. These drugs have the ability to produce a dry, persistent cough in some patients. It is unclear why this occurs. Some patients are able to tolerate the drug despite this, but others find it too bothersome and choose to switch to another medication such as an ARB. ARBs are also capable of producing a dry cough, but to a lesser degree.

As with diuretics, you may feel light headed or dizzy when getting up from a seated position while taking an ACEI. Care must be taken to rise slowly from sitting or lying. Also, diarrhea has been reported while taking ACEIs. In these cases, the diarrhea generally resolves after switching to another medication.

Skin rash, taste disturbances, and neutropenia (low number of neutrophils in the blood) are also possible side effects of ACEIs. Neutropenia can lead to an increased susceptibility to infection.

Another potentially serious side effect of ACEI is called 'angioedema'. Symptoms of this condition include swelling of the face, hands, feet, and possibly the throat. This condition can be life-threatening because it can affect your internal organs and your ability to breathe. ACEI-induced angioedema is up to five times greater in people of African descent.[8-10] If you notice any facial swelling or have trouble breathing while taking an ACEI, seek emergency services immediately. If you've experienced angioedema with ACEIs in the past, do not take an ACEI.

It's important NOT to use an ACEI and an ARB together. These medications are similar in how they work and in their possible side effects. Taking them together could increase the risk of side effects mentioned above. As a result, people are generally prescribed either one or the other.

Finally, ACEIs should not be taken while pregnant as they can cause birth defects.

Angiotensin Receptor Blockers (ARB)

These medications work in a way similar to ACEI. *They are also one of the 4 main classes of medications recommended as a first choice to treat high blood pressure in the general non-black population due to its ability to lower blood pressure in this population. It is also first line in people 18 years or older with chronic kidney disease (regardless of race or diabetes status).[1]* This again is due to the fact that ACEI and ARBs have been shown to improve kidney function in patients with chronic kidney disease. However, potassium levels should be closely monitored with these patients.

Examples of ARBs include:
- Losartan (Cozaar®)
- Valsartan (Diovan®)
- Irbesartan (Avapro®)
- Candesartan (Atacand®)
- Eprosartan (Teveten®)
- Olmesartan (Benecar®)
- Telmisartan (Micardis®)

There were no studies meeting the JNC 8 panel's eligibility criteria that compared diuretics or CCBs to ARBs in black patients. The guidelines say that ARBs are recommended in patients with chronic kidney disease regardless of race. However, there was less evidence to support the use of ARBs in black patients with kidney disease (instead of an ACEI). *Thus, ACEI are recommended for black patients with chronic kidney disease (instead of ARBs).*

As with ACEI, ARBs can cause high levels of potassium in the blood. Make sure you and your doctor closely monitor your potassium levels especially if you have kidney problems, are taking potassium supplements, or are taking other medications that can raise your potassium levels.

Like ACEI, ARBs can also cause 'angioedema'. Symptoms of this condition include swelling of the face, hands, feet, and throat. This condition can be life-threatening because it can affect your internal organs and your ability to breathe. If you notice any facial swelling or have trouble breathing while taking an ARB, seek emergency services immediately. If you've experienced angioedema with ARBs in the past, do not take an ARB.

Other potential side effects of ARBs include dizziness, taste disturbances, and diarrhea. ARBs do not generally cause the same dry, persistent cough that ACEIs often cause, but they are still capable of causing this side effect.

As mentioned before, it's important to **NOT use an ACEI and an ARB together**.

ARBs must also not be used in pregnancy as they can cause birth defects.

Calcium Channel Blockers

Calcium channel blockers (CCBs) decrease the pumping force of the heart. This lowers blood pressure and lessens the work load on the heart. There are two classes of CCBs shown below.

The 2 classes of CCB include:

Dihydropyridine Calcium Channel Blockers

• Amlodipine (Norvasc®)
• Felodipine (Plendil®)
• Isradipine (Dynacirc CR®)
• Nicardipine sustained release and long-acting (Adalat CC®, Procardia XL®, Cardene SR®)
• Long-acting nifedipine (Adalat CC®, Procardia XL®)
• Nisoldipine (Sular®)

Nondihydropyridine Calcium Channel Blockers

• Diltiazem (Cardizem CD®, Cardizem XT®, Dilacor XR®, Tiazac®)
• Verapamil (Calan®, Calan SR®, Isoptin®, Isoptin SR®, Verelan®)

CCBs is one of the 4 major drug classes recommended by the JNC panel for the initial treatment of high blood pressure in the non-black population. CCBs are particularly helpful in the black population as well and are recommended as a first choice along with thiazides in the black population.[1] CCBs provide better stroke prevention and blood pressure reduction in the black population when compared to ACEIs.[1] However, in patients with heart failure, an ACEI should be considered before CCBs.[1]

Calcium channel blockers may be prescribed for a variety of health conditions including high blood pressure, angina (chest pain), heart arrhythmias (abnormal heart rhythm or rate), certain types of heart failure, and pulmonary hypertension (high blood pressure in the blood vessels of the lungs).

Potential side effects of calcium channel blockers include lightheadedness, low blood pressure, slower heart rate, drowsiness, constipation, swelling of feet, ankles and legs, increased appetite, gastroesophageal reflux disease (GERD), tenderness/bleeding of the gums, and sexual dysfunction.

CCBs are generally avoided in certain people with heart failure. If a CCB is required, amlodipine or felodipine may be used, but first discuss it with your doctor.[4]

Nondihydropyridine CCBs should generally be avoided in people taking beta blockers because the combination can increase the risk of bradycardia (slow heart beat) and heart block (condition where the electrical signals that move across the heart are partially or fully blocked, therefore causing an arrhythmia).[4]

High Blood Pressure Medications NOT Recommended as a First Choice for Treating High Blood Pressure

β-blockers (or 'beta blockers')

Beta blockers work by blocking the effects of the hormone epinephrine (AKA adrenaline). Adrenaline is the 'fight or flight' hormone produced by the body when it senses a threat to its survival. Among other actions, adrenaline shunts blood away from the digestive tract, sex organs, and skin and sends it to the heart, muscles, and lungs to prepare the body to fight or run.

By blocking the actions of adrenaline, beta blockers cause the heart to beat slower and with less force. This lowers the blood pressure and decreases the work for the heart. Some beta blockers also help keep the blood vessels dilated so that blood can move through them easier.

Let's look at some examples of beta blockers.

Table 9. **Examples of Beta-blockers**

Beta-blockers that target the heart • **Atenolol (Tenormin®)** **Betaxolol (Kerlone®)** • **Bisoprolol (Zebeta®)** • **Metoprolol (Lopressor®, Toprol-XL®)**	• These drugs focus on the heart • These drugs are preferred in people who have asthma, chronic obstructive pulmonary disease (COPD) and emphysema
Beta blockers that target the heart and also help widen blood vessels • **Nebivolol (Bystolic®)**	• These drugs focus on the heart but also help relax the blood vessels (widen the blood vessels so blood can flow easier)
More beta blockers that target the heart and also help relax blood vessels • **Carvedilol (Coreg®)** • **Labetalol (Normodyne®, Trandate®)**	• These drugs, like nebivolol, focus on the heart and also help relax blood vessels. They work in a slightly different way than nebivolol • Carvedilol is preferred in people with heart failure
Beta-blockers that don't just target the heart (they affect the lungs, too) • **Nadolol (Corgard®)** • **Propranolol (Inderal®)**	• These are generally not prescribed for patients with asthma, chronic obstructive pulmonary disease (COPD) and emphysema because these drugs can affect the lungs as well as the heart
Beta-blockers that block the effects of adrenaline but can also stimulate the heart • **Acebutolol (Sectral®)** • **Penbutolol (Levatol®)** • **Pindolol (Visken®)**	• These are usually avoided for the treatment of high blood pressure, especially in people with cardiovascular disease or heart failure.

Both the JNC 8 and ACC/AHA panels do NOT recommend beta blockers for the initial treatment of hypertension. This is because in one study, beta blockers were associated with a higher rate of heart attack and stroke compared to the use of an ARB. In other studies that compared a β-blocker to the drugs of the 4 recommended drug classes, beta blockers performed similarly to the other drugs.[1]

It's important to remember that beta blockers are often prescribed for other health conditions besides high blood pressure. For example, beta blockers have been shown to decrease the risk of death in patients after a heart attack and in patients with heart failure. *So in people with heart failure or who have had a heart attack, beta blockers may be preferred.*[4]

The most common side effects with beta blockers include cold hands and feet, stomach cramps, dizziness (especially upon standing up from a sitting position), slow heartbeat, low blood pressure, tiredness, and sleep disturbances.

Beta blockers can cause increases in blood sugar. They have also been known to potentially mask the symptoms of low blood sugar, like shakiness, jitteriness, or fast heart rate. Therefore, if you are diabetic or prone to low blood sugar, you may need to test your blood sugar more often because you may not get those symptoms you normally get with low blood sugar.

Key to Success

Remember, beta blockers are often prescribed for other health conditions besides high blood pressure. If you are taking a beta blocker, it is important to continue to take it unless otherwise instructed by your doctor.

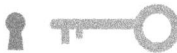

Alpha Blockers

Alpha blockers work by relaxing the smooth muscles throughout the body, including those in the walls of the blood vessels. In this way, they keep the blood vessels more open (keep them from getting narrow). This helps blood move easier through the blood vessels and, in turn, lowers blood pressure.

Because alpha blockers relax the smooth muscles throughout the body, including those in the heart and penis, they are not used that often to treat high blood pressure. When used for high blood pressure, they are typically reserved for emergency situations in the hospital.

Examples of alpha blockers include:

• Doxazosin (Cardura®)
• Prazosin (Minipress®)
• Terazosin (Hytrin®)

Although they are not often used for high blood pressure, they are prescribed for other health conditions such as an enlarged prostate. Therefore, alpha blockers may be a good choice for high blood pressure treatment in men with benign prostatic hyperplasia (BPH).[4]

Side effects of alpha blockers may include orthostatic hypotension (low blood pressure upon standing), dizziness, fatigue, headache, heart palpitations, nausea, and impotence. Pancreatitis (inflammation of the pancreas) and priapism (a persistent and painful penile erection) have also been reported when using alpha blockers, but they are rare.

Centrally-acting Drugs

These drugs are called 'centrally-acting' because they actually work in the brain, the 'central' control center of the body. By acting on certain receptors in the brain, these drugs are able to decrease the output of the heart and decrease the tension in the blood vessels. This lowers blood pressure. Examples of centrally-acting drugs include:

• Clonidine (Catapress®)

• Methyldopa (Aldomet®)

• Guanfacine (Tenex®)

These medications are also NOT recommended as one of the 4 main classes of drugs to treat high blood pressure. They may sometimes be prescribed for other various health conditions like hot sweats.

Centrally-acting drugs are generally considered as a last option for the treatment of high blood pressure, especially in older people, because they have many side effects. Orthostatic hypotension (low blood pressure upon standing) is a common side effect of these medications. Other less common side effects include a dry mouth, slowed heartbeat, constipation, confusion, dizziness, headache, drowsiness, trouble sleeping, erectile dysfunction, and seizure.

If you are currently taking one of these centrally-acting drugs, do not stop it without first talking to your doctor. Stopping clonidine abruptly can cause rebound high blood pressure that can become life threatening.

Vasodilators

Vasodilators dilate the blood vessels in the body, making them wider so blood can flow through them easier. This lowers blood pressure and decreases the work on the heart. Side effects for these medications may include headache, heart palpitations, flushing chest pain, and diarrhea. Here are some examples of vasodilators:

• Hydralazine (Apresoline®)

• Minoxidil (Loniten®)

Most vasodilator drugs are "mixed" vasodilators. This means they dilate both arteries and veins and therefore can have large, unintended consequences on the body if the patient has other conditions like heart failure or angina (chest pain caused by the heart not getting enough oxygen). For this reason they're not used very often to control high blood pressure.

These medications may also cause water and salt retention and a very fast heartbeat. For these reasons they are typically used along with a diuretic and a beta blocker. A unique potential side effect of minoxidil is hirsutism (when the body produces excess hair, sometimes in areas hair does not usually grow). Minoxidil has also been associated with pericardial effusion (fluid around the heart).[4] When taking hydralazine, watch for symptoms of lupus, including achy joints, pain in the chest while breathing (pleurisy), and a butterfly-shaped rash on the cheeks and nose.[4]

Renin Inhibitors

Aliskiren (Tekturna® or Rasilez®) is the first in this new class of medications for high blood pressure. Aliskiren is available by itself or in combination with hydrochlorothiazide. This medication works by preventing vasoconstriction (prevents the blood vessels from getting narrower). Aliskiren also decreases the amounts of water and salt reabsorbed in the body. These actions cause the lowering of blood pressure.

People who have diabetes and are taking an ACE or an ARB should not take aliskiren because in trials these people had a higher rate of stroke, kidney problems, high blood potassium, and low blood pressure.[13]

Which Blood Pressure Medications Should I Take?

Determining which blood pressure medication is right for you will depend on many things like your genetics, your race, and other health conditions (like diabetes or kidney disease). As you will see, there is some disagreement among the different guidelines as to which class of drugs should be used first; however, *the common theme is that, generally, medications that are tried first typically come from one of the 4 main classes of high blood pressure medications (thiazides, CCBs, ACEIs and ARBs).*

Remember, these recommendations are just general guidelines. You and your doctor may find that you require medications outside of these recommendations. As you will see in other sections of this book, patients with other health conditions may require other medications. In these instances, these medications may be the best choice for their high blood pressure treatment. For example, a person who has had a heart attack may be taking a beta blocker because beta blockers have been shown to decrease the risk of death in people who have had a heart attack.[14] For these patients, a beta blocker may be the best blood pressure drug even though it is not one of the 4 main groups of blood pressure lowering medications. Again, do NOT discontinue any medications you are currently taking without first discussing it with your doctor.

STEP 4: Discover Which Blood Pressure Medications May Be Right to You:

As you look over Table 8, checkmark any boxes to the left that may apply to you.

If you wish, take this table (or the table in Appendix III) with you to your next doctor's appointment to discuss which medications you should consider in your blood pressure treatment plan.

Table 10*. **Drugs of Choice for High Blood Pressure[1,4]**

Check all that apply	Population	Drug of Choice	Drugs to Avoid	Comments
☑	Non-black population (including those with diabetes)	JNC 8: CCB, thiazide, ACEI or ARB For age < 60 years old ASH recommends: • 1st line: ACEI or ARB • 2nd line: CCB	In one study beta blockers resulted in a higher rate of cardiovascular death, heart attack and stroke compared to the use of an ARB.	Beta blockers have been shown to decrease the risk of death associated with certain conditions (for example,

Check all that apply	Population	Drug of Choice	Drugs to Avoid	Comments
		or thiazide • 3rd line: CCB plus ACEI **or** ARB plus thiazide For age > 60 years old ASH recommends: • 1st: CCB or thiazide preferred, ACEI or ARB ok too • 2nd line: CCB, thiazide, ACEI or ARB • 3rd line: CCB plus ACEI **or** ARB plus thiazide ACC/AHA: • 1st: thiazide • 2nd line: CCB • 3rd line: ACEI or ARB	In other studies beta blockers performed similarly to the 4 main classes (thiazides, CCB, ACEI, ARB).	after a heart attack and in people with heart failure). *Do not stop taking your beta blocker without consulting your doctor.*
■	Black population (including those with diabetes)	JNC 8: CCB or thiazide ASH recommends: • First line: CCB or thiazide • 2nd line: ACEI or ARB • 3rd line: CCB plus ACEI **or** ARB plus	ACEI are generally not recommended as a first choice in the black population (*unless the patient has chronic kidney disease*) due to a 51% higher rate of stroke in	CCBs provide better stroke prevention and blood pressure reduction in this population compared to ACEIs.

Check all that apply	Population	Drug of Choice	Drugs to Avoid	Comments
		thiazide ACC/AHA: • First line: CCB or thiazide • 2nd line: ACEI or ARB • 3rd line: CCB plus ACEI **or** ARB plus thiazide	this population in one study compared to CCBs. ACEIs were also less effective at lowering blood pressure in the black population in this study.[1]	Thiazides reduce stroke risk better than ACEIs in this population.
▪	Heart failure	JNC 8 recommends: 1st- Thiazide, 2nd- ACEI (regardless of race) ASH, ACC/AHA: recommends: ACEI or ARB plus beta blocker plus diuretic plus spironolactone regardless of blood pressure. Amlodipine can be added for additional blood pressure control.	Verapamil and diltiazem should be avoided in patients with systolic heart failure.[4]	
▪	Age 18 years or older with chronic kidney disease	JNC 8 recommends: ACEI or ARB (all ages, all races)		

105

Check all that apply	Population	Drug of Choice	Drugs to Avoid	Comments
	(regardless of race or diabetes status)	ASH recommends: • 1st line: ACEI or ARB (ACEI for black population) • 2nd line: CCB or thiazide • 3rd line: CCB or thiazide (whichever hasn't been used yet)		
☐	Age 75 years or older with chronic kidney disease	JNC 8 recommends: ACEI or ARB (all ages, all races) ASH recommends: CCBs and thiazide-type diuretic should be used instead of ACEI or ARB due to the risk of high potassium in the blood and further renal impairment		
☐	Coronary artery disease	ASH recommends: • 1st line: beta blocker plus ARB or ACEI		

Check all that apply	Population	Drug of Choice	Drugs to Avoid	Comments
		• 2nd: add CCB or thiazide • 3rd: CCB or thiazide (whichever hasn't been used yet) ACC/AHA: Beta blocker, ACEI, ARB (depending on other conditions. For example: beta blocker for heart attack). Other medications may be added such as dihydropyridine CCB, thiazide, aldosterone antagonist.		
▪	Stroke	JNC8: CCB or thiazide is recommended first for the black population with stroke. ASH recommends for nonblack population: • 1st line: ACEI or ARB • 2nd line: add		

Check all that apply	Population	Drug of Choice	Drugs to Avoid	Comments
		CCB or thiazide • 3rd line: CCB or thiazide (whichever hasn't been used yet) ACC/AHA: ACEIs are more effective than thiazides or CCBs in lowering BP and preventing stroke in nonblack population.		

*CCB = calcium channel blocker

ACEI = angiotensin converting enzyme inhibitors

ARB = angiotensin receptor blockers

How Can I Expect My Treatment to Progress?

The main purpose of treating high blood pressure is to minimize the risk of developing serious health conditions such as heart attack, heart failure, kidney failure, and stroke. This is accomplished by maintaining your goal blood pressure (See Table 4). Keep in mind that many people will require more than one high blood pressure drug to achieve blood pressure control. In fact, ACC/AHA has outlined criteria that tells us when to consider starting with one medication and when to start with two:

Table 11. **When to Start with More Than One Medication**[4]

	Who	Start With...
▪	Adults with stage 1 high blood pressure with a BP goal of 130/80	Start with 1 first line medication (thiazides, CCBs, ACEIs, ARBs). Other agents may be added later if needed
▪	Adults with stage 2 high blood pressure with a BP that is more than 20/10 above their BP goal.	Start with 2 first line medications in different classes (thiazides, CCBs, ACEIs, ARBs)

In general, the guidelines recommend following up monthly until goal blood pressure is achieved. They also recommend following up more often after any change to blood pressure medications. When adjusting your medications to achieve your blood pressure goal, your doctor may decide to increase the dose of the initial drug or add a second drug from one of the other 3 recommended drug classes. [4] If goal blood pressure cannot be reached with 2 drugs, a third drug from the 4 main drug classes may be added, keeping in mind that an ACEI and an ARB should not be used together. If goal blood pressure cannot be reached using only the drugs in the 4 recommended drug classes, antihypertensive drugs from other classes may be used.

STEP 5: Figure Out When You Should Follow-up with Your Doctor Again

Check the boxes below that apply to you. Take this chart with you to your next doctor's appointment so that you can both decide on a follow-up schedule that works for you.

Table 12. **Recommended High Blood Pressure Montitoring**[4]

	Criteria	Recommended Monitoring
■	Adults with normal BP (BP < 120/80)	Reassess in 1 year
■	Adults with elevated blood pressure (SBP 120-129 or DBP 80) with CVD risk < 10%	Reassess within 3 to 6 months.
■	Adults with Stage 1 high blood pressure (SBP 130-139 or DBP 80-89) with CVD or CVD risk > or = to 10%	If using non-drug therapy, reassess in 3-6 months. If using non-drug and drug therapy, reassess in 1 month (if goal met, follow up in 3-6 months. If goal not met, follow up more often than 3-6 months and consider intensifying therapy)
■	Adults with Stage 2 high blood pressure (BP > or = to 140/90)	Reassess in 1 month (if goal met, follow up in 3-6 months. If goal not met, follow up more often than 3-6 months and consider intensifying therapy)
■	Adults with very high blood pressure (SBP > or = to 180 or DBP > or = to 110)	See your doctor right away or go to the Emergency Room/Urgent Care to be evaluated.

If you are finding it difficult to stick with your medication regimen, consider using medications that are dosed only once a day, rather than twice a day or more. Also, using medications that contain a combination of ingredients in one pill (rather than taking each ingredient individually) may help, too.[4]

The Bottom Line

'Blood pressure' refers to the pressure the blood exerts against the artery walls. It tells us how hard the heart is working to pump blood. When your heart has to work too hard (like when your blood pressure is too high), it puts strain on the heart. The heart can deal with this extra work for a while, but long term this strain can weaken the heart and cause health problems.

High blood pressure is also called *hypertension.* When blood pressure is high, this can mean that the arteries are constricting or narrowing. Sometimes this narrowing of the arteries is caused by the build-up of plaques along the inside of the artery walls. This buildup of plaque is called *atherosclerosis or cardiovascular disease (CVD).*

Over time, atherosclerosis causes the arteries to become narrow and stiff, causing high blood pressure. This narrowing of the arteries decreases the amount of blood that can reach vital organs like the kidneys, eyes, heart, and brain.

If left unchecked, high blood pressure can increase your risk of developing other devastating health conditions like dementia, stroke, heart failure, heart attack, blindness and/or kidney failure.

Your blood pressure reading is expressed as two numbers. For example, your blood pressure may be 138/78 mmHg. The top number is called the **systolic blood pressure (SBP)**; the bottom number is called the **diastolic blood pressure (DBP)**.

Proper technique is important when measuring blood pressure. Make sure before you take your blood pressure that you are seated quietly for at least five minutes prior to the reading with both feet on the floor. For best results, the arm on which the reading is taken should be supported at heart level. The bladder of the cuff (the part that fills with air) should be able to wrap at least 80% of the way around your upper arm. The most accurate readings are done over a bear arm and not over the sleeve of a shirt.

Blood pressure goals are as follows:

When to Treat and Treatment Goals*[1,4]

*BP = blood pressure, SBP = systolic blood pressure, DBP = diastolic blood pressure

Check all that apply	Criteria	JNC 8	ACC/AHA	ACC/AAFP	ASH
☐	Age > 60 years old (without diabetes or chronic kidney disease)	**Treat when:** BP > 150/90		**Treat when:** SBP > 150	**Treat when:** BP > 140/90 unless age is > 80 years old, then consider treating when BP > 150/90
		Goal: BP < 150/90		**Goal:** SBP < 150	**Goal:** BP < 140/90 unless age > 80 years old, then consider goal BP < 150/90
☐	Age 18 to 59 years old (without diabetes or chronic kidney disease)	**Treat when:** BP > 140/90			
		Goal: BP < 140/90			
☐	Age 18 or older with no clinical CVD and 10-year		**Treat when:** BP > 140/90		

	ASCVD risk < 10%		**Goal:** BP < 130/80		
■	CVD or 10-year ASCVD risk > or = to 10%		**Treat when:** BP > 130/80		
			Goal: BP < 130/80		
■	Diabetes mellitus	**Treat when:** BP > 140/90	**Treat when:** BP > 130/80		
		Goal: BP < 140/90	**Goal:** BP < 130/80		
■	Chronic kidney disease (includes those with transplant)	**Treat when:** BP > 140/90	**Treat when:** BP > 130/80		
		Goal: BP < 140/90	**Goal:** BP < 130/80		
■	Age 18 years or older with chronic kidney disease or diabetes	**Treat when:** BP > 140/90			
		Goal: BP < 140/90			**Goal:** Consider BP < 130/80 if there is albumin in the urine
■	Age > or = to 65 years old, not in assisted living		**Treat when:** BP > 130/80		

		Goal: BP < 130/80		
■	Heart Failure	**Treat when:** BP > 130/80		
		Goal: BP < 130/80		
■	History of stroke	**Treat when:** BP > 140/90 OR BP > 130/80 if lacunar stroke		
		Goal: BP < 130/80		
■	Peripheral arterial disease	**Treat when:** BP > 130/80		
		Goal: BP < 130/80		

Remember not all of the guidelines agree on what the official blood pressure goals should be. This is why you may see different goals under the different guideline organizations above. If you are 60 years old or older and do not have chronic kidney disease or diabetes, you may want to discuss with your doctor whether you want to go with the recommendation of a blood pressure goal of 130/80, 140/90 or 150/90.

Non-medication Treatment

Weight loss for overweight patients is recommended as part of one's high blood pressure treatment plan. A sensible plan should also include a heart-healthy diet that includes sodium restriction, alcohol restriction, and possibly potassium supplements. Also, men should limit themselves to no more than 2 drinks per day and women to no more than 1 drink per day.[4] Increased physical activity is highly recommended.

Typically lifestyle changes can be expected to lower one's SBP by 4-5 mm Hg and DBP by 2-4 mmHg. However, according to guidelines, a diet full of fruits, vegetables and healthy grains that is low in saturated fat may lower SBP by as much as 11 mm Hg.[4]

Medication Treatment

The **4 major groups** of medications recommended as treatment for high blood pressure are:

1. *Thiazide diuretics*
2. *Calcium channel blockers (CCB)*
3. *Angiotensin converting enzyme inhibitors (ACEI)*
4. *Angiotensin receptor blockers (ARB)*

Depending on other health conditions you may have, your doctor may prescribe you medications for high blood pressure outside of these 4 groups. For example, if you have a history of heart attack, your doctor may want you to take a beta blocker.

Drug Choices for High Blood Pressure

Population	Drug of Choice		
Non-black population (including those with diabetes)	JNC 8: CCB, thiazide, ACEI or ARB		
	For age < 60 years old ASH		

	recommends: • 1st line: ACEI or ARB • 2nd line: CCB or thiazide • 3rd line: CCB plus ACEI **or** ARB plus thiazide For age > 60 years old ASH recommends: • 1st: CCB or thiazide preferred, ACEI or ARB ok too • 2nd line: CCB, thiazide, ACEI or ARB • 3rd line: CCB plus ACEI **or** ARB plus thiazide ACC/AHA: • 1st: thiazide • 2nd line: CCB • 3rd line: ACEI or ARB		
Black population (including those with diabetes)	JNC 8: CCB or thiazide ASH recommends: • First line: CCB or thiazide • 2nd line: ACEI or ARB		

	• 3rd line: CCB plus ACEI **or** ARB plus thiazide ACC/AHA: • First line: CCB or thiazide • 2nd line: ACEI or ARB • 3rd line: CCB plus ACEI **or** ARB plus thiazide		
Heart failure	JNC 8 recommends: 1st- Thiazide, 2nd- ACEI (regardless of race) ASH, ACC/AHA: recommends: ACEI or ARB <u>plus</u> beta blocker <u>plus</u> diuretic <u>plus</u> spironolactone regardless of blood pressure. Amlodipine can be added for additional blood pressure control.		
Age 18 years or older with chronic kidney disease (regardless of race or diabetes	JNC 8 recommends: ACEI or ARB (all ages, all races)		

status)	ASH recommends: • 1st line: ACEI or ARB (ACEI for black population) • 2nd line: CCB or thiazide • 3rd line: CCB or thiazide (whichever hasn't been used yet)		
Age 75 years or older with chronic kidney disease	JNC 8 recommends: ACEI or ARB (all ages, all races) ASH recommends: CCBs and thiazide-type diuretic should be used instead of ACEI or ARB due to the risk of high potassium in the blood and further renal impairment		
Coronary artery disease	ASH recommends: • 1st line: beta blocker plus ARB or ACEI • 2nd: add CCB or thiazide • 3rd: CCB or thiazide (whichever hasn't		

	been used yet) ACC/AHA: Beta blocker, ACEI, ARB (depending on other conditions. For example: beta blocker for heart attack). Other medications may be added such as dihydropyridine CCB, thiazide, aldosterone antagonist.		
Stroke	JNC8: CCB or thiazide is recommended first for the black population with stroke. ASH recommends for nonblack population: • 1st line: ACEI or ARB • 2nd line: add CCB or thiazide • 3rd line: CCB or thiazide (whichever hasn't been used yet) ACC/AHA: ACEIs are more effective than thiazides or CCBs in		

	lowering BP and preventing stroke in nonblack population.		

CCB = calcium channel blocker, ACEI = angiotensin converting enzyme inhibitors, ARB = Angiotensin receptor blockers

Keep in mind that many people will require more than one high blood pressure drug to achieve blood pressure control. In fact, ACC/AHA has outlined criteria that tells us when to consider starting with one medication and when to start with two:

When to Start with More Than One Medication[4]

	Who	Start With…
■	Adults with stage 1 high blood pressure with a BP goal of 130/80	Start with 1 first line medication. Other agents may be added later if needed
■	Adults with stage 2 high blood pressure with a BP that is more than 20/10 above their BP goal.	Start with 2 first line medications in different classes (thiazides, CCBs, ACEIs, ARBs)

Recommended High Blood Pressure Montitoring[4]

	Criteria	Recommended Monitoring
■	Adults with normal BP (BP < 120/80)	Reassess in 1 year
■	Adults with elevated blood pressure (SBP 120-129 or DBP 80) with CVD risk < 10%	Reassess within 3 to 6 months.

	Criteria	Recommended Monitoring
	Adults with Stage 1 high blood pressure (SBP 130-139 or DBP 80-89) with CVD or CVD risk > or = to 10%	If using non-drug therapy, reassess in 3-6 months. If using non-drug plus drug therapy, reassess in 1 month (if goal met, follow up in 3-6 months. If goal not met, follow up more often than 3-6 months and consider intensifying therapy)
	Adults with Stage 2 high blood pressure (BP > or = to 140/90)	Reassess in 1 month (if goal met, follow up in 3-6 months. If goal not met, follow up more often than 3-6 months and consider intensifying therapy)
	Adults with very high blood pressure (SBP > or = to 180 or DBP > or = to 110)	See your doctor right away or go to the Emergency Room/Urgent Care to be evaluated.

If you are finding it difficult to stick with your medication regimen, consider using medications that are dosed only once a day, rather than twice a day or more. Also, using medications that contain a combination of ingredients in one pill (rather than taking each ingredient individually) may help, too.[4]

Remember, the goal of treating your high blood pressure is to minimize your risk for developing serious health conditions such as stroke, heart attack and kidney failure. Thanks to the efforts of organizations like the JNC, ASH, AHA and ACC, we have more information than ever to help us determine the best medication for lowering our blood pressure. Following their recommendations, we can significantly decrease our risk of heart attack, stroke, and even death. If you have high blood pressure, make sure to work closely with your doctor, using the guidelines as a tool, to choose the best medications for your situation.

REFERENCES

1. James PA, Oparil S, Carter BL, et al. 2014 evidence-based guideline for the management of high blood pressure in adults: report from the panel members appointed to the Eighth Joint National Committee (JNC 8). *JAMA* 2013 Dec 18. doi

2. Merai R, Siegel C, Rakotz M, Basch P, Wright J, Wong B; DHSc., Thorpe P. CDC Grand Rounds: A Public Health Approach to Detect and Control Hypertension. *MMWR Morb Mortal Wkly Rep.* 2016 Nov 18;65(45):1261-1264

3. Mozzafarian D, Benjamin EJ, Go AS, et al. Heart Disease and Stroke Statistics-2015 Update: a report from the American Heart Association. *Circulation.* 2015;e29-322.

4. 2017 ACC/AHA/AAPA/ABC/ACPM/AGS/APhA/ASH/ASPC/NMA/PCNA Guideline for the Prevention, Detection, Evaluation, and Management of High Blood Pressure in Adults: A Report of the American College of Cardiology/American Heart Association Task Force on Clinical Practice Guidelines. *J Am Coll Cardiol* 2017;Nov 13:[Epub ahead of print]

5. Salvetti A and Ghiadoni L. Thiazide Diuretics in the Treatment of Hypertension: An Update. *JASN* April 2006 vol. 17 no. 4 suppl 2 S25-S29

6. Barzilay JU et al. ALLHAT Collaborative Research Group. Fasting glucose levels and incident diabetes mellitus in older nondiabetic adults randomized to receive 3 different classes of antihypertensive treatment. *Arch Intern Med* 2006: 166:2191-201.

7. Kostis, JB, Wilson AC, Freudenberger RS, Cosgrove NM, Pressel SK, Davis BR. Long-term effect of diuretic-based therapy on fatal outcomes in subjects with isolated systolic hypertension with and without diabetes. *Am J Cardiol.* 2005, 95: 29-35

8. Kostis JB, Kim HJ, Rusnak J, et al. Incidence and characteristics of angioedema associated with enalapril. Arch Intern Med 2005; 165:1637.

9. Brown NJ, Ray WA, Snowden M, Griffin MR. Black Americans have an increased rate of angiotensin converting enzyme inhibitor-associated angioedema. Clin Pharmacol Ther 1996; 60:8.

10. Gibbs CR, Lip GY, Beevers DG. Angioedema due to ACE inhibitors: increased risk in patients of African origin. Br J Clin Pharmacol 1999; 48:861.

11. Law MR, Morris JK, Wald NJ. Use of blood pressure lowering drugs in the prevention of cardiovascular disease: meta-analysis of 147 randomised trials in the context of expectations from prospective epidemiological studies. *BMJ.* 2009;338:b1665

12. Dong C, Della-Morte D, Rundek T, Wright CB, Elkind MSV, Sacco RL. Evidence to Maintain the Systolic Blood Pressure Treatment Threshold at 140 mm Hg for Stroke Prevention: The Northern Manhattan Study. Hypertension. 2016. doi: 10.1161/HYPERTENSIONAHA.115.06857.

13. Harel Z et al. The effect of combination treatment with aliskiren and blockers of the renin-angiotensin system on hyperkaliemia and acute kidney injury: Systematic review and meta-analysis. BMJ 2012 Jan 9; 344:e42.

14. Ibanez B, James S, Agewall S, et al. 2017 ESC Guidelines for the Management of Acute Myocardial Infarction in Patients Presenting With ST-Segment Elevation: The Task Force for the Management of Acute Myocardial Infarction in Patients Presenting With ST-Segment Elevation of the European Society of Cardiology (ESC). *Eur Heart J* 2017; Aug 26:[Epub ahead of print].

CHAPTER 3

CHRONIC OBSTRUCTIVE PULMONARY DISEASE (COPD)

The Empowered Medicine Guide to COPD

How to Use This Chapter

This chapter is arranged in a step-by-step fashion. First, we will go over the basics of chronic obstructive pulmonary disease (COPD) such as what it is and why treating it is important. Then we will follow a step-by-step process for figuring out what COPD medications may be best for you. Feel free to write your own information in the blanks provided to aid in your calculations. Finally, we will look at the different medications recommended (and NOT recommended) for treating COPD.

If you wish, use Appendix IV in the back to log your own information for easy calculations and sharing with your doctor. Also, at the end of this chapter you will find a section called 'The Bottom Line'. This box sums up the main points of the chapter

COPD: The Basics

Chronic obstructive pulmonary disease (COPD) is a condition that makes it very hard to breath. In the United States, COPD refers to a combination of two conditions: emphysema and chronic bronchitis. People with COPD may wheeze, have shortness of breath, and have tightness in their chest. They may also have a chronic cough that produces a lot of mucus.

When the lungs are functioning normally, air goes down the ıdpipe) and into tubes in your lungs called bronchi. These tubes branch out into thousands of smaller tubes called bronchioles. At the end of these bronchioles are many small air sacs called alveoli [al-**vee**-*uh*-lahy]. These alveoli fill up with air like little balloons each time you breathe.

Small blood vessels called capillaries collect oxygen from the air in the alveoli. Oxygen is a vital element in our body. The cells in our bodies must have oxygen to function properly. The oxygen passes from the air sacs into the blood while carbon dioxide (CO_2) passes from the blood into the air sacs. CO_2 is a waste product that our bodies produce. Our bodies must get rid of the CO_2, thus CO_2 is blown out of the lungs when one exhales.

HUMAN LUNG

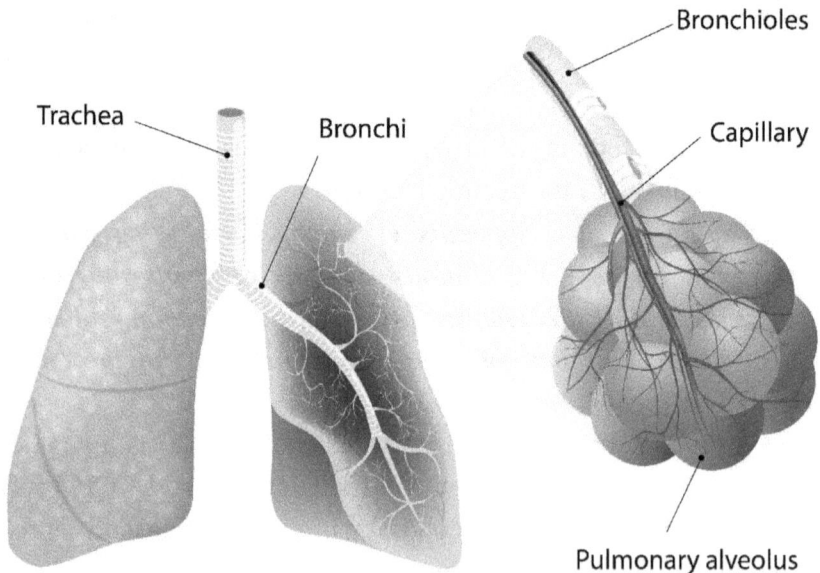

Trachea

Bronchi

Bronchioles

Capillary

Pulmonary alveolus

Figure 1

When someone has COPD, it generally means the air sacs have lost their elasticity. The walls of the air sacs may be damaged, thick, swollen, and have lost their shape. When this happens, it makes it very difficult for the lungs to exchange oxygen and CO_2. Mucus glands may also start working overtime producing more mucus than normal. This can cause the airways to become clogged.

What are the Symptoms of COPD?

Symptoms of COPD may include a chronic cough, often called a 'smoker's cough'. One may also have shortness of breath, wheezing, and chest tightness. As the disease progresses, one may find their lips and/or nails turn gray or blue. This is a sign that your tissues are not getting enough oxygen and should promptly be reported to your doctor. Finally, your heartbeat may be faster than usual. This is the heart's attempt to pump blood faster to deliver more oxygen to the oxygen-deprived tissues of the body. Some medications used to treat COPD can make your heart beat faster.

The symptoms of COPD generally tend to worsen over time and can limit your ability to perform normal everyday tasks like walking or cooking. The severity of COPD differs from person to person. COPD is not contagious, meaning it cannot be passed from person to person.

What Causes COPD?

COPD is caused by the long-term inhalation of lung irritants. The most common irritant that causes COPD is tobacco smoke. Tobacco smoke from cigarettes, pipes, and cigars can all cause COPD. Air pollution, chemical fumes, and the burning of wood or cooking fuels can also cause COPD, although these are less common. Furthermore, a rare disease called alpha-1 antitrypsin deficiency can also cause COPD.

As of the date of this writing, there is not enough evidence to say for sure if e-cigarettes or vaping cause COPD. Although initial research does suggest they can contribute to COPD.

Approximately 75% of people with COPD are current or previous smokers.[1] However, that leaves 25% of people with COPD who have never smoked. It is best to never start smoking if you want to avoid developing COPD. If you smoke, quitting can dramatically decrease your risk of developing COPD. Also, make sure to burn wood and cooking fuels in well-ventilated areas. Finally, the avoidance of vaping, dusts, chemical agents, and fumes might also help one avoid COPD.

Why is it Important to Prevent COPD?

Chronic lower respiratory diseases like COPD is the 3rd leading cause of death in the United States.[2] COPD develops slowly over time. Many people don't realize they have COPD until they can't perform routine activities like walking or cooking without becoming unusually out of breath.

It's important to recognize symptoms when they start to occur and seek treatment when needed. The goal of managing COPD is to improve exercise tolerance (your ability to exercise) and reduce how often and how severe your COPD exacerbations are (COPD exacerbations are a temporary worsening of your symptoms). Diligently managing your COPD can help keep you out of the hospital and improve your quality of life.

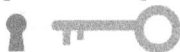

Key to Success

The goal of managing COPD is to improve exercise tolerance (your ability to exercise) and reduce how often and how severe your COPD exacerbations are (COPD exacerbations are a temporary worsening of your symptoms). Diligently managing your COPD can help keep you out of the hospital and improve your quality of life.

How is COPD Diagnosed?

Guidelines for the diagnosis and treatment of COPD have been put out by an organization called the Global Initiative for Obstructive Lung Disease (Also known as 'GOLD'). GOLD is an international collaboration of COPD experts. Periodically, GOLD releases an update of their COPD guidelines.

According to the 2017 GOLD COPD guidelines, COPD should be considered in any patient who has trouble breathing, has chronic cough or sputum production, and a history of exposure to risk factors for the disease (like long-term exposure to smoke or fumes).[3]

The GOLD COPD guidelines recommend that your doctor diagnose your condition and ask you a series of questions about your symptoms as follows:

Table 1: GOLD Recommendations for the Diagnosis and Assessment of COPD Symptoms

1. **Spirometry**: First, using spirometry, your doctor will confirm the diagnosis of COPD (see Table 3 below).

2. **Assessment Questions**: Second, it's recommended that your doctor use the Modified British Medical Research Council (mMRC) questionnaire **OR** the COPD Assessment Test (CAT) to determine how severe your symptoms are.

3. **Exacerbations and Hospitalizations:** Next, the guidelines recommend that your doctor ask you how many COPD exacerbations you've had in the last 12 months and how many of those resulted in hospitalizations.

4. **ABCD Scoring**: Finally, it's recommended that your doctor uses the GOLD ABCD scoring system to figure out what group your COPD falls into. This will determine what medications will likely work best for you.

Let's take a closer look at each of the 4 steps above:

STEP 1: Spirometry: Use Your Spirometry Results to Diagnose COPD

Spirometry is a common test done at your doctor's office. It is used to assess how well your lungs work. It involves breathing into a handheld device. The device measures how much air you inhale, how much you exhale and the speed of your breath. Spirometry is used to diagnose several health conditions including COPD and asthma. It may also be used to monitor your progress during the treatment of these health conditions.

The spirometry results will tell your doctor how the lungs are functioning compared to other people of the same age, height, weight, sex, and ethnicity. To do this your doctor will calculate a predicted normal value before you take the spirometry test. Then he/she will compare your test results with the predicted normal value that was calculated before the test.

Before we talk about how to read your spirometry results, we need to look at what the different parts of your spirometry test mean.

1. The first value, forced vital capacity (FVC), is the total amount of air you can forcefully breathe out after breathing in as deeply as possible.

2. The second value, the forced expiratory volume (FEV1) is the amount of air you can force out of your lungs in one second.

If either of these values is abnormal, there may be something restricting your breathing.

Your doctor will likely look at your FEV1 and FVC separately and also look at your FEV1/FVC ratio. If this ratio is less than 0.7, then a diagnosis of restrictive lung disease may be made. Your doctor will evaluate your symptoms and spirometry results and will determine if your symptoms are being caused by a condition such as COPD, asthma, congestive heart failure, or tuberculosis.

You can get an idea of what your predicted values are at the Centers for Disease Control's (CDC) online calculator at https://www.cdc.gov/niosh/topics/spirometry/refcalculator.html. Once you know your FEV1 and FVC values from your spirometry test, you can plug them into the calculator and see how your spirometry results compare to the predicated normal values. You can also see if your FEV1/FVC is less than 0.7.

Let's break down this process so you can plug your own numbers in.

STEP 1a: Obtain your FEV1 and FVC from your latest spirometry test (you may need to ask for these results from your doctor's office):
Write in your FEV1 and FVC here:

My FEV1 is _____
My FVC is _____

STEP 1b: Plug your FEV1 and FVC values into the CDC's online calculators at
https://www.cdc.gov/niosh/topics/spirometry/refcalculator.html. The calculator will calculate your FEV1 ÷ FVC, then it will multiply it by 100 to give you a percentage. Enter this value in the blank below **(this number will be calculated on the CDC online tool so you can just look and write it in here; no math required).**

FEV1/FVC% is _____ %

Note: if your FEV1/FVC% is less than 0.7, then your doctor might diagnose you with COPD.

Step 1c: Determine Which GOLD Group You are In

If you've been diagnosed with COPD, your doctor can use your spirometry results to figure out how to classify your condition. To do this, your doctor will divide your FEV1 by the predicted FEV1 (from the CDC website).

Your FEV1 ÷ predicted FEV1 (on CDC website) = _____

Then multiply this answer this answer by 100 to get the percent you need.

= _____ %

You and your doctor will use this percentage to see which GOLD class you fall into.

Table 3: **Classification of COPD Based on Spirometry Results**[3]

Check the box next to the GOLD group that applies to you:

☐	**GOLD 1**: Very mild COPD with a FEV1 about 80% or more of normal
☐	**GOLD 2**: Moderate COPD with a FEV1 between 50 and 80 percent of normal
☐	**GOLD 3**: Severe emphysema with FEV1 between 30 and 50 percent of normal
☐	**GOLD 4**: Very severe COPD with a lower FEV1 than Stage 3, or those with Stage 3 FEV1 *and* low blood oxygen levels

Classification based on spirometry numbers can give you an idea of how severe your condition is. The down side is it only captures one piece of the COPD puzzle. Studies show that looking at symptoms actually give a better idea of how you are doing and can help determine which medications to use to treat your COPD. After all, two patients with similar spirometry numbers can have very different symptoms and tolerate exercise very differently. For this reason, the GOLD COPD Guidelines recommend using a one of two tests (sets of assessment questions) to determine how severe your symptoms are: the mMRC and the CAT (see below).

STEP 2: Assessment Questions

The Modified British Medical Research Council (mMRC) questionnaire **OR** the COPD Assessment Test (CAT) can help determine how severe your symptoms are. The results of these tests can help give a better idea of which treatment options may be more effective.

Table 4: **The Modified British Medical Research Council (mMRC) questionnaire[3]**

Grade	Description of Breathlessness
0	I only get breathless with strenuous exercise.
1	I get short of breath when hurrying on level ground or walking up a slight hill.
2	On level ground, I walk slower than people of the same age because of breathlessness or have to stop for breath when walking at my own pace.
3	I stop for breath after walking about 100 yards or after a few minutes on level ground.
4	I am too breathless to leave the house, or I am breathless when dressing.

Table 5: **COPD Assessment Test (CAT)**[3]

	1 2 3 4 5	
I never cough	1 2 3 4 5	I cough all the time
I have no phlegm (mucus) in my chest at all	1 2 3 4 5	My chest is full of phlegm
My chest does not feel tight at all	1 2 3 4 5	My chest feels very tight
When I walk up a hill or up one flight of stairs I am not breathless	1 2 3 4 5	When I walk up hill or up one flight of stairs I am very out of breath
I am not limited doing any activities at home	1 2 3 4 5	I am very limited doing any activities at home
I am confident leaving home despite my lung condition	1 2 3 4 5	I am not at all confident leaving home because of my lung condition
I sleep soundly	1 2 3 4 5	I don't sleep soundly because of my lung condition
I have lots of energy	1 2 3 4 5	I have no energy at all

Note your mMRC and/or your CAT test here:

My mMRC score is:_____

My CAT score is: _____

Hang onto your mMRC and CAT scores for now. We will look at them later.

STEP 3: Exacerbations and Hospitalizations

The GOLD guidelines recommend that your doctor ask how many COPD exacerbations you've had in the last 12 months and how many of those had resulted in a hospitalization. This information will be combined with the information you provide about your symptoms to determine which ABCD group (see below) you fall into for treatment purposes.

Note your hospital admission information here:

In the last 12 months, I have had _____ number of COPD exacerbations
In the last 12 months, I have had _____ number of hospitalizations due to my COPD

STEP 4: ABCD Scoring

This is the last step of scoring your COPD. The GOLD COPD "ABCD" grading system is used to figure out the severity of your condition. The ABCD system combines information you provide about your symptoms, looks at how many exacerbations you are having, and how many of them have landed you in the hospital. This information is used to help determine the right medication therapy for you.

You can use Figure 2 or Table 6 below to figure out which ABCD group you fall into.

Exacerbation
History

More than 1
exacerbation not
requiring a hospital
admission
OR at least 1
exacerbation requiring
hospital admission

C Less symptoms High Risk	**D** More Symptoms High Risk

1 or less
exacerbations not
requiring a hospital
admission

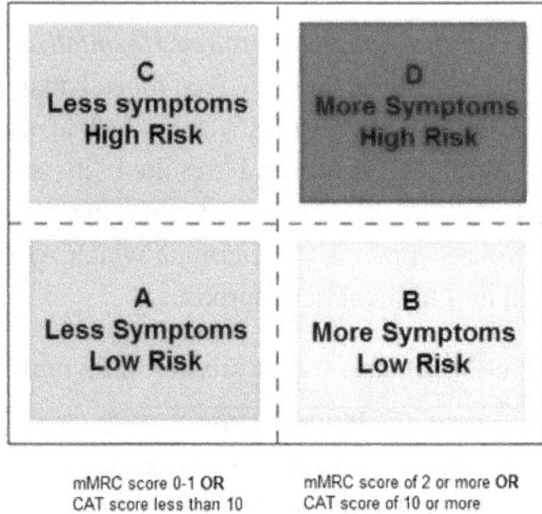

A Less Symptoms Low Risk	**B** More Symptoms Low Risk

mMRC score 0-1 OR   mMRC score of 2 or more OR
CAT score less than 10   CAT score of 10 or more

Figure 2: GOLD COPD ABCD Grading System

As you can see, the lower your mMRC or CAT score, the less risk you have. A lower number of exacerbations and hospital visits also means you're at a lower risk. Here's another way to look at it:

Table 6: **GOLD COPD ABCD Grading System**

ABCD Group	Symptoms	Exacerbations/Hospitalizations *(in the past 12 months)*
Group A: Less symptoms, low risk	mMRC score of 0-1 OR CAT score of less than 10	1 or less exacerbations not requiring a hospital visit
Group B: More symptoms, low risk	mMRC score of 2 or more OR CAT score of 10 or more	1 or less exacerbations not requiring a hospital visit

ABCD Group	Symptoms	Exacerbations/Hospitalizations *(in the past 12 months)*
Group C: Less symptoms, high risk	mMRC score of 0-1 OR CAT score of less than 10	More than 1 exacerbation not requiring a hospitalization **OR** at least 1 exacerbation requiring a hospitalization
Group D: More symptoms, high risk	mMRC score of 2 or more OR CAT score of 10 or more	More than 1 exacerbation not requiring a hospitalization **OR** at least 1 exacerbation requiring a hospitalization

Based on which group you fall into above, your doctor will be able to categorize your condition into group A, B, C, or D. This will determine which medications may best treat your COPD.

Note your COPD grade here:

My COPD grade is:

☐ **Grade A**
☐ **Grade B**
☐ **Grade C**
☐ **Grade D**

Let's take a look at the treatment options for COPD now. Here is a quick rundown of medications used to treat COPD.

Medications for COPD

Medications for COPD include:

• **SABAs** (short acting beta agonist)-examples: albuterol, levalbuterol, terbutaline

• **SAMAs** (short acting muscarinic antagonist)-example: ipratropium

• **LABAs** (long acting beta agonist)-examples: salmeterol, formoterol, arformoterol, indacaterol, olodaterol

- **LAMAs** (long acting muscarinic antagonist)-examples: tiotropium, aclidinium, glycopyrronium, umeclidinium
- **ICSs** (inhaled corticosteroid)-examples: beclomethasone, budesonide, ciclesonide, flunisolide, fluticasone, mometasone
- **PDE4 Inhibitors**-example: roflumilast
- **Methylxanthines**-examples: theophylline, aminophylline
- **Mucolytics**-example: acetylcysteine
- **Opioids**- examples: morphine, hydrocodone, oxycodone
- **Antibiotics**-examples: azithromycin, erythromycin
- Various combinations of medications in inhalers

Which Medications are Best for My COPD?

As you can see there are many medication choices available. How does one know which medication will best treat their COPD? Thankfully, the GOLD guidelines have compiled data from the most recent studies and have outlined which medications appear to work the best depending on what group (group A, B, C, or D) you fall into.

Table 7: **COPD Therapy based on GOLD ABCD Groups**

ABCD Group	Drug Therapy	Alternative Therapy
Group A: Less symptoms, low risk	SABA or SAMA	LABA or LAMA or SABA plus SAMA
Group B: More symptoms, low risk	LABA or LAMA	LABA plus LAMA
Group C: Less symptoms, high risk	ICS plus LABA or LAMA	LAMA plus LABA or LABA plus PDE4 inhibitor or LAMA plus PDE4 inhibitor
Group D: More symptoms, high risk	ICS plus LABA plus/or LAMA	ICS plus LABA plus LAMA or ICS plus LABA plus PDE4 inhibitor or LABA plus LAMA or LAMA plus PDE4 inhibitor

Currently there is no cure for COPD, and unfortunately there is currently no quality data from trials that demonstrates that any medication can keep your lung function from decreasing over time.[3] However, there are several medications that can be used to help control symptoms and keep you out of the hospital. These medications for COPD are used to decrease symptoms and improve exercise tolerance so you can feel better.

STEP 5: Determine Which Medications May be Best for You

Using your COPD grade, note which group of medications may be best for you. **Check the box below that applies:**

☐ **Grade A:**
- SABA or SAMA or…
- LABA or LAMA or…
- SABA + SAMA

☐ **Grade B:**
- LABA or LAMA or…
- LABA + LAMA

☐ **Grade C:**
- ICS + LABA + LAMA or…
- LAMA + LABA or…
- LABA + PDE4 inhibitor or…
- LAMA + PDE4 inhibitor

☐ **Grade D:**
- ICS + LABA +/or LAMA or…
- ICS + LABA + LAMA or…
- ICS + LABA + PDE4 inhibitor or…
- LABA + LAMA or…
- LAMA + PDE4 inhibitor

Here we will discuss all of the medications used to treat COPD. You will notice that each medication has at least 2 names: the generic name and the brand name. The generic is its basic, scientific name. The brand name is the name given to the drug by the drug company that makes it. So for example, acetaminophen is the generic name of the popular pain reliever and Tylenol® is the brand name.

Short-acting bronchodilators -- These types of medications widen the airways in the lungs allowing more air to flow in. These medications are short-acting. Their effect may last 4-6 hours or so.

Short-acting beta agonist (SABA) – These medications are used as rescue therapy for fast relief of COPD symptoms. Examples of these medications include terbutaline (Brethine®), albuterol (salbutamol, ProAir®, ProAir HFA, Ventolin HFA, Accuneb®, VoSpire ER®, Proventil®, Proventil HFA®), levalbuterol (Xopenex®). More common side effects include headache, dizziness, nausea, vomiting, diarrhea, anxiety, and shakiness.

Short-acting muscarinic antagonist (SAMA) – These are also called 'short-acting anticholinergics'. An example of this medication includes ipratropium (Atrovent®). Inhaled anticholinergic drugs are not absorbed very well, so side effects with these medications are somewhat limited. Some may experience dryness of the mouth, skin flushing, rapid heartbeat, heart palpitations, worsening of glaucoma, nausea, headache, and urinary retention (trouble urinating). This trouble with urination may be increased in men with enlarged prostates.

Long-acting bronchodilators -- These types of medications also widen the airways in the lungs allowing more air to flow in. These medications are long-acting. Their effect may last 12 hours or longer. Examples of long-acting bronchodilators include:

Long-acting beta agonist (LABA) -- Examples of these medications include salmeterol (Serevent®, Advair®) formoterol (Foradil®), arformoterol (Brovana®), indacaterol (Arcapta Neohaler®), olodaterol (Striverdi Respimat®). Potential side effects of these medications include headache, muscle or skeletal pain, tremors, and/or cardiac arrhythmia (abnormal rate or rhythm of the heart). If you experience palpitations or lightheadedness/fainting while taking these medications, seek medical attention immediately.

Long-acting muscarinic antagonist (LAMA) --These are also called 'long-acting anticholinergics'. In addition to dilating the airways to let more oxygen into the lungs, they work with certain receptors in the body to help dry up secretions (like mucous). Examples of these medications include tiotropium (Spiriva®, Spiriva Respimat®), aclidinium (Tudorza Pressair®), glycopyrronium bromide (Robinul®, Robinul Forte®, Cuvposa®, Glycate®), and umeclidinium (Incruse Ellipta®). As mentioned in the SAMA section above, inhaled anticholinergic drugs are not absorbed very well so side effects with these medications are somewhat limited. Some may experience dryness of the mouth, skin flushing, rapid heartbeat, heart palpitations, worsening of glaucoma, nausea, headache, and urinary retention (trouble urinating). The trouble with urination may be increased in men with enlarged prostates.

Inhaled corticosteroids (ICS) and systemic corticosteroids- ICSs work by reducing inflammation in the airways. They also help reduce the amount of mucous in the lungs. This helps clear out airways so it is easier to breathe. Systemic corticosteroids (corticosteroids that you can take in pill form by mouth or as an injectable form) can improve lung function, improve oxygenation, shorten recovery time, and shorten hospitalization duration.[3] Oral and Intravenous corticosteroids are only recommended for treating hospitalized COPD patients or in the case of an emergency situation.

Long term therapy with an ICS (where the ICS is the only medication) is not recommended. Duration of ICS therapy should not be more than 5-7 days.[3]

ICSs are generally found in combination with LABAs in a single inhalation device. Examples of inhalers that include an ICS plus another medication include formoterol/beclomethasone (Fostair®), formoterol/budesonide (Symbicort®), formoterol/

mometasone (Dulera®), salmeterol/fluticasone (Advair®, Advair HFA), vilanterol/fluticasone (Breo Ellipta®).

Potential side effects of ICSs include sore mouth/throat, hoarseness, cough, airway spasms, thrush (fungus infection of the mouth), slight reduction in growth, decreased bone thickness in adults, cataracts, and increased risk of pneumonia.[3]

There are a couple of things you can do to help decrease the risk of developing thrush while taking inhaled corticosteroids.

1. Use the lowest dose possible needed to control your symptoms.

2. Use a spacer (see Figure 3) with your meter dosed inhaler (MDI). A spacer is a handheld device that attaches to your inhaler. You first spray the medication into the spacer then inhale from the spacer. This helps make sure you inhale most of the vapor instead of accidently spraying it on your tongue.

3. Always rinse your mouth out with water after each use of your ICS inhaler. Do not swallow the water. The idea is to spit out any medicine left in the mouth that could cause thrush. Spitting it out will also help ensure less medication gets into the blood stream where it may contribute to more side effects.

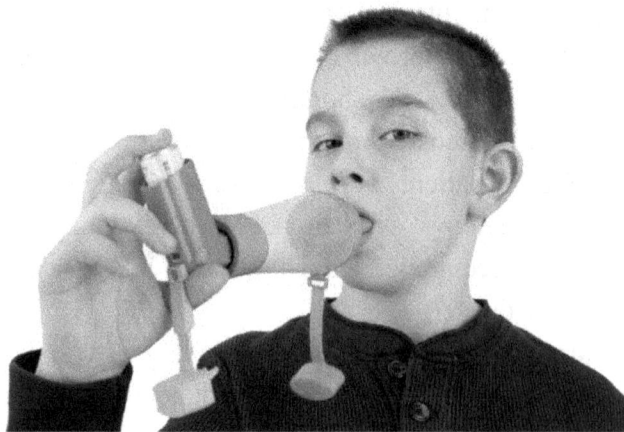

Figure 4: Boy with Inhaler and Spacer

Oral PDE4 inhibitors – An example of this group of medications is roflumilast (Daliresp®). Roflumilast is an add-on therapy for patients with severe COPD symptoms who experience exacerbations while taking a combination of a bronchodilator with an ICS. Possible side effects of roflumilast include weight loss, decreased appetite, diarrhea, nausea, backache, dizziness, headache, and insomnia. Suicidal thoughts have also been reported with this medication. If you experience suicidal thoughts while taking roflumilast, seek medical attention immediately.

Methylxanthines – Examples of this group of medications include theophylline (Theo-Dur®) and aminophylline (Norphyl®, Phyllocontin®, Tryphylline®). Studies show that these drugs have modest lung-dilating effects. There is also limited data on the effects of these medications on COPD exacerbation rates.[3] Blood levels of these medications must be monitored to prevent toxicity. Unfortunately, much of the benefit occurs only when near-toxic doses are given.[3] Methylxanthines are not generally recommended due to increased side effect profiles. Potential side effects of these medications include nausea, vomiting, headache, insomnia, tremor, irritability, restlessness, heart arrhythmias, seizure, and severe allergic reactions.

Mucolytics – Mucolytics break down excess mucous that may be plugging up the lungs. Acetylcysteine is most often used for this purpose. Acetylcysteine also has antioxidant properties. It is being researched for its role in helping to heal lung damage caused by cigarette smoke which contains a great deal of free radicals. Free radicals are unstable molecules that damage cells. Due to its antioxidant and anti-mucous properties, acetylcysteine has been shown to decrease the number of COPD exacerbations you have.[3]

Acetylcysteine is not available in an inhaler. Instead it in available as a nebulizer solution. Nebulizer solutions are put into a nebulizer machine which turns the medication into a mist that you inhale. Acetylcysteine is recommended in selected patients. We will talk a little more about nebulizer solutions in a moment.

Potential side effects of acetylcysteine include nausea, vomiting, fever, runny nose, drowsiness, clamminess, chest tightness, coughing, wheezing and shortness of breath.

Antibiotics – The use of antibiotics, when an infection is present in the lungs, can shorten recovery time and reduce the risk of treatment failure. Two antibiotics in particular: azithromycin and erythromycin, were shown to reduce COPD exacerbations over one year. But treatment with azithromycin is associated with an increased risk of bacterial resistance and hearing impairment.[3]

Potential side effects depend on which antibiotic is prescribed. Consult your doctor or pharmacist for possible side effects of the particular antibiotic you are prescribed.

Opioids – The GOLD guidelines mention that daily oral opioids may be helpful in the relief of severe COPD symptoms that haven't responded to other medications.[3] Opioids can be effective in providing relief from muscle and bone pain, aid with sleep, and may help one breathe easier. However, care must be taken when dosing opioids because too much opioid can cause respiratory depression (can decrease your ability to breathe on your own). It's important that the lowest possible dose to obtain relief is prescribed. This is especially important in patients who are opioid naïve (haven't had opioids before). These patients are at an especially high risk for serious respiratory depression and even death from opioids.

Potential side effects of opioids include sedation, nausea, vomiting, dizziness, constipation, physical dependence, tolerance, and trouble breathing.

Empowered U

In the medical world, a LAMA is:

a. A domesticated woolly animal in the camel family

b. A teacher in Tibetan Buddhism

c. A type of long-acting medication that dilates airways and helps decrease mucous secretions in the lungs

d. I don't know but "llama" think about it for a bit.

Answer: c

It's important to mention that proper technique is extremely important when using an inhaler. One might think that all inhalers are created equally. After all, how hard can it be? Well, contrary to popular belief there are many different types of inhalers including metered dose inhalers (MDI) dry powder inhalers (DPI), and soft mist inhalers (SMI):

• **Metered dose inhaler (MDI)**-Liquid medication that is inhaled slowly. A spacer may help ensure that more medication is inhaled

• **Dry powder inhaler (DPI)**-A dry powder medication that is inhaled by placing your lips around the mouthpiece. A spacer is NOT used with these inhalers.

• **Soft mist inhaler (SMI)**-Medication in slow mist form. The SMI forms a soft cloud of mist that is easy to inhale.

Below is a summary of the medications used for the treatment of COPD including those inhalers that may contain a combination of drugs.

Table 8: **Medications for the Treatment of COPD***

Short-acting beta-agonists (SABA)	
Albuterol (MDI or DPI)	Salbutamol, ProAir®, ProAir HFA®, Ventolin®, Ventolin HFA, Accuneb®, VoSpire ER®, Proventil®, Proventil HFA®
Levalbuterol (MDI)	Xopenex®
Terbutaline (DPI)	Brethine®
Long-acting beta-agonists (LABA)	
Salmeterol (MDI or DPI)	Serevent®, Advair®
Formoterol (DPI)	Foradil®
arformoterol	Brovana®
Indacaterol (DPI)	Arcapta Neohaler®
Olodaterol (SMI)	Striverdi Respimat®
Short-acting muscarinic antagonist (SAMA) -- AKA short-acting antiholinergics	
ipratropium (MDI)	Atrovent®
Long-acting muscarinic antagonist (LAMA) – AKA long-acting anticholinergics	
Tiotropium (DPI or SMI)	Spiriva®, Spiriva Respimat®
Aclidinium MDI or DPI)	Tudorza Pressair®
glycopyrronium bromide (DPI)	Robinul®, Robinul Forte®, Cuvposa®, Glycate®
Umeclidinium (DPI)	Incruse Ellipta®
Inhaled Corticosteroids (ICS)	
Beclomethasone	QVAR®, Beclovent®, Beconase®, Vancenase®, QNASL®, Qvar Redihaler®
Budesonide	Pulmicort®, Pulmicort Flexhaler®, Pulmicort Respules®, Pulmicort Turuhaler®, Rhinocort®, Rhinocort Aqua®, Uceris®
Ciclesonide	Alvesco®, Omnaris®, Zetonna®

Flunisolide	Aerospan®, Aerobid®, Aerobid-M®, Nasalide®, Nasarel®
Fluticasone furoate	Veramyst®, Arnuity Ellipta®
Fluticasone propionate	Flovent®, Flovent Rotadisk®, Flovent Diskus®, Cutivate®, Flonase®, Armonair Respiclick®, Xhance®
Mometasone	Elocon®, Nasonex®, Propel®,Asmanex Twisthaler®
Oral PDE4 inhibitors	
Roflumilast	Daliresp®
Methylxanthines	
Theophylline	Theo-Dur®
Aminophylline	Norphyl®, Phyllocontin®, Tryphylline®
Mycolytics	
Acetylcysteine	Mucomyst®
Combination short-acting beta-agonist (SABA) plus anticholinergic in one device	
Generic	**Brand Name**
Albuterol/ipratropium (MDI)	Combivent®
Combination of long-acting beta-agonist (LABA) plus anticholinergic in one device	
Formoterol/aclidinium (DPI)	Duaklir®, Brimica®
Formoterol/glycopyrronium (MDI)	Bevespi®
Indacaterol/glycopyrronium (DPI)	Utibron®
Vilanterol/umeclidinium (DPI)	Anoro Ellipta®
Olodaterol/tiotropium (SMI)	Stiolto Respimat®
Combination of long-acting beta-agonist (LABA) plus corticosteroids (ICS) in one device	
Formoterol/beclomethasone (MDI or DPI)	Fostair®
Formoterol/budesonide (MDI or DPI)	Symbicort®
Formoterol/mometasone (MDI)	Dulera®
Salmeterol/fluticasone (DPI or MDI)	Advair®, Advair HFA®

147

Vilanterol/fluticasone (DPI)	Breo Ellipta®
Opioids	
Morphine	Avinza®, Kadian®, MS Contin®, Morphabond ER, Oramorph SR, Roxanol
hydrocodone	Norco®, Hysingla ER®, Zohydro ER®, Vantrela ER®
Oxycodone	OxyContin®, Percocet®, Percodan®, Xtampza ER®
Antibiotics	
Azithromycin	Zithromax®
Erythromycin	Ery-Tab®

*MDI – metered dose inhaler, DPI = dry powder inhaler, SMI = soft mist inhaler

---

Key to Success

If this whole scoring system seems confusing, don't worry. I've included a lot of information here, but as always there will be a section at the end of this chapter that recaps and highlights the main points you may want to know if you have COPD.

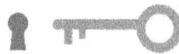

Nebulizers

Some COPD medications are available in the form of an inhalation liquid that is used with a machine called a small volume nebulizer (SVN or simply 'nebulizer'). These medications are provided in a liquid form which is poured into the SVN machine. The machine uses electricity or batteries to turn the medication into a mist over several minutes. The mist is then inhaled through a mouthpiece or mask. Because it delivers the medication in a mist over an extended period of time it is thought that more of the medication reaches the patient's lungs through a nebulizer (vs. inhalers).

Here is a list of the medications above available as a nebulizer solution:

Table 9. **COPD Medications Available as a Nebulizer Solution**

Generic Name	Brand Name
Albuterol	Accuneb®
Levalbuterol	Xopenex®
Ipratropium bromide	Atrovent®
Albuterol and ipratropium	Duoneb®
Budesonide	Pulmicort®
Formoterol fumarate	Performist®
Arformoterol tartrate	Brovana®
Acetylcysteine	Mucomyst®

One drawback to SVN machines is that they are not as portable as inhalers (even though there are 'portable' sized nebulizer machines available). Thus they are often used at home or at the hospital.

Nebulizer tubing, masks, and mouthpieces are made of plastic that degrades over time. They can also harbor bacteria that can make you sick. Therefore they need to be replaced periodically. If you use a nebulizer machine at home, it is imperative that you follow the instructions that come with the machine with regard to use, cleaning, and changing the tubing and other parts.

Always follow the manufacturer's instructions for cleaning and replacing nebulizer parts. With that in mind, here are some general guidelines:

General Instructions for nebulizer Use:
1. Plug in the nebulizer unit
2. Make sure the mouth piece or mask is clean.
3. Wash your hands

4. Place the medication into the nebulizer medication cup

a. If your medication is premixed, open up the ampule and squeeze the medicine into the cup

b. If your medication is not premixed, measure the correct amount of medication and add saline to make a minimum of 3 mL (3 cc) in the cup.

5. Connect the tubing to the nebulizer unit

6. Connect the mouthpiece or mask

7. Turn on the nebulizer machine

8. After observing that the mist is coming out of the mouthpiece or mask, put the mouthpiece in your mouth and close your lips around it. If using a mask, put the mask over your nose and mouth making sure there are no gaps between the mask and your skin as it hugs your face.

9. Breath slowly, inhaling the medicine. Continue breathing in and out slowly until the medicine is all gone. This may take around 10-15 minutes.

Immediately After Use:

1. Wash your hands.

2. Disconnect the mouthpiece or mask from the t-shaped piece.

3. Remove the tubing. Set aside. Do not wash or rinse the tubing or compressor.

4. Rinse the mask or mouthpiece and t-shaped part in warm running water for 30 seconds.

5. Shake off excess water and allow to air dry on a clean cloth or paper towel.

6. Put the mouth piece or mask back together with the tubing and t-shaped part. Connect back to the machine. Run the machine for about 10-20 seconds. This is to help dry everything off.

7. Disconnect the tubing from the machine and store in a zip lock bag to keep it clean and dry.

Deep Cleaning (Do This Once or Twice a Week – Check with Manufacturer):

1. Remove the mouthpiece or mask from the cup. Remove the tubing and set it aside. Do not wash the tubing.

2. Wash the mouthpiece or mask and the t-shaped part in warm, soapy water (dishwashing soap is recommended). Do NOT wash the tubing or compressor unit.

3. Rinse the washed parts in running water for at least 30 seconds.

4. Soak the t-shaped part, cup, and mask or mouthpiece in a solution that is 1 part distilled white vinegar and 2 parts distilled water for 30 minutes.

5. Rinse these parts off for one minute. Use distilled or sterile water, if possible.

6. Shake off excess water and allow parts to air dry on a clean cloth or paper towel.

7. When dry, put these parts back together and connect them to the machine. Let the machine run for 10-20 seconds to help dry everything off.

8. Disconnect the tubing and store in a zip lock bag.

Other Therapies

Influenza vaccine

Influenza vaccination (AKA the "flu shot") can reduce serious illness (such as lower respiratory tract infections requiring hospitalization) and death in COPD patients.[3] A flu shot can be obtained at many doctors' offices. Many pharmacies now also offer flu shots.

Pneumococcal vaccine

There are two pneumococcal vaccines: PCV13 and PPSV23. They differ in that PCV13 is active against 13 serotypes and PPSV23 is active against 23 serotypes. A serotype is a genetic variation within a species of bacteria or virus. PCV13 plus a dose of PPSV23 (at least 1 year later) is recommended for all patients 65 years of age and older. PPSV23 is also recommended for younger patients with other significant health problems, including chronic heart or lung disease. PPSV23 has been shown to reduce the incidence of community-acquired pneumonia in certain COPD patients who are less than 65 years old.[3]

Supplemental Oxygen

It should be noted that the 2017 GOLD guidelines advise against the routine use of oxygen by stable COPD patients who do not have severe resting hypoxemia (low level of oxygen in the blood at rest). This is due to the results of a recent trial that showed oxygen did NOT improve outcomes or quality of life in the patients being tested[3] The guidelines do say that doctors should think about the needs of the individual patient when considering whether to prescribe oxygen.

The guidelines also go on to say that *patients with severe resting hypoxemia (oxygen in the blood less than 88%) should all continuously receive supplemental oxygen*. Long-term oxygen therapy has been shown to improve survival in patients with severe resting chronic hypoxemia.[3] Supplemental oxygen should be adjusted to improve the patient's hypoxemia with a target saturation of 88-92%. Blood gases should be checked frequently (at least every 60-90 days) after oxygen is started to ensure good oxygenation without carbon dioxide build up in the blood, and to make sure the blood is not becoming too acidic.[3]

Ventilatory Support

Noninvasive ventilation (NIV) is a form of noninvasive positive pressure ventilation.

(NPPV) is used in hospitalized COPD patients. This is basically when oxygen is supplied by a mask that 'pushes' the oxygen into your lungs by positive pressure. It has been shown to decrease morbidity (sickness) and mortality (death) in patients who have a severe COPD exacerbation. [3]

Also, patients with both COPD and obstructive sleep apnea have benefited from the use of continuous positive airway pressure (CPAP). CPAP provides oxygen by gentle positive pressure to help keep airways open and improve oxygenation. CPAP has been shown to improve survival and the risk of hospital admissions. [3]

Surgical and Non-surgical Interventions

Getting rid of non-functioning lung tissue through non-surgical procedures may improve exercise tolerance and lung function in certain COPD patients who have not responded well to medical therapy.[3] These types of procedures involve removing non-functioning lung tissue by inserting instruments through the trachea and bronchi while the patient is comfortably sedated.

Lung volume reduction surgery (LVRS) has been shown to improve survival in certain patients with decreased exercise tolerance. [3] This type of procedure involves making incisions in the chest wall. Lung transplant surgery has been shown to improve quality of life and lung function in appropriate patients. [3]

Palliative Care and Hospice

Palliative care is a type of care that focuses on improving one's quality of life and providing comfort to people with serious life-threatening illnesses. Palliative care is similar to hospice care. Both focus on keeping the patient comfortable and pain free. This may mean addressing physical, emotional, and/or spiritual pain. However, hospice is comfort care without a focus on treatment that can cure diseases. Patients on hospice have chosen not to pursue further curative treatment and instead want to focus on being comfortable. They may have received curative treatment but it may no longer be effective. Palliative care, on the other hand, may or may not involve curative treatment.

Private insurance generally pays for hospice but most hospice care for seniors is paid for by Medicare. Thus patients considering hospice care must meet Medicare's eligibility requirements if they are planning on Medicare paying for it. Medicare requires that 2 doctors certify that the patient has less than six months to live. In contrast, palliative care may be started at any time, regardless of if the patient is terminal or not.

Hospice services include 24/7 medications, medical equipment, nursing, social services, and emotional support. Hospice care may be delivered at a medical facility or in the patient's home.

If you are considering palliative care or hospice care, talk with your doctor. He/she will be able to help you obtain the proper resources you'll need to make the best decision.

The Bottom Line

Refer to Appendix IV for a step-by-step worksheet that will help you determine what COPD therapy may be right for you.

COPD is a condition that makes it very hard to breathe. COPD makes it very difficult for the lungs to exchange oxygen and carbon dioxide. Mucus glands may also produce more mucus than normal. Symptoms of COPD may include chronic cough, shortness of breath, wheezing, chest tightness, bluish/gray toe or fingernails, and rapid heartbeat. Note: if your toes or fingernails are bluish/gray, let your doctor know immediately, especially if this is a change from your normal skin color.

COPD is caused by the long-term inhalation of lung irritants like tobacco smoke. Diligently managing your COPD can help reduce symptoms, keep you out of the hospital, and improve your quality of life.

Medications for COPD include:

- **SABAs** (short acting beta agonist)-albuterol, levalbuterol, terbutaline

- **SAMAs** (short acting muscarinic antagonist)-ipratropium

- **LABAs** (long acting beta agonist)-salmeterol, formoterol, arformoterol, indacaterol, olodaterol
- **LAMAs** (long acting muscarinic antagonist)-tiotropium, aclidinium, glycopyrronium, umeclidinium
- **ICSs** (inhaled corticosteroid)-beclomethasone, budesonide, ciclesonide, flunisolide, fluticasone, mometasone
- **PDE4 Inhibitors**-roflumilast
- **Methylxanthines**-theophylline, aminophylline
- **Mucolytics**-acetylcysteine
- **Opioids**-morphine, hydrocodone, oxycodone
- **Antibiotics**-azithromycin, erythromycin
- Various combinations of medications in inhalers

It is recommended that your doctor follow these general steps to diagnose and manage your COPD:

1. **Spirometry**: First, the doctor uses this to verify the diagnosis of COPD.

2. **Assessment Questions**: Second, it's recommended that your doctor use the Modified British Medical Research Council (mMRC) questionnaire **OR** the COPD Assessment Test (CAT) to determine how severe your symptoms are.

3. **Exacerbations and Hospitalizations:** Next, your doctor will ask you how many COPD exacerbations you've had in the last 12 months and how many of those resulted in a hospitalization.

4. **ABCD Scoring**: Finally, your doctor will use the GOLD ABCD scoring system to figure out what group your COPD falls into. The GOLD guidelines recommend different medications depending on which group you fall into.

Spirometry to Diagnose COPD

Spirometry is required to make the diagnosis of COPD. Spirometry is a common test done at your doctor's office. It is used to assess how well your lungs work. It involves breathing into a small handheld device. The device measures how much air you inhale, how much you exhale, and how quickly you exhale.

Your spirometry results will tell your doctor how your lungs are functioning compared to other people of the same age, height, weight, sex, and ethnicity. Your spirometry results will be used to help determine which COPD GOLD group you fall into.

Classification of COPD Based on Spirometry Results[3]

- **GOLD 1**: Very mild COPD with a FEV1 about 80 percent or more of normal

- **GOLD 2**: Moderate COPD with a FEV1 between 50 and 80 percent of normal

- **GOLD 3**: Severe COPD with FEV1 between 30 and 50 percent of normal

- **GOLD 4**: Very severe COPD with a lower FEV1 than Stage 3, or those with Stage 3 FEV1 *and* low blood oxygen levels

Assuming you have been diagnosed with COPD based on your spirometry results, the next step is to determine which medications will be right for you. This is accomplished by answering some assessment questions and questions about how many COPD exacerbations ('flare-ups') you've had in the last 12 months. Check Appendix IV for instructions on plugging your spirometry results into the CDC calculator. Note them in Appendix IV.

Assessment Questions

The Modified British Medical Research Council (mMRC) questionnaire **OR** the COPD Assessment Test (CAT) can help determine how severe your symptoms are. You can check out these tests in Appendix IV. You can make note of your score there.

Exacerbations and Hospitalizations

The GOLD guidelines recommend that your doctor ask how many COPD exacerbations you've had in the last 12 months and how many of those had resulted in a hospitalization. This information will be combined with the information you provide about your symptoms to determine which ABCD group (see below) you fall into for treatment purposes. You can note the number of exacerbations and hospitalizations you've had in the last 12 months in Appendix IV.

ABCD Scoring

The GOLD COPD "ABCD" grading system is used to figure out how severe your COPD is. The ABCD system combines information you provide about your symptoms, your exacerbations and your hospitalizations, and assigns you an A, B, C, or D score.

GOLD COPD ABCD Grading System

Exacerbation History

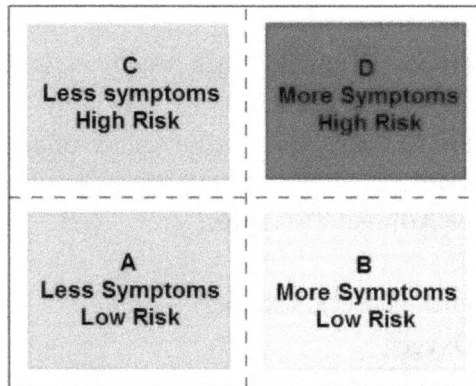

	mMRC score 0-1 OR CAT score less than 10	mMRC score of 2 or more OR CAT score of 10 or more
More than 1 exacerbation not requiring a hospital admission OR at least 1 exacerbation requiring hospital admission	**C** Less symptoms High Risk	**D** More Symptoms High Risk
1 or less exacerbations not requiring a hospital admission	**A** Less Symptoms Low Risk	**B** More Symptoms Low Risk

Symptoms

Your ABCD score will let the doctor know which ABCD group you fall into and which medications may best manage your COPD:

Grade A:
- SABA or SAMA or...
- LABA or LAMA or...
- SABA + SAMA

Grade B:
- LABA or LAMA or...
- LABA + LAMA

Grade C:
- ICS + LABA + LAMA or...
- LAMA + LABA or...
- LABA + PDE4 inhibitor or...
- LAMA + PDE4 inhibitor

Grade D:
- ICS + LABA +/or LAMA or...
- ICS + LABA + LAMA or...
- ICS + LABA + PDE4 inhibitor or...
- LABA + LAMA or...
- LAMA + PDE4 inhibitor

REMEMBER:
- Proper technique when using an inhaler helps ensure you receive all of your medication.
- Proper cleaning and maintenance of your nebulizer machine is very important.

Other Adjunct Therapies:
- Flu shot
- Pneumococcal vaccine
- Oxygen
- Ventilatory support
- Surgical and nonsurgical interventions
- Palliative care and hospice

Outlook

COPD has no cure yet, and doctors do not know how to reverse the damage to the lungs caused by COPD. The medicines talked about in this chapter have not been shown to prevent the decline in lung function over time. However, these treatments and lifestyle changes can help you feel better and stay more active. Staying as active as you can and staying compliant with COPD therapy can help improve symptoms and your quality of life.

It's important to take the information above with you to your next doctor's appointment to discuss your COPD treatment, especially if your COPD is not controlled. The hope is that the information above will aid in the discussion of your COPD therapy with your doctor.

REFERENCES

1. United States, 2011.Centers for Disease Control and Prevention. "Chronic Obstructive Pulmonary Disease Among Adults". *Morbidity and Mortality Weekly Report* 2012; 61(46):938–43 [accessed 2015 Nov 11].

2. National Center for Health Statistics. Health, United States, 2016: Chartbook on Long-term Trends in Health. Hyattsville, Maryland. 2017.

3. Global Initiative for Chronic Obstructive Lung Disease. 2017 Pocket guide to COPD diagnosis, management, and prevention; a guide for health care professionals. GOLD website. http://goldcopd.org/wp-content/uploads/2016/12/wms-GOLD-2017-Pocket-Guide.pdf. Published January 2017. Accessed April 26, 2017.

4. Nicholas T. Vozoris, Xuesong Wang, Hadas D. Fischer, Chaim M. Bell, Denis E. O'Donnell, Peter C. Austin, Anne L. Stephenson, Sudeep S. Gill, Paula A. Rochon. "Incident opioid drug us and adverse respiratory outcomes among older adults with COPD". *European Respiratory Journal* 2016; DOI: 10.1183/13993003.01967-2015.

CHAPTER 4

TYPE 1 AND TYPE 2 DIABETES MELLITUS

The Empowered Medicine Guide to Diabetes Mellitus

How to Use This Chapter

Welcome to the Empowered Medicine Guide to Diabetes. This chapter is arranged in a step-by-step fashion. First, we will go over the basics of diabetes such as what it is and why treating it is important. Then we will follow a step-by-step process for figuring out what your treatment goals should be. Feel free to write your own information in the blanks provided to aid in your calculations. Finally, we will look what medications may work best for you.

If you wish, use Appendix V in the back to log your own information for easy calculations and sharing with your doctor. Also, at the end of this chapter you will find a section called 'The Bottom Line'. This box sums up the main points of the chapter.

Diabetes: The Basics

Diabetes mellitus is often referred to as 'sugar diabetes' or just 'diabetes'. Diabetes is a serious condition. However, thanks to modern medicine (and the information available in this book!), you can improve your blood sugar control and minimize complications.

If you have diabetes, you know that it can be a major inconvenience. Most people with diabetes take pills or shots to control their blood sugar. But did you know that having diabetes can put you at a higher risk for heart attack and stroke? It also increases your risk for developing kidney failure and blindness. Finally, it can cause nerve damage and decrease blood circulation in the legs. Nerve and circulation problems can lead to serious infections and possible amputation (removal of limbs like feet or toes). This may all sound rather gloomy, but it is true and it is meant to get your attention.

There is a true diabetes epidemic in the U.S. As many as 2 out of 5 Americans are expected to develop type 2 diabetes in their lifetime.[2] The Centers for Disease Control also tell us this[2]:

- 30.3 million Americans have diabetes (this is 1 in 10 people or 9.4% of the population).

- Over half of new cases are diagnosed between the ages of 45 and 64.

- Diabetes remains the 7th leading cause of death in the United States as of 2015.

To be clear, diabetes is not a disease that you 'catch'. Rather, there is a combination of heredity, lifestyle, eating, and exercise habits that contribute to its development. So how does one get diabetes? To answer this we need to know a little something about carbohydrates.

What are Carbohydrates?

When we eat, we usually eat some form of carbohydrates ('carbs'). Carbs include starches and fibers found in grains, fruits, and vegetables. Carbs are broken down in the body to give us the energy we need to function properly.

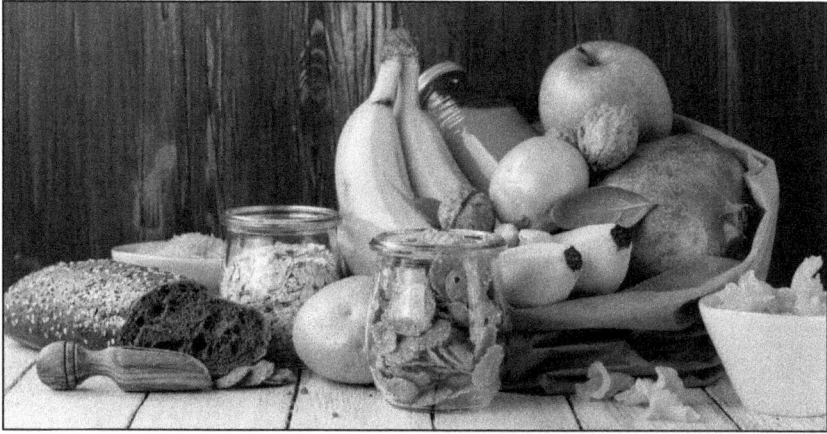

Figure 1: **Examples of Carbohydrates**

Sugar is a refined carb. Sugar breaks down in the body almost right away to be used. Other carbs break down slower. Sugar is included in many of the foods you might eat. Here are some places you might find carbs in the form of sugar.

Places You Might Find "Sugar"

Fruits and fruit juices, jams, smoothies

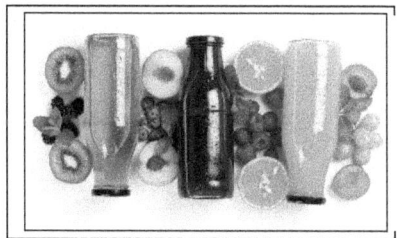

Regular soft drinks and fruit drinks (not diet)

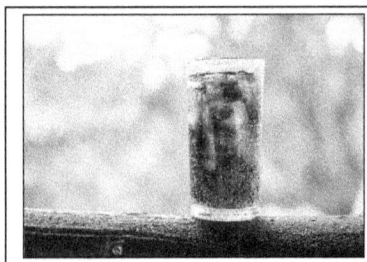

'Sweets' like ice cream, candy, donuts, cookies, pie, cake, muffins

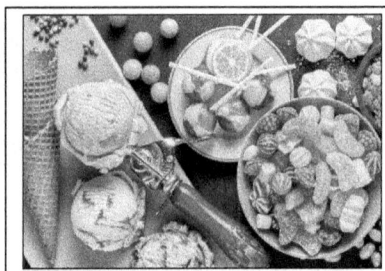

Dairy products like milk and yogurt

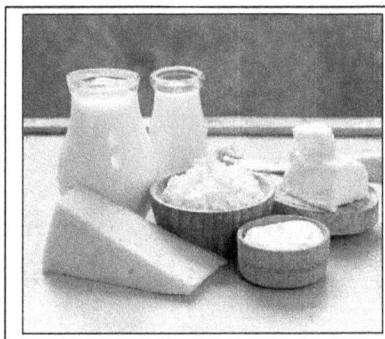

Many condiments like ketchup, barbeque sauce,

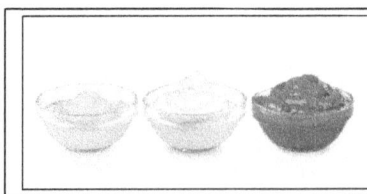

When looking at a nutrition label on a food item, notice they list the grams of carbohydrates and grams of sugar (see Figure 2). Knowing how many grams of sugar are in a food is good because sugar is used very quickly by the body and tends to 'spike' your blood sugar levels very quickly. This means that your blood sugar number is quick to rise (and may be quick to fall). These foods are also referred to as 'high glycemic index' foods. It is thought by many experts that sticking to foods that don't spike your blood sugar levels ('low glycemic index' foods) helps one from gaining weight.

So you see, it's nice to know how many grams of sugar are in a food. However, ***if you are taking insulin for your diabetes, you will use the "carbohydrate" value on the food label to figure out how much insulin you should take***. What is insulin? I'm glad you asked!

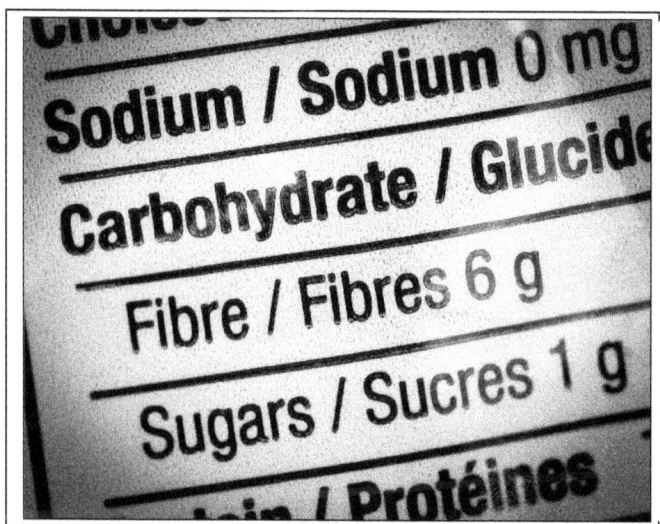

Figure 2: **Nutrition Label**

What Is Insulin?

After we eat, the carbs in that meal are absorbed from the intestines into the blood stream as glucose. We often refer to this glucose in the blood as 'blood sugar' or 'blood glucose'. This glucose is used by the brain, muscles, and other tissues for energy.

Insulin is a substance secreted by an organ in the body called the pancreas. Insulin is released into the blood stream when you eat a meal with carbs. Insulin is needed for the tissues to use glucose produced from the carbs.

The body's tissues have insulin receptors on them (we'll think of these receptors as little 'doorways'). These 'doorways' allow the glucose to enter into the tissues so it can be used. **Insulin acts as the 'key' that opens these 'doorways' and allows the glucose to enter the tissues.**

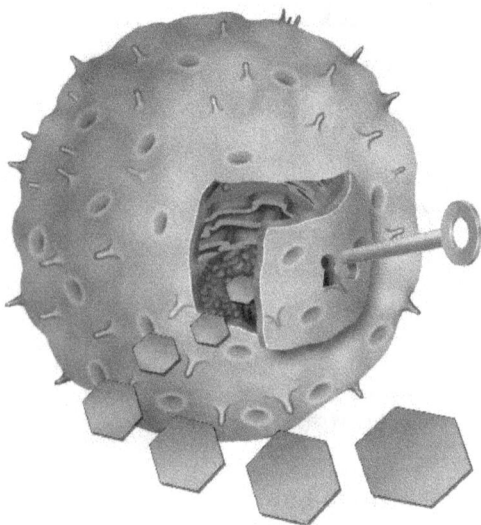

Figure 3: **Insulin (the Key) Unlocking Doorway for Glucose to Enter the Tissues**

Are you still with me? It may be a little confusing at first. It helps to keep in mind that insulin is a 'key' of sorts.

In addition to receiving glucose from the foods we eat, our liver stores glucose and releases it into the blood stream from time to time.

This is one of our body's defense mechanisms. Our livers were designed to store glucose and release it in case of famine. So when there is a shortage of food, the liver can release some of the glucose it has stored so the body doesn't starve.

With the help of insulin, our bodies can use glucose from the foods we eat to get energy to function properly. When your body uses all of the glucose in the blood stream and in the liver, it can start breaking down fats to get energy.

Now that we understand what carbs, sugar, and insulin are, we can look at the main types of diabetes that affect our aging population. We will then see what the guidelines have to say about treating diabetes.

Prediabetes

Prediabetes is a condition that indicates one is at high risk for developing type 2 diabetes. It describes someone who doesn't meet the criteria for type 2 diabetes but whose glucose levels are too high to be considered normal.

Like type 2 diabetes, prediabetes is associated with obesity, especially in those who carry a disproportionate amount of weight in their abdomen. Those with high triglycerides and/or low HDL cholesterol and those with high blood pressure are also at higher risk.[4]

It is thought that 'prediabetes' develops when the insulin-producing cells of the pancreas begin to fail and/or insulin resistance starts to take place. Prediabetes management is generally focused on diet changes and weight loss. Lifestyle changes with or without medications and/or surgery can prevent prediabetes from progressing to type 2 diabetes. It should be noted that prediabetes does **not** lead to type 1 diabetes, which seems to appear unprovoked.

Currently there are no medications that are approved by the FDA for use in prediabetes to manage blood sugar or prevent type 2 diabetes. However, medications such as metformin and acarbose have been shown to decrease the risk of developing type 2 diabetes in this population by 25 to 30%.[1]

Like diabetes, prediabetes increases the risk of heart attack and stroke. Because of this, the guidelines state that patients with prediabetes should utilize lifestyle changes and diabetes medications to get their blood sugar (and blood pressure and their cholesterol, if needed) under control. [1]

Type 1 Diabetes

Type 1 diabetes accounts for only about 5% to 10% of all diabetes cases.[2] The old idea that type 1 diabetes only happens in children and young adults is no longer accurate. Type 1 diabetes can occur in children or adults.[4]

Type 1 diabetes is when the body can't produce its own insulin. Without insulin to process the glucose in your blood, your blood sugar starts to rise. It is thought that type 1 diabetes is caused when your immune system attacks the cells in the pancreas that make insulin. Experts are not sure why the immune system decides to attack the pancreas; however, some evidence suggests that viruses play a role. As a result, your pancreas loses the ability to make insulin.

Key to Success

With type 1 diabetes, the body cannot produce any of its own insulin. Without insulin, your body can not use the glucose from the foods you eat. This causes your blood sugar to rise.

High blood sugar is a serious problem. Over time, it can wreak havoc on your body. Through complicated mechanisms, it can affect your cholesterol and damage your arteries. As mentioned earlier, this increases your risk for heart attack and stroke. It also increases the risk of damage to your eyes, kidneys, and lower limbs. Extremely high blood sugar can cause dehydration, coma, and even death.

Empowered U

Which is a true statement about diabetes?
a. Diabetes **decreases** our risk of stroke
b. Diabetes **increases** our risk of heart attack
c. Type 1 diabetes makes up the majority of diabetes cases
d. None of the above

Answer: b

In general, people with type I Diabetes need to use insulin shots to control their blood sugar. This is because their bodies have lost the ability to produce insulin, so it has to be replaced. These insulin shots provide the body with the insulin it cannot make anymore.

When the body cannot produce enough insulin, a complication called diabetic ketoacidosis (DKA) can happen. DKA is when there is a buildup of acids in the blood called ketones. Ketones are produced when the body is forced to break down fat for fuel instead of glucose. If not treated promptly, DKA can lead to brain swelling, kidney failure, and trouble breathing.

Testing Urine for Ketones

If you have type 1 diabetes, you should know how to test your urine for ketones so you can be proactive and correct the problem before it becomes troublesome. Ketones present in the urine let you know that the body is at risk for DKA.

Ketone tests are available at your local pharmacy. The tests typically include test strips that are used to test your urine for ketones. You can either collect a urine sample in a clean container and dip the strip into the urine in the cup **OR** pass the strip through the stream of urine. You will then wait for the strip to change color. Compare the color that appears on the strip to the color chart on the strip bottle. This will give you an idea of how many ketones are in your urine.

Small amounts of ketones in the urine can mean that you are at risk for ketone buildup. Moderate or large amounts of ketones in the urine is a sign that you need to seek medical help. ***You should talk to you doctor to come up with a plan of what to do when you detect small, moderate, or large amounts of ketones in your urine.***

According to the American Diabetes Association (ADA) website, one should check their ketones[3] when:

- Your blood sugar is more than 300 mg/dl
- You feel nauseated, are vomiting, or have abdominal pain
- You are sick (for example, with a cold or flu)
- You feel tired all the time
- You are thirsty or have a very dry mouth
- Your skin is flushed
- You have a hard time breathing
- Your breath smells "fruity"
- You feel confused or "in a fog"

Type 2 Diabetes

Type 2 diabetes (the most common type) typically results when one of the following happens:

1. the body can't produce insulin ('keys')
2. the body's tissues stop responding to insulin (it gets rid of receptors or 'doorways')
3. a combination of both of these problems

It is thought that in most people with type 2 diabetes, the problems listed above cause the tissues to develop insulin resistance. *Insulin resistance is a condition where the body's tissues stop responding to insulin. This causes blood sugar to rise.*

Key to Success

So with type 2 diabetes, the body becomes insulin resistant (unable to use the glucose in the blood). This causes blood sugar to rise

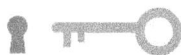

Let's take a closer look at how insulin resistance happens. When we constantly consume significant quantities of food, it causes our pancreas to continually pump out insulin to process the carbs we eat. As a result, some experts think the body decides there is too much insulin in the blood stream. Because of the surplus of insulin, the body then decides it doesn't need as many insulin receptors. Remember, these insulin receptors are the 'doorways' on the tissues that let the glucose in.

The body then gets rid of some of the insulin receptors. Recall that insulin is the 'key' to these doorways. When there are fewer 'doorways' for these 'keys' to work on, the tissues aren't able to let as much glucose in. Blood sugar begins to rise. Because there are fewer insulin receptors, the body is said to be 'insulin resistant'.

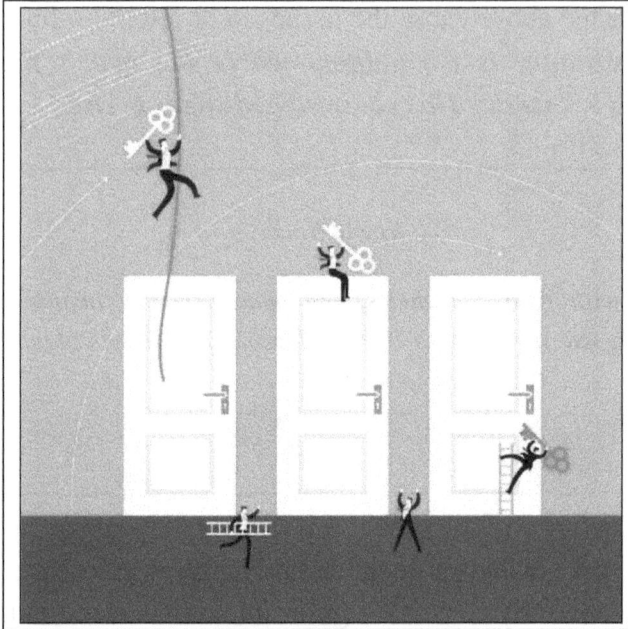

Figure 4: **Keys (Insulin) and Doorways (Receptors)**

As a result of this insulin resistance, some believe the pancreas tries to pump out more and more insulin to compensate. Unfortunately, this doesn't help. In fact it makes matters worse! Because the body sees more insulin in the blood stream, it decides to get rid of even more receptors. Some experts think that the pancreas may eventually burn itself out and lose the ability to produce insulin. They refer to this process as 'beta cell burnout'. It is called this because the cells in the pancreas that make insulin are types of cells called beta cells.

So at this point, not only has the body stopped responding to insulin, but it may have also lost the ability to produce it. This is a problem because if the body stops producing insulin, one is at risk for DKA. DKA does happen in people with type 2 diabetes, but it is not seen as often as it is seen in type 1 diabetes.

Type 2 diabetes frequently occurs in people who are overweight and in people who have fat that is predominantly distributed in the abdominal region.[4] This is probably due to the fact that eating more calories than you can use not only causes you to gain weight, it causes your pancreas to pump out more insulin. Over time this can result insulin resistance and type 2 diabetes.[4]

When type 2 diabetes is observed in someone who is not overweight and does not have the abdominal fat distributed as described above, it is usually seen in association with another illness-like infection or with the use of certain drugs, like steroids. The risk of type 2 diabetes does increases with age and lack of physical activity. Certain ethnic groups are also more likely to experience type 2 diabetes, like African Americans, American Indians, Hispanic/Latinos, and Asian Americans. Finally, having a family history of diabetes is associated with type 2 diabetes. [4]

Gestational Diabetes

Gestational diabetes is diabetes that happens during pregnancy in a patient who does not previously have diabetes. It usually happens during the second or third trimester. Most of the time, this type of diabetes goes away after the baby is born. However, if you've had gestational diabetes, you have a greater chance of developing type 2 diabetes later in life.

The majority of this chapter will be a discussion on type 1 and type 2 diabetes. However here is a summary of recommendations for Gestational Diabetes from the ADA:

Table 2: **Gestational Diabetes Recommendations**[4]

---

1. Women are screened for undiagnosed diabetes at the first prenatal doctor's visit

2. A test for gestational diabetes at 24-28 weeks of gestation be performed (if the woman hasn't been previously diagnosed with diabetes)

3. Women diagnosed with gestational diabetes are tested again 4-12 weeks postpartum utilizing an oral glucose tolerance test (OGTT) (this test will be explained in a bit)

4. Women with a history of gestational diabetes should be screened for type 2 diabetes every 3 years after pregnancy

5. Women with a history of gestational diabetes who are diagnosed with prediabetes postpartum should use lifestyle interventions and/or metformin therapy to prevent the development of type 2 diabetes

---

Other Types of Diabetes

There are other types of diabetes including cystic fibrosis-related diabetes and neonatal diabetes. We will be restricting our discussion in this chapter primarily to type 1 and type 2 diabetes. For more information on other types of diabetes, visit www.cff.org or www.niddk.nih.gov.

Screening for Prediabetes and Diabetes

The ADA recommends people over the age of 45 get screened every 3 years for prediabetes and diabetes.[4] They also recommend using an assessment tool for screening. They offer the ADA risk test for this purpose (located at: www.diabetes.org/socrisktest). This tool takes into consideration your age, sex, ethnicity, personal history of gestational diabetes, family history, blood pressure, physical activity level, and weight status. *A score of 5 or higher indicates a higher risk for prediabetes or diabetes.*

Testing for prediabetes or diabetes should be considered in adults who are overweight or obese (BMI of 25 kg/m or more, Asian Americans with a BMI greater than 23 kg/m) and have one or more of the risk factors below (see Table 3).

Table 3: **Risk factors for Diabetes**[4]

- First degree relative with diabetes
- African American, Latino, Native American, Asian American, Pacific Islander
- History of cardiovascular disease (for example, a history of heart attack)
- High blood pressure (140/90 or more, or are on medication therapy for high blood pressure)
- HDL cholesterol less than 35 mg/dL (0.90 mmol/L) and/or a triglyceride level of 250 mg/dL (2.82 mmol/L) or more.
- Women with polycystic ovary syndrome
- Physical inactivity

STEP 1: If you are over 45 years old and have not been diagnosed with prediabetes or diabetes, take the ADA risk test at the web address above and write your score in below.

My ADA Diabetes Risk Score is = _____

STEP 2: Is this number more than 5? If so, contact your health care provider to get tested for prediabetes and diabetes.

I need to be tested for diabetes at my doctor's office	☐ **Yes** (my risk score is more than 5)	☐ **No** (my risk score is less than 5)

Diagnosis of Prediabetes and Diabetes

There are actually several ways to be diagnosed with prediabetes or diabetes. Each of these ways should be repeated on a different day to make the diagnosis of diabetes. If your blood sugar is really high or if you have symptoms in addition to high blood sugar, your doctor may decide that retesting on another date is not necessary. Whether you retest or not, these tests should be carried out in a doctor's office or lab to be considered for diagnosis.

Before we look at how to diagnose prediabetes and diabetes, let's take a look at a few tests and what they mean:

Table 4: **Tests Used to Test for Prediabetes and Diabetes**

Test	What is It?
A1C	A1C is an estimate of your **average blood sugar over the last few months.** This is done by looking at hemoglobin (a protein in the blood that is coated in sugar).
Fasting Blood Glucose (FBG or 'fasting blood sugar')	A blood sugar reading that is taken after at least 8 hours with no food.
Oral Glucose Tolerance Test (OGTT)	An OGTT is a reading of your blood sugar 2 hours after you are given 75 gm of sugar to eat.

Now that we have an understanding of the different tests that are used, let's look at how prediabetes and diabetes are diagnosed.

Table 5: **Diagnosis of Prediabetes and Diabetes[4]***

		A1C	**Fasting Blood Sugar (FBG)**	**Oral Glucose Tolerance Test (OGTT)**	**Other**
	Prediabetes	A1C of 5.7-6.4%	FBG of 100 mg/dL (5.6 mmol/L) to 125 mg/dL (6.9 mmol/L	Blood glucose of 140 mg/dL (7.8 mmol/L) to 199 mg/dL (11 mmol/L) after a 2-hour OGTT	
	Diabetes	A1C of 6.5% or more	FBG of 126 mg/dL (7 mmol/L) or greater after no food for at least 8 hours.	Blood glucose of 200 mg/dL (11.1 mmol/L) or more during a 2 hour OGTT test. The test should use 75 gm of glucose dissolved in water	Classic symptoms of high blood sugar with a random blood sugar of 200 mg/dL (11.1 mmol/L) or more.

*NOTE: FBG should be used to diagnose type 1 diabetes (instead of A1C). A panel of autoantibodies may also be ordered.

STEP 3: After visiting your doctor to get tested for prediabetes and type 2 diabetes, circle any symptoms in Table 5 that apply. If you have anything circled in the prediabetes row, check the prediabetes box. If you have anything circled in the type 2 diabetes row, check that box. Did the boxes checked indicate that you may have prediabetes, type 2 diabetes, or neither?

☐ **Prediabetes**	☐ **Type 2 Diabetes**	☐ **Neither**

Estimated Average Glucose (eAG)

When reading about blood sugar levels, you might come across a term called the "Estimated average glucose (eAG)". This is a term that you might hear sometimes instead of A1C because it is a little easier to understand than A1C. An eAG tells you how high your blood sugar is on average. To better help patients understand how their A1C relates to an eAG, the ADA has created a conversion tool that can be accessed online by going to: https://professional.diabetes.org/diapro/glucose_calc. For a general idea of how A1C and eAG numbers compare, you can review the chart below.

Table 6: **A1C and Estimated Average Blood Sugar Level (eAG)**[17]

A1C Level	Estimated Average Blood Sugar
5%	97 mg/dL (5.4 mmol/L)
6%	126 mg/dL (7 mmol/L)
7%	154 mg/dL (8.5 mmol/L)
8%	183 mg/dL (10.2 mmol/L)
9%	212 mg/dL (11.8 mmol/L)
10%	240 mg/dL (13.3 mmol/L)
11%	269 mg/dL (14.9 mmol/L)
12%	298 mg/dL (16.5 mmol/L)
13%	326 mg/dL (18.1 mmol/L)
14%	355 mg/dL (19.7 mmol/L)

I've Been Diagnosed with Prediabetes or Diabetes; Now What?

Once you've been diagnosed with prediabetes or diabetes, it is recommended that your doctor do a complete medical evaluation for you to:

- Confirm the diagnosis
- Check for diabetes complications and other conditions that need to be addressed (like cardiovascular disease or high blood pressure)
- A medical evaluation which may include medical history, allergies, past side effects, physical exam, and lab assessment
- Determine a plan for initial and ongoing care for the management of your prediabetes or diabetes
- Determine the need for referrals to other doctors, immunizations, and other health screenings

STEP 4: Check the appropriate box below when you have set up a complete medical evaluation with your doctor.

I have been diagnosed with prediabetes or diabetes and have scheduled a complete medical evaluation with my doctor	☐ **Yes**	☐ **No**

Immunizations

Your doctor may also want to make sure you are up on your immunizations. The ADA contends that people with diabetes have a higher risk of hepatitis B infection (a severe illness affecting the liver that is caused by a virus spread by sexual contact or blood), influenza

(AKA 'the flu'), and pneumococcal disease (an infection that causes pneumonia, meningitis, middle ear and sinus infections).

The ADA recommends that adults and children with diabetes receive vaccinations as recommended by the CDC. The schedule of recommended vaccinations can be found at: www.cdc.gov/vaccines/schedules/hcp/imz/child-adolescent.html, and www.cdc.gov/vaccines/schedules/hcp/imz/adult.html

Here is a summary of the ADA Guidelines for Immunizations for people with diabetes:

Table 7: **ADA Immunization Recommendations for People with Diabetes**[4]

• Obtain recommended vaccinations for children and adults with diabetes by age
• All people 6 months of age or older should get vaccinated against influenza annually
• Children before age 2 should get vaccinates with PCV 13 (Brand name Prevnar 13®)
• People with diabetes ages 2 through 64 years old should also receive PPSV23 (Brand name Pneumovax 23®)
• At age 65 years of age or older, regardless of vaccination history, a PPSV23 (Pneumovax 23®) should be given
• A 3-dose series of hepatitis B vaccine to unvaccinated adults with diabetes ages 19 through 59 years old is recommended.
• A 3-dose series of hepatitis B vaccine to unvaccinated adults with diabetes ages 60 years and older is recommended.

Assessing Other Health Conditions

There are several health conditions that have been associated with diabetes that your doctor may want to assess you for. You should be screened for each of these conditions soon after being diagnosed with diabetes.

You may have heard that diabetics should manage their ABCs (A1C, blood pressure, and cholesterol). People with diabetes are more prone to high blood pressure and high cholesterol. So it is emphasized that people with diabetes need to pay close attention to these conditions. As we'll discuss in a moment, the ADA recommends shooting for a goal of an A1C less than 7%. They also recommend a ***blood pressure goal of less than 130/80 and LDL (AKA "bad cholesterol") less than 100 mg/dL (but less than 70 mg/dL if one has cardiovascular disease).*** [4]

There are other conditions your doctor may want to screen for. Managing these health conditions can help make managing your diabetes much easier. Here is a list of some of these conditions.

- Autoimmune Conditions – your body's immune system attacks certain parts of the body
  o Autoimmune thyroid disease - thyroid gets attacked
  o Celiac disease - small intestine gets attacked
  o Autoimmune gastritis - stomach gets attacked
  o Dermatomyositis - affects muscles and skin
  o Autoimmune hepatitis - liver gets attacked
  o Myasthenia gravis - nerves get attacked
- Cancer
- Dementia
- Hypoglycemia (low blood sugar)
- Fatty liver
- Pancreatitis (inflammation of the pancreas)
- Bone fractures
- Hearing problems
- HIV (certain medications used to treat HIV can put you at a high risk for diabetes)
- Low testosterone in men
- Obstructive sleep apnea
- Anxiety disorders
- Periodontal disease-disease of the teeth and gums

- Psychosocial/emotional disorders
- Disordered eating behavior (abnormal eating)
- Serious mental illness

Other Considerations; Foot Care

It is imperative that people with diabetes practice proper foot care. Proper foot care can decrease the risk of amputations for people with diabetes. This is because diabetes can lead to decreased circulation and nerve problems in the feet and legs. As a result, people with diabetes often experience numbness and/or tingling in the feet and legs. This is called 'neuropathy'. This can be a problem.

We are meant to feel pain in our feet for a reason. For example, when you step on a thorn or cut your foot, the pain tells you that the foot needs attention. When we realize we are wounded, we can clean it, dress it, and protect it from further injury. If your foot is numb, you may not feel that there is a wound that needs attention. This can lead to serious infections that, if not taken care of, can lead to amputation.

To lessen the risk of amputation, it's recommended that people with diabetes check their feet every day for swelling, cuts, and blisters. Tend to injuries promptly. Wear comfortable shoes and never go outside without shoes.

Key to Success

When you have diabetes, you should manage your ABCs (A1C, blood pressure, and cholesterol). Aim for:

- *Blood pressure goal of less than 130/80*
- *LDL (AKA "bad cholesterol") less than 100 mg/dL (but less than 70 mg/dL if one has cardiovascular disease).* [4]

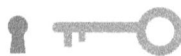

Diabetes Self-Management Education and Support

It is recommended that all people with diabetes take part in diabetes self-management education and support (DSMES). The goal of DSMES is to improve health and quality of life through education. It is hoped that through DSMES, people can gain the skills they need to be able to maintain their diabetes care at home.

It is recommended that people with diabetes take part in DSMES at least at these 4 critical times[4]:

1. At diagnosis
2. Every year
3. When problems arise
4. When a change occurs

DSMES programs are offered by various health care professionals. DSMES can be done in a group setting or on an individual basis. It can even be done via technology (via webinars or skype meetings, for example). Accredited DSMES programs are generally covered by Medicare and may be covered by most private insurances as well. However, note that *Medicare and private insurances generally cover in-person DSMES visits.* Phone, skype, or other alternative forms of meeting may not be covered. Check with your insurance.

STEP 5: Contact your doctor's office to find a DSMES program near you. Check the box below when you have made your first DSMES appointment:

My DSMES appointment is scheduled for: _____

Nutrition Therapy

Proper nutrition should be at the center of one's diabetes management strategy. Some people with type 2 diabetes are able to manage their high blood sugar with diet alone. People with type 1 diabetes will not be able to manage their diabetes with diet alone and will require insulin. This is because their body no longer makes its own insulin.

The Mediterranean diet represents one model of healthful eating that people have been enjoying for centuries. It is a suitable diet plan just about anyone can adapt, including people with type 1 or type 2 diabetes. It's a healthy diet made of fruits, vegetables, legumes, nuts, whole grains, olive oil, fatty fish, and a small amount of red wine per day. Some studies show that the Mediterranean diet decreases fasting blood sugar levels or A1C for people with diabetes.[10-15]

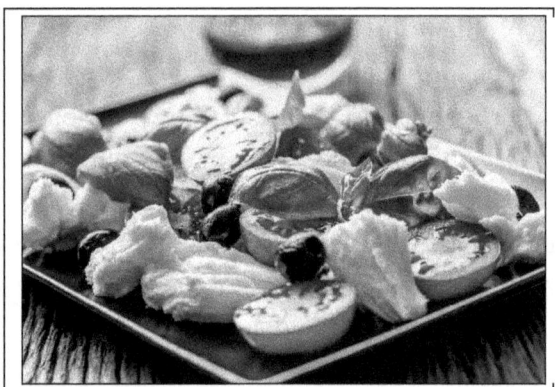

Figure 5: **Example of Food on the Mediterranean Diet**

In addition to the Mediterranean diet, there are several other diets to choose from. Learning which foods to choose can help prevent unwanted weight gain and the progression of diabetes. Meal planning works best when its individualized. To help create a plan that's right for you, *it's recommended that all people with diabetes be offered a referral to a Registered Dietician (RD).* RD referrals have been shown to decrease A1C in people with diabetes.[4]

A Registered Dietician can help you:

1. Learn how to plan your own meals
2. Learn healthful eating patterns
3. Discover how to incorporate a variety of nutritious food into your meal plan

4. Manage your weight
5. Delay or prevent diabetes and its complications
6. Identify your individual nutrition needs

STEP 6: Contact your doctor's office to find a RD near you. Check the box below when you have made your first appointment:

My first RD consultation is scheduled for: _____

How to test your blood sugar

If you've been diagnosed with prediabetes or diabetes, it's important to know how to correctly test your blood sugar at home. This will be an important skill that you will need to learn. Without knowing your blood sugar, it may be hard to know if you are running too high or too low. If you will be taking insulin, learning how to test your blood sugar is a must.

Keeping your blood sugar in a safe range is important. Blood sugar that is too low deprives your body of the energy it needs to function. For example, your brain, heart, and muscles all require the energy in your blood sugar to function properly. Blood sugar that is too low can cause shakiness and trouble thinking. Blood sugar that is too high can lead to damage in the body if sustained over many years. Finally, remember that severely-high or severely-low blood sugar can cause coma and death.

It's recommended that you keep a log of your blood sugar results from testing your blood sugar at home. This will help you and your doctor adjust your therapy.

To test your blood sugar, you will need a blood glucose meter from the drug store. There are many different kinds of meters, from very basic to more complicated. Be sure to follow the instructions that come with your meter.

If you need help choosing a meter or help learning how to use one, ask your pharmacist to help you. Some meters allow you to check blood sugar at your forearm, thigh, or back of your hand. Check your device. Checking at these sites, if your machine is NOT made to do this, may result in inaccurate results.

Most meters work the same way. Basically you will:

1. Wash your hands with soap and water

2. Insert a test strip into the meter

3. Prick your finger (or other site if meter allows you to test somewhere else) using the lancing device provided to get a small bead of blood

4. Touch the glucose strip tips to the bead of blood so the strip can absorb some of the blood

5. In a few moments your result will appear on the display of the meter.

A continuous glucose monitor (AKA insulin pump) is also available through your doctor. This is a monitor you wear all of the time. A tiny sensor goes under your skin so the device can take a blood sugar reading every few minutes or so. This data can be wirelessly transmitted to a remote receiver that you keep in your purse or pocket.

Continuous glucose monitors are a great option for people that have to test frequently or have trouble testing their own blood (due to dementia or arthritis in the hands, for example).

Who Should Test Their Blood Sugar?

Keeping track of your blood sugar results at home is important. This is information that can be used to adjust your food intake, exercise, and medications so you can achieve your goals and feel better. Whether you use continuous glucose monitoring or are testing yourself throughout the day, it is recommended that you test your blood sugar regularly if you:

- Are taking insulin
- Have a hard time controlling your blood sugar
- Are prone to low blood sugar levels (especially if you don't usually have the symptoms of low blood sugar like shakiness, sweating, fainting, fatigue, or heart palpitations)
- Are pregnant
- Have ketones in your urine

What Should Be My Blood Sugar Goal Be?

Blood sugar targets are very individualized. Factors like life expectancy, history of low blood sugar and other health conditions may influence how stringently you manage your blood sugar (see Figure 6). You should talk to you doctor about specific blood sugar goals that are right for you. In general, however, it is recommended that one *aim for a goal of 80-130 mg/dL (4.4 to 7.2 mmol/L) right before meals and less than 180 mg/dL (10 mmol/L,) 1 to 2 hours after meals.*[4]

When Should One Test Their Blood Sugar?

It's recommended that people using insulin shots or who have an insulin pump test their blood sugar[4]:

- Prior to each meal and snack
- At bedtime
- Prior to exercise
- When they think their blood sugar might be too low or too high
- After treating themselves due to low blood sugar
- Occasionally after meals

It's important to use good technique when testing your blood sugar at home. Your doctor, pharmacist, or registered dietician can help you with your technique, if needed.

What Can Cause Low Blood Sugar?

Typically low blood sugar happens when:
1. You skip or delay eating a meal of snack
2. You take too much insulin
3. You exercise
4. You drink alcohol
5. You're sick and not eating much

See the 'Treating Low Blood Sugar at Home' section toward the end of the chapter for tips on how to avoid low blood sugar, especially when taking insulin.

A1C Testing

After being diagnosed with diabetes, it is recommended that *people who are meeting their treatment goals test their A1C at least two times a year. People who are not meeting their treatment goals should test every 3 months.*[4] Remember, A1C is a reflection of your blood sugar over the last 3 months. It's a helpful way for you and your doctor to see if you are at risk for diabetes complications.

What Should My A1C Goal Be?

The ADA notes that if you are diabetic, your *A1C goal should be less than 7%* (53 mmol/mol) or *eAG less than 154 mg/dL* for most nonpregnant adults. However, your doctor may suggest a lower A1C goal if he/she feels you are at a higher risk of diabetes complications. Your doctor may also suggest an A1C goal higher than 7% if you are prone to bouts of very low blood sugar, have limited life expectancy, or have health conditions that make it hard to achieve an A1C less than 7%. [4]

Figure 6 gives you an idea of the different health conditions that your doctor may take into consideration when determining an A1C goal for you.

Figure 6: **Health Conditions and How Stringent Blood Sugar Control May Be[4]***

Very Stringent	Less stringent
Newly diagnosed diabetes	Have had diabetes for a long time
Long life expectancy	Short life expectancy
No other health conditions	Many other health conditions
Fewer Bouts of Seriously Low Blood Sugar	Many Bouts of Seriously Low Blood Sugar
Very motivated, very capable	Not very motivated, poor self-care
Have resources and support	Few resources and support

*Everyone is different. This table represents a suggestion only

Now, without further delay, let's look at the medications used to treat type 1 and type 2 diabetes.

Insulin for the Treatment of Diabetes

Insulin

Most people with type 1 diabetes (and some with type 2 diabetes) will need to be treated with multiple doses of insulin throughout the day. Insulin is given via a small injection into the fatty layer just below the top layer of skin.

An insulin pump can be used instead, if preferred. Insulin pumps are programmed to deliver the insulin automatically. They attach to the body via a thin cannula which is kind of like a needle but softer and more flexible. Bolus doses of insulin can be given through the pump before meals as well. Many of these pumps are very small and can be put into a pocket.

When trying to figure out how much insulin to give yourself, you should take into consideration:[4]

1. How active you intend to be
2. How many carbohydrates you plan to eat
3. What your blood sugar reading is before your meal

Types of Insulin

There are different types of insulin. They are classified depending on how long they last. Rapid/regular/short-acting insulin are usually used in combination with an intermediate/long-acting insulin.

As an alternative, one can use a premixed insulin which is a combination of an intermediate-acting insulin PLUS a rapid/regular/short-acting insulin.

- **Intermediate/long-acting insulin** - is given less often and helps keep blood sugar levels nice and even throughout the day.
- **Rapid/regular/short-acting insulin** - is usually given before each meal, to help the body use the energy from the food you eat.

Table 8: *Types* of Insulin

	Type of Insulin	How it's Different	Examples
Usually given prior to meals	**Rapid-acting insulin**	Starts to work in about 15 minutes (take no more than 15 minutes before a meal), effects peak in 1 hour and lasts for 2 to 4 hours.	Insulin glulisine (Apidra®), insulin lispro (Humalog®) insulin aspart (Novolog®)
	Regular or short-acting insulin	Starts to work in about 30 minutes (take no more than 30 minutes before a meal), effects peak in about 2 to 3 hours and lasts for 3 to 6 hours.	(Humulin R®, Novolin R®)
Usually given once or twice daily to control evenly throughout the day	**Intermediate-acting insulin**	Starts to work in 2 to 4 hours, effects peak in about 4 to 12 hours and lasts for 12 to 18 hours	NPH insulin-isophane (Humulin N®, Novolin N®)
	Long-acting insulin	Starts to work in several hours then lowers blood sugar pretty evenly over 24 hours.	Insulin detemir (Levemir®) insulin glargine (Lantus®)
	Various premixed insulins	A combination of NPH insulin and a short or rapid acting insulin that can be helpful for someone who has trouble drawing up two different insulins due to dexterity or poor eyesight. Humulin	Humulin 70/30, Humalog Mix 50/50, Humalog Mix 75/25, Novolin 70/30, Novolog Mix 70/30

	Type of Insulin	How it's Different	Examples
		70/30, for example, means there is 70% intermediate-acting insulin PLUS 30 % regular-acting insulin.	
	Inhaled insulin	Rapid-acting. Starts to work within 12 to 15 minutes, effects peak around 30 minutes and it's out of your system in about 180 minutes. Given before each meal. Must be used in combination with long-acting insulin	Afrezza®

Sliding Scale

You may hear the term "sliding scale". Sliding scale means you adjust the dose of your rapid/regular/short-acting insulin before meals based on how many grams of carbohydrates you will be eating in that meal. ***Generally, 1 unit of insulin will take care of 1 serving of carbs (1 serving of carbs is about 12-15 grams of carbohydrate).*** For example, if you eat two pieces of toast (each piece has 15 grams of carbs, or 30 grams total), then you will need about 2 units of rapid-acting insulin before your meal.

Let's take a look at a food label and see how many carbs are in the food:

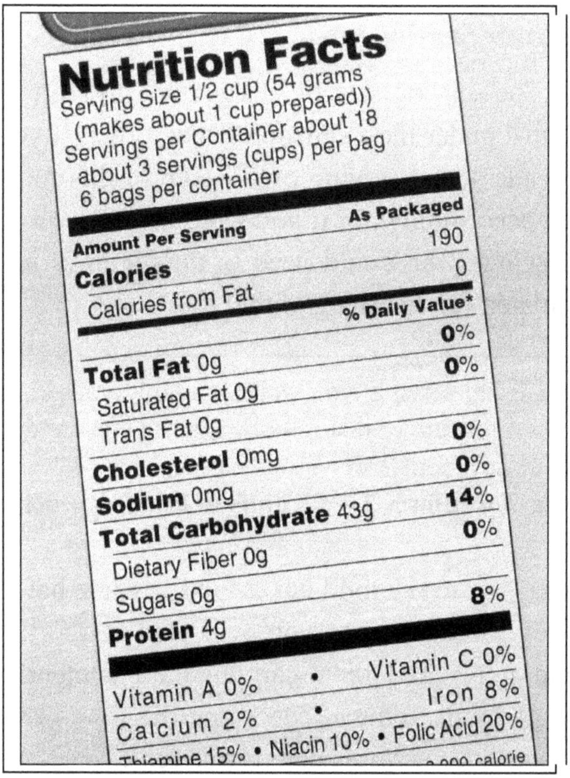

Figure 7: **Food Nutrition Label**

You can see on this nutrition label where 1 serving of this food has a total carbohydrate of 43 grams. Here are the steps you would use to figure out how much insulin to take:

STEP 1: Find out how many servings of carbs you have to cover with your insulin (remember each serving of carbs is 15 gm of carbs):
To do this, divide: 43 gm total ÷ 15 g per serving = 2.87 servings of carbs
STEP 2: Find out how many units of insulin you need. If you are taking 1 unit of insulin for every serving of carbs then you multiply:
2.9 servings X 1 unit per servings = **2.9 units of insulin needed**

So, if you are going to eat food for a meal that contains 43 grams of carbs, you would need to take 2.9 units of insulin.

Watch Your Serving Sizes!

NOTE: The serving size of this particle food in Figure 7 is ½ cup (see that just under the 'Nutrition Facts' title?) If you're going to eat more than the stated serving of a ½ cup of this food, you would have to adjust accordingly. So if you were going to eat 1 cup (double the ½ cup serving) you would need to double your insulin amount that you calculated for 1 serving of that food.

So for a 1 cup serving, you would multiply your units of insulin you needed for 1 serving of that food by 2 since you are doubling your carb servings of this food:

2.9 units of insulin X 2 = 5.8 units of insulin needed

Of course, not every food has a food label. What about a piece of fruit or vegetable? Below you will find a short list of some common food items and their carbohydrate content. For a more complete list of foods you can check out the Empowered Medicine Carb Counter at http://www.empoweredmedicine.com/Carb-Counter.php or download an app on your phone that allows you to look up the carb content of foods on the go. A great app that I personally use myself is "My Fitness Pal".

Table 9: **Foods and Their Carbohydrate Content**

Food	Grams of Carbohydrate
1 slice of bread	15 g
3 cups of popcorn	15 g
1 small fruit	15 g
1 cup milk	12 g
1 cup cooked pasta	45 g
1 ½ cup cooked veggies	15 g
1 medium potato	30 g
½ cup vanilla ice cream	15 g

Sugar-free Products

There are products that claim to be 'sugar free' out there. These products might use sugar-alternatives to give the product a sweet flavor instead of sugar. However, even though there is no 'sugar' listed on the nutrition label, there may still be carbohydrates. Check out the carbohydrate listing on the nutrition label. You will still need to use insulin to cover these carbohydrates.

Even if You Don't Take Insulin…

Even if you don't take insulin, you should learn how to read food labels. It will help you make sure you are eating enough food to get the energy you need but not eating too much to where you are using too much insulin. Using too much insulin can lead to weight gain.

It's ideal to work with an RD who can help you figure out how many calories you need per day based on your individual needs. The 2015-2020 Dietary Guidelines for Americans gives recommendations for how many calories one needs in a day based on their age and activity level.

For example, the average 60-year-old female who is not very active needs to take in about 1800 calories per day. According to the guidelines, men and women should get about 45 to 65% of their calories from carbohydrates. [18]

If you know how many calories you need a day and know that 45 to 65% of those calories should be from carbs, you can figure out how many grams of carbs you can have per day.

Let's look at an example and the steps you would take to figure out how many grams of carbs you can have per day. In this example, we will calculate the grams of carbs needed to provide 45% of calories in an 1800 calorie per day diet.

STEP 1: Find out how many carb calories are equal to 45% by multiplying 0.45 by the total number of calories you are able to have:

Multiply 0.45 X 1800 calories = 810 calories

STEP 2: Find out how many grams of carbs is equal to 810 calories (HINT: there are 4 calories in 1 gram of carbs, so you must divide the total number of calories by 4):

810 calories ÷ 4 calories per gram = 202.5 grams of carbs

So, if you are able to take in 1800 calories per day, you are able to eat 202.5 grams of carbs

If you were to divide this up into 3 big meals and 2 snacks in a day, it may look something like this:

Three larger meals at about 45 g carbs each (breakfast, lunch, supper) plus,

Two snacks at 35 g carbs each.

When dosing insulin, most people will have a dose of basal insulin (intermediate/long-acting insulin) once or twice a day. They also usually will take rapid/regular/short-acting insulin with each larger meal (breakfast, lunch, supper). Many do not give any insulin with snacks, but sometimes people do, depending on their doctor's recommendations. It's important not to skip meals, especially when you are taking insulin. Work with your doctor and dietician to find out how much of each type of insulin you should be taking throughout the day.

Mixing Insulins

There is a way to decrease the number of times you have to inject yourself each day. If you find yourself taking a dose of NPH insulin and a dose of short/rapid acting insulin at the same time, you can draw them both up in one syringe for one injection. However, you have to follow proper technique to avoid over or under-dosing insulin. Let's go over that technique now.

NOTE: You CAN mix NPH insulin with rapid, regular or short-acting insulin (insulin aspart, insulin glulisin, insulin lispro, or regular insulin). You **CAN NOT** mix insulin glargine or insulin detemir (Lantus® or Levemir®) with other insulins.

Let's take a look at which insulins can be mixed together. Note which insulins are 'clear' and which are 'cloudy' when you look at the vial.

Figure 8: **Mixing Guide for Insulin**

Type of Insulin	Name of Insulin	Cloudy or Clear?	Can you Mix with Other Insulin?
Rapid-acting insulin	Insulin glulisine (Apidra®) insulin lispro (Humalog®) insulin aspart (Novolog®)	Clear	Yes
Regular or short-acting insulin	(Humulin R®, Novolin R®)	Clear	Yes
Intermediate-acting insulin	NPH insulin (Humulin N®, Novolin N®)	Cloudy	Yes
Long-acting insulin	Insulin detemir (Levemir®) insulin glargine (Lantus® Toujeo®), insulin degludec (Tresiba®)	Do NOT mix	No. Do NOT mix

Directions for Mixing Insulin

If you find yourself getting ready to take a dose of intermediate-acting insulin and rapid, regular, or short-acting insulin at the same time, you can combine the insulins in the same syringe.

1. Test your blood sugar. If it's not too low, you may proceed.

2. Gather your supplies: vial of cloudy (intermediated-acting) insulin, vial of clear (rapid/regular/short-acting) insulin, 1 insulin syringe, alcohol wipes.

3. Wash your hands.

4. Calculate how many units of clear insulin, how many units of cloudy insulin and how many TOTAL insulin units (clear plus cloudy) you will need.

5. Pick up the cloudy insulin vial. Mix it gently by rolling it between your hands.

6. Set the cloudy vial back onto the table.

7. Take the lid off of each insulin vial and wipe the stopper of each vial with an alcohol swab. Let dry.

8. Remove the caps from each end of the insulin syringe. Draw the plunger back to correct unit mark for your CLOUDY insulin.

9. Insert the needle into the CLOUDY insulin vial.

10. Keeping the insulin vial upright, push the syringe plunger down to inject this amount of air into the cloudy vial.

11. With the plunger still pushed down, withdraw the needle from the vial. Set the vial aside.

12. Pull the plunger of the syringe down to the correct unit mark for the CLEAR insulin dose.

13. Insert the needle into the CLEAR bottle.

14. Push the plunger down to inject the air into the vial.

15. Leave the needle inserted in the vial.

16. Carefully turn the bottle upside down with the needle still inserted in the bottle.

17. With the needle still inserted, pull the plunger of the syringe back to the correct unit mark for the CLEAR insulin dose.

18. Look for air bubbles in the syringe.

19. If there are air bubbles, push the insulin back into the vial and try pulling the plunger back to the correct unit mark again. Keep checking for air bubbles and pushing the insulin back into the vial until you get the right amount of insulin into the syringe. NOTE: these air bubbles won't hurt you, but they do take up space that

should be occupied by insulin and therefore could cause you to get less insulin into the syringe than you need.

20. With this CLEAR dose of insulin in the syringe, pull the needle out of the vial and set the vial of CLEAR insulin aside. Be careful not to move the plunger.

21. Pick up the CLOUDY bottle of insulin.

22. Turn the CLOUDY bottle upside down and push the needle into the bottle. Be very careful not to move the plunger (you don't want to inject any of the clear insulin in the syringe into the cloudy vial).

23. Pull the plunger down and withdraw the correct number of TOTAL insulin units you need (clear plus cloudy).

24. The plunger should now be on the unit mark showing the total units of both the CLEAR and CLOUDY types of insulin.

25. Pull the needle out of the vial. Set both bottles on the table.

26. Look for air bubbles in the syringe.

27. If you see air bubbles, discard the dose and begin again.

28. If you set the syringe down. Do not let the needle touch anything.

29. Wipe the chosen injection site with an alcohol prep pad. Let the alcohol dry.

30. Pinch the skin at the chosen injection site.

31. Pick up the syringe.

32. Insert the needle straight into the skin at a 90-degree angle. Make sure the needle is all the way through the skin.

33. Push the plunger down to inject the insulin.

34. Pull the needle out of the skin.

35. Apply pressure to the injection area with an alcohol swab.

36. Discard the needle and syringe as advised.

Use the Right Syringe

When drawing up insulin it is VERY important to actually use an *insulin* syringe. *Do NOT use a non-insulin syringe*. Syringes that are not insulin syringes mark the units on the syringe in milliliters (mL) instead of insulin units (units). Insulin syringes are marked in units. *Using an insulin syringe decreases the risk of measuring errors since you just pull the syringe plunger back to the number of units of insulin you want to give.*

Strengths of Insulin

There are also different strengths of insulin. It appears as though the population overall is becoming more and more insulin-resistant. This may be due to an increasing over-abundance of processed foods that contain more carbs and sugars than ever before. This phenomenon has paved the way for more concentrated insulins to enter the market.

Table 9: *Strengths* of Insulin

Strength of Insulin	How it's Different	Examples
U-100	100 units/mL – This is the typical strength that most insulins come in	Rapid/regular/short-acting insulin, intermediate-acting insulin and long-acting insulin like: Tresiba® 100 unit/mL- (insulin glargine like Lantus®) Lantus® *insulin glargine) Levemir®(insulin detemir)
U-200	200 units/mL – Rapid acting	insulin lispro Tresiba® 200 unit/mL
300 units/ml	300 units/mL – Long acting	Toujeo® 300 units/mL- (insulin glargine like Lantus® but 300 units/mL)

Typically insulin vials contain insulin that have a concentration of 100 units per milliliter (100 units/mL). More concentrated insulins are available. For example, Toujeo® is a long-acting insulin that is 3 times as potent (300 units/mL).

It's EXTREMELY important to note what strength your insulin is. If you accidently took 1 mL of 300 unit/mL insulin instead of 1 mL of 100 unit/mL insulin, you would be taking 3 times the dose of insulin you need. It's very possible you could experience dangerously low blood sugar. So, make sure to check the strength of insulin you are taking and ***make sure you see the section at the end of this chapter called "Treating Low Blood Sugar at home".***

How Much Insulin?

You will need to work with your doctor and your RD to figure out how much insulin you should be taking. Insulin dosing is something that needs to be tailored for each person.

When first starting insulin, most people with type 1 diabetes are started on 0.4 to 1 unit per kilogram of body weight per day (units/kg/day). With type 2 diabetes, it's common to be started at 0.6 to 1 units/kg/day. 50% of this calculated daily dose is typically given as basal insulin (AKA immediate or long-acting insulin). The other 50% is given with meals (divided among the days' meals as rapid, regular or short-acting insulin).

For example:

Let's say you weigh 70 kg. Your doctor wants to start you on 1 unit/kg/day. If you ate 3 meals a day, how much long-acting insulin and how much rapid-acting insulins would you need?

Answer:

1. Find out total number of units needed:
a. 70 kg X 1 unit/kg = 70 units of insulin needed
2. 50% (half) of this dose will be given as **long acting insulin**:
a. ½ of 70 = 35 units to be given once daily as long-acting insulin

3. 50% (half) will be given divided up amongst meals as **rapid-acting insulin**:

    a. ½ of 70 = 35 units

    b. 35 units divided up between 3 meals = 11.6 units of rapid-acting insulin (we'll go with 11 units) at each meal

Other Treatments Besides Insulin

Medications for the Treatment of Diabetes

The choice of medications to treat diabetes is very individualized. When choosing medications, you and your doctor should take into consideration:

- How effective the medication is
- Risk of causing low blood sugar
- Risk of weight gain
- Tolerability
- Other side effects
- Cost
- Ease of use

There are medications you inject (besides insulin) and medications you take by mouth. These medications are sometimes available not only by themselves, but also in combination with another drug. This can be very helpful if you want to decrease the number of pills you have to take per day. It is also a better deal. For the price of one copay you are getting two medications.

The downside is that combination products only come in a few options with fixed doses, so adjusting your doses can be a challenge at times.

You will see in Table 10 that combination products are mentioned where available. Let's take a look at what the AACE/ACE guidelines and Micromedex (a trusted source health professionals use to obtain medication information) say about these medications.

Table 10: Summary of Treatments Used for the Treatment of Type 1 and Type 2 Diabetes[1,16]

Metformin

Effectiveness: High
Chance of causing low blood sugar: Low
Weight change?: Loss

Metformin (Glucophage®, Metformin®, Glumetza®, Riomet®, Fortamet®) is a type of medication called a biguanide. It is a medication that is taken orally. It is available by itself or in a combination product that contain more than two medications:

- Repaglinide and metformin (Prandimet®)
- Metformin and glipizide (Metaglip®)
- Metformin and pioglitazone (ACTOplus Met®)
- Metformin and glyburide (Glucovance®)
- Metformin and rosiglitazone (Avandamet®)
- Metformin and sitagliptin (Janumet®)

Metformin decreases how much sugar your liver makes and decreases how much sugar is absorbed from the intestines. It also makes your body more sensitive to insulin. This means it takes less insulin to get the same effect.

Metformin can promote weight loss and reduce blood sugar. There is a very low risk of experiencing low blood sugar with metformin. Some evidence suggests that metformin has cardioprotective ('heart protecting') properties.

Metformin should be used with caution in patients with chronic kidney disease (CKD) and should NOT be started in people with an estimated glomerular filtration rate (eGFR) less than 45 mL/min (this is a calculation your doctor uses to assess your kidney function).

Side effects of metformin include an increased risk of lactic acidosis (a potentially life-threatening condition where there is too much acid in the body). Metformin can also cause vitamin B12 absorption problems, so talk to your doctor about taking vitamin B12 supplements while taking metformin. Metformin can also cause anemia and peripheral neuropathy (nerve damage to the nerve endings, usually noticed in hands and feet).

Insulin-secretagogues

Effectiveness: High
Chance of causing low blood sugar: Yes (High)
Weight change?: Gain

'Insulin-secretagogues' is a big word that basically means 'those medications that cause the pancreas to produce more insulin'. These medications are taken orally. This class includes 2 groups of drugs: 1) sulfonylureas, and 2) glinides. These medications can lower your blood sugar, and therefore can lower A1C.

As far as side effects go, both groups are associated with weight gain and low blood sugar. In fact, sulfonylureas are associated with the second-highest risk for dangerously low blood sugar (next to insulin).

Sulfonylureas
- Glimepiride (Amaryl®)
- Glyburide (DiaBeta®, Micronase®)
- Glipizide (Glucotrol®)
- Chlorpropamide
- Tolazamide (Tolinase®)
- Tolbutamide
- Glipizide and metformin (Metaglip®)
- Glimepiride and rosiglitazone (Avandaryl®)
- Glyburide and metformin (Glucovance®)
- Glimepiride and pioglitazone (Duetact®)

Glinides
- Nateglinide (Starlix®)
- Repaglinide (Prandin®)
- Repaglinide and metformin (Prandimet®)

Pramlintide (Symlin®, SymlinPen®) for type 1 and type 2 diabetes

Effectiveness: High
Chance of causing low blood sugar: Yes
Weight change?: Loss

Pramlintide is a medication that you inject subcutaneously (into the fatty under-layer of skin tissue). It has been approved by the Food and Drug Administration (FDA) for the treatment of type 1 and type 2 diabetes in patients who take rapid-acting insulin before meals. It delays emptying of the stomach and enhances the feeling of "feeling full after a meal". Pramlintide is given in fixed doses before meals. It is used in addition to insulin, however, it CANNOT be mixed in the same syringe. Two separate syringes must be used.

It may take some experimenting to find the right dose of pramlintide that works for you. You may want to start out trying it at one meal every day. You can work with your doctor to adjust the dose up or down until you figure out what dose will work for you. Waiting 3 days before increasing the dose may help decrease the amount of nausea you feel.

When you figure out what dose works for you at that meal, then replicate that at other meals (the dose of pramlintide is the same at every meal). Some report that the 'right' dose will produce a 'full feeling' after you eat and/or reduce the spike of insulin that tends to happen after meals. If you do not experience this, you may need to increase your dose.

Pramlintide can cause weight loss and usually decreases the amount of insulin one has to use. Nausea is a common side effect but usually goes away. Other potential side effects include redness at the injection site, stomach pain, tiredness, dizziness, cough, sore throat, and joint pain.

When starting this medication, it's important to work with your doctor on lowering your insulin dose from the start to prevent your blood sugar from going too low. When starting pramlintide, your insulin doses should be cut in half then adjusted from there.

Sodium-glucose Cotransporter 2 Inhibitors (SGLT2)

Effectiveness: Intermediate
Chance of causing low blood sugar: Low
Weight change?: Loss

Sodium-glucose Cotransporter 2 Inhibitors (SGLT2) and combination products that contain SGLT2 inhibitors include:

- Canagliflozin (Invokana®)
- Dapagliflozin (Farxiga®)
- Empagliflozin (Jardiance®)
- Empagliflozin and linagliptin (Glyxambl®)
- Empagliflozin and metformin (Synjardy®)
- Dapagliflozin and metformin (Xigduo XR®)

These medications are taken by mouth and are FDA-approved to help lower blood sugar in people with type 2 diabetes. SGLT2s can decrease blood sugar, A1C, weight, and blood pressure. Medications in this category have also been shown to decrease the risk of death in patients with type 2 diabetes, especially in those with a history of cardiovascular disease and/or heart failure. They may also decrease the risk of heart attack and stroke. On the downside, one trial showed that they may increase the risk of amputation, increase LDL cholesterol, and increase the risk of bone fractures and certain genital infections.

SGLT2s do not work well in patients with decreased kidney function. Side effects of these medications stem from the fact that these drugs can cause dehydration. As a result, they can cause kidney impairment, low blood pressure, fainting, and falls. There have also been reports of these medications causing DKA (diabetic ketoacidosis) in patients with type 1 and type 2 diabetes.

It is recommended that people taking one of these medications stop the medication 24 hours before a scheduled surgery and before intense physical activity (like intense sport activities). When taking medications from this class of drugs, one should avoid very low carbohydrate meal plans and avoid drinking too much alcohol. Doing these things while taking a medication from this class of drugs can increase the risk of experiencing dangerously low blood sugar levels.

Thiazolidinediones [TZDs] or "Glitazones"

Effectiveness: High
Chance of causing low blood sugar: No
Weight change?: Gain

Examples of thiazolidinediones (TZDs or "glitazones") include:
- Pioglitazone (Actos®)
- Rosiglitazone (Avandia®)
- Rosiglitazone and glimepiride (Avandaryl®)
- Pioglitazone and metformin (ACTOplus Met®)
- Rosiglitazone and metformin (Avandamet®)
- Pioglitazone and glimepiride (Duetact®)

Glitazones have been shown to decrease the risk of future development of diabetes in 60 to 75% of people with prediabetes. They can lower A1C and have a low risk of causing low blood sugar. However, these drugs have been associated with the development of weight gain, water retention, and possible heart failure (especially in people with pre-existing heart dysfunction). There is also an increased risk of bone fractures. For these reasons, many doctors prefer to reserve them for those people who don't respond to other therapies.

Glucagon-like peptide 1 (GLP1) receptor agonists

Effectiveness: High
Chance of causing low blood sugar: No
Weight change?: Loss

Examples of these medications include:
- Exenatide (Byetta® and Bydureon®)
- Liraglutide (Victoza® and Saxenda®)
- Lixisenatide (Lyxumia®)
- Albiglutide (Tanzeum®)
- Dulaglutide (Trulicity®)
- Semaglutide (Ozempic®)

These medications are given as a subcutaneous injection (like insulin and pramlintide). They stimulate insulin production and suppress glucagon production. They may be effective in preventing diabetes in people with prediabetes. These drugs have been associated with a decrease in weight, blood lipids, and blood pressure. They have been shown to decrease the risk of kidney problems and death from cardiovascular problems (like heart attack and stroke) in people with type 2 diabetes who have cardiovascular disease.

GLP1 medications should be avoided by people with a family history of thyroid cancer. Exenatide should not be used in those with very low kidney function. Liraglutide, albiglutide and dulaglutide may be used in certain people with kidney disease. All of the drugs in this class should be used with caution, if at all, in people with a history of pancreatitis as these drugs can aggravate or cause pancreatitis. They also can delay emptying of the stomach and therefore should be used with caution in people with severe gastro-esophageal reflux disease (GERD) and/or gastroparesis (a condition where the stomach is slow to move food out of the stomach and into the intestines). These medications have a very low risk of causing blood sugar that is dangerously low. However, there is a lack of long-term safety data with these drugs.

Dipeptidyl peptidase 4 (DPP4) inhibitors (the "gliptins")

Effectiveness: Intermediate
Chance of causing low blood sugar: No
Weight change?: Neutral

Examples of peptidyl peptidase 4 (DPP4) inhibitors (AKA the gliptins) include:
- Sitagliptin (Januvia®)
- Saxagliptin (Onglyza®)
- Linagliptin (Tradjenta®)
- Alogliptin (Nesina®)
- Vildagliptin (Galvus®)
- Alogliptin (Nesina® Vipidia®)
- Metformin and alogliptin (Kazano®)
- Sitagliptin and metformin (Janumet®)

DPP4 inhibitors increase the production of insulin and suppress the production of glucagon in the body. They can lower A1C but do not tend to cause either weight gain or weight loss. Unlike some other diabetes medications, these medications have not been shown to decrease the risk of death from cardiovascular disease.

There is little risk of low blood sugar with DPP4 inhibitors. They should be used with caution in people with kidney disease (a dose adjustment may be necessary) and/or pancreatitis (they can aggravate or cause pancreatitis). Also, saxagliptin and alogliptin have been shown to increase the risk of heart failure.

Alpha-glucosidase Inhibitors

Effectiveness: Intermediate
Chance of causing low blood sugar: no
Weight change?: Loss

Examples of these medications include:
- Acarbose (Precose®)
- Miglitol (Glyset®)

These medications are taken before meals. They slow down carbohydrate digestion so glucose is absorbed from the food at a slower rate. This lessens the spike in blood sugar that can happen after meals.

It's best to take these medications before meals. Side effects of these medications include bloating, diarrhea, nausea, stomach pain and flatulence.

Pancreatic Surgery

There is a surgical procedure available called "Islet transplantation". This type of procedure involves replacing the cells in the pancreas that make insulin so your body can make insulin again. The down side of this procedure is that it requires the patient to be on life-long immunosuppressive medications to prevent their body's immune system from attacking the newly implanted cells.

Which Medications Should I Use?

When it comes to figuring out which medications to use, the ADA makes the following recommendations:[4]

For people with type 1 diabetes:

• Most people with type 1 diabetes should be treated with multiple daily injections of insulin before meals and basal (intermediate or long-acting) insulin or continuous subcutaneous insulin infusion

• Most people with type 1 diabetes should use rapid-acting insulin

• People with type 1 diabetes should learn to take into consideration one's carbohydrate intake, premeal blood sugar levels, and physical activity

• People with type 1 diabetes who have been successfully using continuous subcutaneous insulin infusion should have continued access to this therapy after they turn 65 years of age

People with type 2 diabetes:

Metformin is the preferred initial medication that should be used for treatment of type 2 diabetes (as long as it is tolerated and not contraindicated (strong recommendation NOT to use)).

Long-term use of metformin may be associated with biochemical vitamin B12 deficiency. Vitamin B12 levels should be considered in metformin-treated patients, especially in those with anemia or peripheral neuropathy.

Consider initiating insulin therapy (with or without additional agents) if you have newly-diagnosed type 2 diabetes and:

• Are symptomatic and/or
• Have A1C ≥10% (86 mmol/mol) and/or
• Blood glucose levels ≥300 mg/dL (16.7 mmol/L)

- Patients with newly-diagnosed type 2 diabetes who have A1C ≥ 9% (75 mmol/mol) may consider starting with two medications (instead of one)

In people without cardiovascular disease, if using one or two medications does not achieve or maintain the A1C goal over 3 months, an additional medication may be used.

Consideration when choosing a medication to treat diabetes should include efficacy, risk of low blood sugar, history of cardiovascular disease, impact on weight, potential side effects, effects on the kidneys, cost, and how it is given (oral vs. injection)

In people with type 2 diabetes AND established atherosclerotic cardiovascular disease:

- Medication therapy should begin with lifestyle management and metformin
- A medication proven to reduce major adverse cardiovascular events and death from cardiovascular disease should be considered as an additional medication (empagliflozin or liraglutide)
- After lifestyle management and metformin, canagliflozin may be considered to reduce major adverse cardiovascular events.

Continuous reevaluation of the medication regimen and adjustment is recommended. For patients with type 2 diabetes who are not achieving their blood sugar goals, drug intensification, including consideration of insulin therapy, should be promptly considered. Metformin should be continued when used in combination with other medications, including insulin, if not contraindicated and if tolerated.

Treating Low Blood Sugar at Home

People taking insulin are especially prone to having bouts of very low blood sugar. *Make sure you talk to your doctor about having a plan for when your blood sugar is too high, too low, or if you feel the symptoms of low blood sugar coming on.* Symptoms of low blood sugar may include shakiness, confusion, fast heart rate, irritability, and hunger. Severely low blood sugar may cause loss of consciousness, coma, or death.

About 15-20 grams of glucose is the preferred treatment for someone who is conscious with a blood sugar less than or equal to 70 mg/dL (3.9 mmol/L).[4] However, 70 mg/dL may be considered low for someone with diabetes whose body is accustom to higher sugar levels. This means these people may have symptoms of hypoglycemia below levels of 80, 90 or evern 120 mg/dL. You may have to repeat giving 15-20 grams of glucose if the blood sugar is not rising to above 100-120 mg/dL. You should carry a monitor and a small bag of low-fat candies (like Skittles®) or glucose tablets (available at the drug store) with you for when you have blood sugar that is too low.

Table 11: **Carbohydrates That Can Be Used for Treating Low Blood Sugar**

Quick carbohydrates that can be used for treating low blood sugar include (each provides 15-30 grams of carbohydrate):
- 12 gummy bears
- 6 large jelly beans
- 5 Life Savers®
- 15 Skittles®
- 4 Starburst®
- ½ cup of soda (not diet)
- 1 cup fat free milk
- ½ cup of orange juice
- ½ banana
- 1 small apple
- 3 to 4 glucose tablets
- 1 tube of glucose gel

Each of these choices above provides 15 to 30 grams of low-fat carbohydrate. After eating one of these options, wait 15 minutes then check your blood sugar again. If your blood sugar is still less than 100 mg/dL, take another serving of one of the options above.

It's important that the candy you carry for this purpose be <u>low fat.</u> Fat slows the absorption of sugar. When treating low blood sugar you need to treat it quickly. Therefore you don't want any fat in the candy you choose to slow absorption. So candy bars, ice cream, and cookies are NOT an option.

After you eat the candy to treat your low blood sugar and your blood sugar has returned to normal, a well-balanced snack (preferably containing protein, fat and carbohydrates) is recommended. If you need help choosing some well-balanced snacks for this purpose, talk to your doctor, pharmacist or RD.

If not treated promptly, severely low blood sugar can be deadly. Eating a small handful of candies when you are too low can help bring your sugar up and get rid of the symptoms of low blood sugar until you can have a balanced snack.

It is recommended that people with diabetes who are prone to bouts of low blood sugar *(less than 54 mg/dL (93 mmol/L))* carry a glucagon pen with them. A glucagon pen can be obtained at your retail pharmacy. Family, friends, and school personnel should be trained on how to use the pen. In the event that your blood sugar dips so low that you become unconscious, someone will be able to use the pen to give you a glucagon injection.

Glucagon is a hormone in the body that caused the liver to release glucose into the blood stream. This raises your blood sugar. It has the opposite action of insulin which lowers blood sugar.

After a normal blood glucose is achieved, a balanced snack should follow, preferably one with protein, carbohydrates, and fat.

Note: if you blood sugar is consistently low, talk to your doctor. You may need to change the doses of the medications you are taking.

> ### *Key to Success*
>
> It is recommended that people with diabetes who are prone to bouts of low blood sugar *(less than 54 mg/dL (93 mmol/L))* carry a glucagon pen with them.

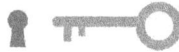

What Types of Things Affect Blood Sugar Levels?

Besides, insulin, many things can affect your blood sugar levels. That's why testing is so important. Things that can affect your blood sugar levels include:

- Activity/ exercise
- Food intake
- Alcohol intake
- Illness

How to Avoid Low Blood Sugar

Check your blood sugar if you have any of these symptoms:

- Weakness
- Dizziness
- Headache
- Sweating
- Anxiety
- Shaking
- Increased heartbeat or heart palpitations

As mentioned before, low blood sugar typically happens when:

1. You skip or delay eating a meal of snack
2. You take too much insulin
3. You exercise
4. You drink alcohol

Special Occasions

It's important to avoid bouts of low blood sugar. Not only do you not feel or function well when you have low blood sugar; it's can be very dangerous. Here are some circumstances where trying to avoid low blood sugar while dosing your insulin can be tricky.

Eating Out: Sometimes dosing your rapid/regular/short-acting insulin while eating out can be tricky. For example, when you're some place (like a restaurant) where you don't know how long it will take for your food to arrive, consider not giving your rapid/regular/short-acting insulin dose until you *see* your food. This will avoid any potentially serious dips in blood sugar.

Exercise: Exercise naturally lowers your blood sugar, so it's important to dose and time your insulin so your blood sugar doesn't go too low. Always check your blood sugar before you exercise and talk to your doctor about having a plan of what to do if your blood sugar is low, normal, or high.

The following is an example 'plan'. *NOTE: this is only one example of how one's plan could look*. Talk to your doctor about tailoring an exercise plan that is right for you.

My Exercise Plan (example)*

Before exercise, check blood sugar (If exercising before a meal, do not take pre-meal insulin yet):

o **If it's critically low (less than 55 mg/dL),** eat at least 30-60 grams of carbohydrates (2-3 servings) to get your blood sugar up. Test again and eat another 15 to 40 grams (1-2 servings) if needed. Then once blood sugar is 100 mg/dL to 120 mg/dL, consider eating a snack that contains at least 30-60 grams of carbohydrates (2-3 servings), some protein and some fat. Consider exercising only after blood sugar is above 150 mg/mL. Don't take any insulin yet. Call an ambulance if feel faint, dizzy, have blurred vision, are confused, feel like fainting, or are extremely weak.

o **If it's 56 mg/dL to 99 mg/dL,** eat at 30-60 grams of carbohydrates (2-3 servings) to get your blood sugar up. Test again and eat another 15

---

to 40 grams (1-2 servings) if needed. Once blood sugar is between 100 mg/dL to 120 mg/dL, consider eating a snack that contains at least 30-60 grams of carbohydrates (2-3 servings), some protein and some fat. Don't take any insulin yet. Call an ambulance if feel faint, dizzy, have blurred vision, are confused, feel like fainting, or are extremely weak. Consider exercising only after blood sugar is above 150 mg/mL.

o **If it's 100 mg/dL to 120 mg/dL),** Consider eating a snack that contains at least 30-60 grams of carbohydrates (2-3 servings), some protein and some fat. Consider exercising only after blood sugar is above 150 mg/mL. Don't take any insulin yet. Call an ambulance if feel faint, dizzy, have blurred vision, are confused, feel like fainting, or are extremely weak.

o **If it's 150 mg/dL to 199 mg/dL,** can go ahead and exercise or consider having a snack of about 30-60 grams of carbohydrates (1-2 servings) about ½ hour before you exercise but don't take any insulin yet. Unless blood sugar is more than 250 mg/dL.

o **If it's 200 mg/dL to 250 mg/,** do not eat a snack. Do not take insulin yet. Proceed to exercising.

o **If it's very high (251 mg/dL or more),** follow your 'Low Blood Sugar Plan'. Talk to your doctor ahead of time about a plan for what to do when your blood sugar is very high. Decide together how much insulin you will take. Seek medical attention if you feel faint, dizzy, have blurred vision, are confused, feel like fainting, or are extremely weak.

Then after you are finished exercising, test your blood sugar again.

or are extremely weak. Do not take any meal-time insulin.

*This plan is only a suggestion and may not work for everyone. Talk to

your doctor about coming up with a plan that works for you.

In general, it takes about 1 unit of short/rapid insulin to lower blood sugar by 45 mg/dL, however this ratio may very from person to person. After you get a feel for how your blood sugar will react to exercise, you will be able to adjust your pre-exercise insulin dose going forward; but proceed cautiously. How much you eat before exercising should be taken into consideration. The amount of carbs you eat before exercise on how strenuous your workout will be.

When in doubt, error on the side of giving LESS insulin because the more insulin you give, the higher the chance you could overshoot your goal and end up with dangerously low blood sugar. Blood sugar that is too low poses more of an immediate danger than blood sugar that is a little too high.

When in doubt, error on the side of giving LESS insulin because the more insulin you give, the higher the chance you could overshoot your goal and end up with dangerously-low blood sugar. Blood sugar that is too low poses more of an immediate danger than blood sugar that is a little too high.

The Bottom Line

Diabetes mellitus is often referred to as 'sugar diabetes' or just 'diabetes'. Diabetes can put you at a higher risk for heart attack and stroke. It also increases your risk for developing kidney failure and blindness. Finally, it can cause nerve damage and decrease blood circulation in the legs. Diabetes is not a disease that you 'catch'. Rather, there is a combination of heredity, lifestyle, eating, and exercise habits that contribute to its development.

To understand how we get diabetes, we need to understand what 'carbs' are. Carbs include starches and fibers found in grains, fruits, and vegetables. Carbs are broken down in the body to give us the energy we need to function properly. 'Sugar' is a refined carb that's found in items like muffins, cakes, cola (not diet), and candy. All carbs we eat are broken down and enter the blood stream to provide us energy. Insulin is a hormone that helps us use blood sugar as energy by helping it enter receptors in our body. Insulin acts as a 'key' to open the 'doors' (receptors). Type 2 diabetes (the most common type) typically results when one of the following happens:
1. the body can't produce insulin ('keys')
2. the body's tissues stop responding to insulin (it gets rid of receptors or 'doorways')
3. a combination of both of these problems

Type 1 diabetes is when the body can't produce its own insulin.

Without insulin to process the glucose in your blood, your blood sugar starts to rise. When the body cannot produce enough insulin, a complication called diabetic ketoacidosis (DKA) can happen. DKA is when there is a buildup of acids in the blood called ketones. Ketones are produced when the body is forced to break down fat for fuel instead of glucose. If not treated promptly, DKA can lead to brain swelling, kidney failure, and trouble breathing. **If you have type 1 diabetes, you should know how to test your urine for ketones** so you can be proactive and correct the problem before you get into trouble. You can obtain a ketone testing kit at your local pharmacy which can test for ketones using a urine sample.

Prediabetes is a condition that indicates one is at high risk for developing type 2 diabetes. It describes someone who doesn't yet meet the criteria for type 2 diabetes but whose glucose levels are too high to be considered normal. Gestational diabetes is diabetes that happens during pregnancy in a patient who did not previously have diabetes. It usually happens during the second or third trimester.

Screening for Prediabetes and diabetes

The ADA recommends people over the age of 45 get screened every 3 years for prediabetes and diabetes.[4] They also recommend using an assessment tool for screening. They offer the ADA risk test for this purpose (located at: www.diabetes.org/socrisktest). **A score of 5 or higher indicates a higher risk for prediabetes or diabetes.**

Testing for prediabetes or diabetes should be considered in adults who are overweight or obese (BMI of 25 kg/m or more, Asian Americans with a BMI greater than 23 kg/m) and have one or more of the risk factors below.

Risk factors for Diabetes[4]

• First degree relative with diabetes
• African American, Latino, Native American, Asian American, Pacific Islander
• History of cardiovascular disease (for example, a history of heart attack)
• High blood pressure (140/90 or more, or are on medication

therapy for high blood pressure)
- HDL cholesterol less than 35 mg/dL (0.90 mmol/L) and/or a triglyceride level of 250 mg/dL (2.82 mmol/L) or more.
- Women with polycystic ovary syndrome
- Physical inactivity

STEP 1: If you are over 45 years old and have not been diagnosed with prediabetes or diabetes, take the ADA risk test at the web address above and write your score in below.

My ADA Diabetes Risk Score is = _____

STEP 2: Is this number more than 5? If so, contact your health care provider to get tested for prediabetes and diabetes.

I need to be tested for diabetes at my doctor's office	■ **Yes** (my risk score is more than 5)	■ **No** (my risk score is less than 5)

Diagnosis of Prediabetes and Diabetes

There are several tests used to test for prediabetes and diabetes.

Tests Used to Test for Prediabetes and Diabetes

Test	What is It?
A1C	A1C is an estimate of your **average blood sugar over the last few months.** This is done by looking at hemoglobin (a protein in the blood that is coated in sugar).
Fasting Blood Glucose (FBG or 'fasting blood sugar')	A blood sugar reading that is taken after at least 8 hours with no food.
Oral Glucose Tolerance Test (OGTT)	An OGTT is a reading of your blood sugar 2 hours after you are given 75 gm of sugar to eat.

Let's look at how these tests can be used to diagnose prediabetes and diabetes.

Diagnosis of Prediabetes and Diabetes[4]*

		A1C	Fasting Blood Sugar (FBG)	Oral Glucose Tolerance Test (OGTT)	Other
■	**Prediabetes**	A1C of 5.7-6.4%	FBG of 100 mg/dL (5.6 mmol/L) to 125 mg/dL (6.9 mmol/L	Blood glucose of 140 mg/dL (7.8 mmol/L) to 199 mg/dL (11 mmol/L) after a 2-hour OGTT	
■	**Diabetes**	A1C of 6.5% or more	FBG of 126 mg/dL (7 mmol/L) or greater after no food for at least 8 hours.	Blood glucose of 200 mg/dL (11.1 mmol/L) or more during a 2 hour OGTT test. The test should use 75 gm of glucose dissolved in water	Classic symptoms of high blood sugar with a random blood sugar of 200 mg/dL (11.1 mmol/L) or more.

*NOTE: FBG should be used to diagnose type 1 diabetes (instead of A1C). A panel of autoantibodies may also be ordered.

STEP 3: After visiting your doctor to get tested for prediabetes and type 2 diabetes, circle any symptoms in Table 5 that apply. If you have anything circled in the prediabetes row, check the prediabetes box. If you have anything circled in the type 2 diabetes row, check that box. Did the boxes checked indicate that you may have prediabetes, type 2 diabetes or neither?

■ **Prediabetes**	■ **Type 2 Diabetes**	■ **Neither**

I've Been Diagnosed with Prediabetes or Diabetes. Now What?

If you've been diagnosed with prediabetes or diabetes, it is recommended that your doctor do a complete medical evaluation for you to:

• Confirm the diagnosis
• Check for diabetes complications and other conditions that need to be addressed (like cardiovascular disease or high blood pressure)
• A medical evaluation which may include: medical history, allergies, past side effects, physical exam, and lab assessment
• Determine a plan for initial and ongoing care, for the management of your prediabetes or diabetes
• Determine the need for referrals to other doctors, immunizations, and other health screenings

STEP 4: Check the appropriate box below when you have set up a complete medical evaluation with your doctor.

I have been diagnosed with prediabetes or diabetes and have scheduled a complete medical evaluation with my doctor	☐ **Yes**	☐ **No**

Part of this comprehensive medical evaluation should include an assessment of your blood pressure and cholesterol levels.
When you have diabetes, you should manage your ABCs (A1C, blood

pressure, and cholesterol). Aim for:

- **Blood pressure goal of less than 130/80**
- **LDL (AKA "bad cholesterol") less than 100 mg/dL (but less than 70 mg/dL if one has cardiovascular disease).** [4]

Diabetes Self-Management Education and Support

It is recommended that all people with diabetes take part in diabetes self-management education and support (DSMES). The goal of DSMES is to improve health and quality of life through education. It is hoped that through DSMES, people can gain the skills they need to be able to maintain their diabetes care at home.

It is recommended that people with diabetes take part in DSMES at least at these four critical times[4]:

1. At diagnosis
2. Every year
3. When problems arise
4. When a change occurs

DSMES programs are offered by various health care professionals. DSMES can be done in a group setting or on an individual basis. It can even be done via technology (via webinars or skype meetings for example). Accredited DSMES programs are generally covered by Medicare and may be covered by most private insurances as well. However, note that **Medicare and private insurances generally cover in-person DSMES visits**. Phone, skype, or other alternative forms of meeting may not be covered. Check with your insurance.

STEP 5: Contact your doctor's office to find a DSMES program near you. Check the box below when you have made your first DSMES appointment:

My DSMES appoint is scheduled for: _____

Nutrition Therapy

It's recommended that all people with diabetes be offered a referral to a Registered Dietician (RD). RD referrals have been shown to decrease A1C in people with diabetes.[4]

An RD can help you:

1. Learn how to plan your own meals
2. Learn healthful eating patterns
3. Discover how to incorporate a variety of nutritious food into your meal plan
4. Manage your weight
5. Delay or prevent diabetes and its complications
6. Identify your individual nutrition needs

STEP 6: Contact your doctor's office to find an RD near you. Check the box below when you have made your first appointment:

My first RD consultation is scheduled for: _____

How to test your blood sugar

To test your blood sugar, you will need a blood glucose meter from the drug store.

If you need help choosing a meter or help learning how to use one, ask your pharmacist to help you. Some meters allow you to check blood sugar at your forearm, thigh, or back of your hand. Check your device. Checking at these sites, if your machine is NOT made to do this, may result in inaccurate results.

Most meters work the same way. Basically you will:

1. Wash your hands with soap and water
2. Insert a test strip into the meter
3. Prick your finger (or other site if meter allows you to test somewhere else) using the lancing device provided to get a small bead of blood
4. Touch the glucose strip tips to the bead of blood so the strip can absorb some of the blood
5. In a few moments your result will appear on the display of the meter. A continuous glucose monitor (AKA insulin pump) is also available through your doctor. This is a monitor you wear all of the time. A tiny sensor goes under your skin so the device can take a blood sugar reading every few minutes or so. This data may be wirelessly transmitted to a remote receiver that you keep in your purse or pocket.

Who Should Check Their Blood Sugar?

Whether you use continuous glucose monitoring or are testing yourself throughout the day, it is recommended that you test your blood sugar regularly if you:

- Are taking insulin
- Have a hard time controlling your blood sugar
- Are prone to low blood sugar levels (especially if you don't usually have the symptoms of low blood sugar like shakiness, sweating, fainting, fatigue, or heart palpitations
- Are pregnant
- Have ketones in your urine

What Should My Blood Sugar Goal Be?

You should talk to you doctor about specific blood sugar goals that are right for you. In general, however, it is recommended that one **aim for a goal of 80-130 mg/dL (4.4 to 7.2 mmol/L) right before meals and less than 180 mg/dL (10 mmol/L,) 1 to 2 hours after meals.**[4]

When Should One Test Their Blood Sugar?

It's recommended that people using insulin shots or who have an insulin pump test their blood sugar[4]:

- Prior to each meal and snack
- At bedtime
- Prior to exercise
- When they think their blood sugar might be too low or too high.
- After treating themselves due to low blood sugar
- Occasionally after meals

What Can Cause Low Blood Sugar

Typically low blood sugar happens when:
1. You skip or delay eating a meal of snack
2. You take too much insulin
3. You exercise
4. You drink alcohol
5. You're sick and not eating much

A1C Testing

After being diagnosed with diabetes, it is recommended that **people who are meeting their treatment goals test their A1C at least two times a year. People who are not meeting their treatment goals should test every 3 months.**[4] Remember, A1C is a reflection of your blood sugar over the last 3 months. It's a helpful way for you and your doctor to see if you are at risk for diabetes complications.

What Should My A1C Goal Be?

The ADA notes that if you are diabetic, your **A1C goal should be less than 7%** (53 mmol/mol) or **eAG less than 154 mg/dL** for most nonpregnant adults.

Insulin for the Treatment of Diabetes

Most people with type 1 diabetes (and some with type 2 diabetes) will need to be treated with multiple doses of insulin throughout the day. Insulin is given via a small injection into the fatty layer just below the top layer of skin.

Types of Insulin

There are different types of insulin. They are classified depending on how long they last.

Types of Insulin			
	Type of Insulin	**How it's Different**	**Examples**
Usually given prior to meals	**Rapid-acting insulin**	Starts to work in about 15 minutes (take no more than 15 minutes before a meal), effects peak in 1 hour and lasts for 2 to 4 hours.	Insulin glulisine (Apidra®) insulin lispro (Humalog®) insulin aspart (Novolog®)
	Regular or short-acting insulin	Starts to work in about 30 minutes (take no more than 30 minutes before a meal), effects peak in about 2 to 3 hours and lasts for 3 to 6 hours.	(Humulin R®, Novolin R®)
Usually given once or twice daily to control evenly throughout the day	**Intermediate-acting insulin**	Starts to work in 2 to 4 hours, effects peak in about 4 to 12 hours and lasts for 12 to 18 hours	NPH insulin-isophane (Humulin N®, Novolin N®)

226

	Long-acting insulin	Starts to work in several hours then lowers blood sugar pretty evenly over 24 hours.	Insulin detemir (Levemir®) insulin glargine (Lantus®)
	Various premixed insulins	A combination of NPH insulin and a short or rapid acting insulin that can be helpful for someone who has trouble drawing up two different insulins due to dexterity or poor eyesight. Humulin 70/30, for example, means there is 70% intermediate-acting insulin PLUS 30 % regular-acting insulin.	Humulin 70/30, Humalog Mix 50/50, Humalog Mix 75/25, Novolin 70/30, Novolog Mix 70/30
	Inhaled insulin	Rapid-acting. Starts to work within 12 to 15 minutes, effects peak around 30	Afrezza®

		minutes and it's out of your system in about 180 minutes. Given before each meal. Must be used in combination with long-acting insulin	

Sliding Scale

You may hear the term "sliding scale". Sliding scale means you adjust the dose of your rapid/regular/short-acting insulin before meals based on how many grams of carbohydrates you will be eating in that meal. **Generally, 1 unit of insulin will take care of 1 serving of carbs (1 serving of carbs is about 12-15 grams of carbohydrate)**. So for example, if you eat 2 pieces of toast (each piece has 15 grams of carbs, or 30 grams total) then you will need about 2 units of rapid-acting insulin before your meal.

For a list of foods and their carbohydrate content you can download an app on your phone that allows you to look up the carb content of foods on the go. A great app that I personally use myself is "**My Fitness Pal**".

Mixing Insulins

You CAN mix NPH insulin with rapid, regular or short-acting insulin (insulin aspart, insulin glulisin, insulin lispro or regular insulin). You **CANNOT** mix insulin glargine or insulin detemir (Lantus® or Levemir®) with other insulins.

Let's take a look at which insulins can be mixed together. Note which insulins are 'clear' and which are 'cloudy' when you look at the vial.

Mixing Guide for Insulin			
Type of Insulin	**Name of Insulin**	**Cloudy or Clear?**	**Can you Mix with Other Insulin?**
Rapid-acting insulin	Insulin glulisine (Apidra®) insulin lispro (Humalog®) insulin aspart (Novolog®)	Clear	Yes
Regular or short-acting insulin	(Humulin R®, Novolin R®)	Clear	Yes
Intermediate-acting insulin	NPH insulin (Humulin N®, Novolin N®)	Cloudy	Yes
Long-acting insulin	Insulin detemir (Levemir®) insulin glargine (Lantus® Toujeo®), insulin degludec (Tresiba®)	Do NOT mix	No. Do NOT mix

Directions for Mixing Insulin

If you find yourself getting ready to take a dose of intermediate-acting insulin and rapid, regular or short-acting insulin at the same time, you can combine the insulins in the same syringe.

1. Test your blood sugar. If it's not too low, you may proceed.

2. Gather your supplies: vial of cloudy (intermediated-acting) insulin, vial of clear (rapid/regular/short-acting) insulin, 1 insulin syringe, alcohol wipes.

3. Wash your hands.

4. Calculate how many units of clear insulin, how many units of cloudy insulin and how many TOTAL insulin units (clear plus cloudy) you will need.

5. Pick up the cloudy insulin vial. Mix it gently by rolling it between your hands.

6. Set the cloudy vial back onto the table.

7. Take the lid off of each insulin vial and wipe the stopper of each vial with an alcohol swab. Let dry.

8. Remove the caps from each end of the insulin syringe. Draw the plunger back to correct unit mark for your CLOUDY insulin.

9. Insert the needle into the CLOUDY insulin vial.

10. Keeping the insulin vial upright, push the syringe plunger down to inject this amount of air into the cloudy vial.

11. With the plunger still pushed down, withdraw the needle from the vial. Set the vial aside.

12. Pull the plunger of the syringe down to the correct unit mark for the CLEAR insulin dose.

13. Insert the needle into the CLEAR bottle.

14. Push the plunger down to inject the air into the vial.

15. Leave the needle inserted in the vial.

16. Carefully turn the bottle upside down with the needle still inserted in the bottle.

17. With the needle still inserted, pull the plunger of the syringe back to the correct unit mark for the CLEAR insulin dose.

18. Look for air bubbles in the syringe.

19. If there are air bubbles, push the insulin back into the vial and try pulling the plunger back to the correct unit mark again. Keep checking for air bubbles and pushing the insulin back into the vial until you get the right amount of insulin into the syringe. NOTE: these air bubbles won't hurt you, but they do take up space that should be occupied by insulin and therefore could cause you to get less insulin into the syringe than you need.

20. With this CLEAR dose of insulin in the syringe, pull the

needle out of the vial and set the vial of CLEAR insulin aside. Be careful not to move the plunger.

21. Pick up the CLOUDY bottle of insulin.

22. Turn the CLOUDY bottle upside down and push the needle into the bottle. Be very careful not to move the plunger (you don't want to inject any of the clear insulin in the syringe into the cloudy vial).

23. Pull the plunger down and withdraw the correct number of TOTAL insulin units you need (clear plus cloudy).

24. The plunger should now be on the unit mark showing the total units of both the CLEAR and CLOUDY types of insulin.

25. Pull the needle out of the vial. Set both bottles on the table.

26. Look for air bubbles in the syringe.

27. If you see air bubbles, discard the dose and begin again.

28. If you set the syringe down. Do not let the needle touch anything.

29. Wipe the chosen injection site with an alcohol prep pad. Let the alcohol dry.

30. Pinch the skin at the chosen injection site.

31. Pick up the syringe.

32. Insert the needle straight into the skin at a 90-degree angle. Make sure the needle is all the way through the skin.

33. Push the plunger down to inject the insulin.

34. Pull the needle out of the skin.

35. Apply pressure to the injection area with an alcohol swab.

36. Discard the needle and syringe as advised.

Strengths of Insulin

There are different strengths of insulin. Some insulins are more concentrated.

Strengths of Insulin		
Strength of Insulin	**How it's Different**	**Examples**
U-100	**100 units/mL--This is the typical strength that most insulins come in**	rapid/regular/short-acting insulin, intermediate-acting insulin and long-acting insulin Tresiba® 100 unit/mL-(insulin glargine like Lantus®) Lantus® *insulin glargine) Levemir®(insulin detemir)
U-200	200 units/mL – Rapid acting	insulin lispro Tresiba® 200 unit/mL
300 units/ml	300 units/mL – Long acting	Toujeo® 300 units/mL-(insulin glargine like Lantus® but 300 units/mL)

It's EXTREMELY important to note what strength your insulin is. If you accidently took 1 mL of 300 unit/mL insulin instead of 1 mL of 100 unit/mL insulin, you would be taking 3 times the dose of insulin you need. It's very possible you could experience dangerously low blood sugar. So, make sure to check the strength of insulin you are taking and **make sure you see the section at the end of this chapter called "How to Treat Low Blood Sugar at home".**

How Much Insulin Do I Need?

You will need to work with your doctor and RD to figure out how much insulin you should be taking. Insulin dosing is something that needs to be tailored for each person.

When first starting insulin, most people with type 1 diabetes are started on 0.4 to 1 unit per kilogram of body weight per day (units/kg/day). With type 2 diabetes, it's common to be started at 0.6 to 1 units/kg/day. 50% of this calculated daily dose is typically given as basal insulin (AKA immediate or long-acting insulin). The other 50% is given with meals (divided among the days' meals as rapid, regular or short-acting insulin).

For example:

Let's say you weigh 70 kg. Your doctor wants to start you on 1 unit/kg/day. If you ate 3 meals a day, how much long-acting insulin and how much rapid-acting insulins would you need?

Answer:

1. Find out total number of units needed:
a. 70 kg X 1 unit/kg = 70 units of insulin needed
2. 50% (half) of this dose will be given as **long acting insulin**:
a. ½ of 70 = 35 units to be given once daily as long-acting insulin
3. 50% (half) will be given divided up amongst meals as **rapid-acting insulin**:
a. ½ of 70 = 35 units
b. 35 units divided up between 3 meals = 11.6 units of rapid-acting insulin (we'll go with 11 units) at each meal

Other Treatments Besides Insulin

Medications for the Treatment of Diabetes

The choice of medications to treat diabetes is very individualized. When choosing medications, you and your doctor should take into consideration:

- How effective the medication is
- Risk of causing low blood sugar
- Risk of weight gain
- Tolerability
- Other side effects
- Cost
- Ease of use

Summary of Treatments Used for the Treatment of Type 1 and Type 2 Diabetes

Metformin

Effectiveness: High
Chance of causing low blood sugar: Low
Weight change?: Loss
How to take it: oral

Metformin (Glucophage®, Metformin®, Glumetza®, Riomet®, Fortamet®) is a type of medication called a biguanide. It is a medication that is taken orally. It is available by itself or in a combination product that contain more than two medications:

- Repaglinide and metformin (Prandimet®)
- Metformin and glipizide (Metaglip®)
- Metformin and pioglitazone (ACTOplus Met®)
- Metformin and glyburide (Glucovance®)
- Metformin and rosiglitazone (Avandamet®)
- Metformin and sitagliptin (Janumet®)

Metformin decreases how much sugar your liver makes and decreases how much sugar is absorbed from the intestines. It also makes your body more sensitive to insulin. This means it takes less insulin to get the same effect.

Metformin can promote weight loss and reduce blood sugar. There is a very low risk of experiencing low blood sugar with metformin. Some evidence suggests that metformin has cardioprotective ('heart protecting') properties.

Metformin should be used in caution with patients with chronic kidney disease (CKD) and should NOT be started in people with an estimated glomerular filtration rate (eGFR) less than 45 mL/min (this is a calculation your doctor uses to assess your kidney function).

Side effects of metformin include an increased risk of lactic acidosis (a potentially life-threatening condition where there is too much acid in the body). Metformin can also cause vitamin B12 absorption problems so talk to your doctor about taking vitamin B12 supplements while taking metformin. Metformin can also cause anemia and peripheral neuropathy (nerve damage to the nerve endings, usually noticed in the hands and feet).

Insulin-secretagogues

Effectiveness: High
Chance of causing low blood sugar: Yes (High)
Weight change?: Gain
How to take them: oral

'Insulin-secretagogues' is a big word that basically means 'those medications that cause the pancreas to produce more insulin'. These medications are taken orally. This class includes 2 groups of drugs: 1) sulfonylureas, and 2) glinides. These medications can lower your blood sugar and therefore, can lower A1C.

As far as side effects go, both groups are associated with weight gain and low blood sugar. In fact, sulfonylureas are associated with the second-highest risk for dangerously low blood sugar (next to insulin).

Sulfonylureas
- Glimepiride (Amaryl®)
- Glyburide (DiaBeta®, Micronase®)
- Glipizide (Glucotrol®)
- Chlorpropamide
- Tolazamide (Tolinase®)
- Tolbutamide
- Glipizide and metformin (Metaglip®)
- Glimepiride and rosiglitazone (Avandaryl®)
- Glyburide and metformin (Glucovance®)
- Glimepiride and pioglitazone (Euetact®)

Glinides

- Nateglinide (Starlix®)
- Repaglinide (Prandin®)
- Repaglinide and metformin (Prandimet®)

Pramlintide (Symlin®, SymlinPen®) for type 1 and type 2 diabetes

Effectiveness: High
Chance of causing low blood sugar: Yes
Weight change?: Loss
How to take it: subcutaneous injection

Pramlintide is a medication that you inject subcutaneously (into the fatty under-layer of skin tissue). It has been approved by the Food and Drug Administration (FDA) for the treatment of type 1 and type 2 diabetes in patients who take rapid-acting insulin before meals. It delays emptying of the stomach and enhances the feeling of "feeling full after a meal". Pramlintide is given in fixed doses before meals. It is used in addition to insulin, however, it can NOT be mixed in the same syringe. Two separate syringes must be used.

It may take some experimenting to find the right dose of pramlintide that works for you. You may want to start out trying it at one meal every day. You can work with your doctor to adjust the dose up or down until you figure out what dose will work for you. Waiting 3 days before increasing the dose may help decrease the amount of nausea you feel.

When you figure out what dose works for you at that meal, then replicate that at other meals (the dose of pramlintide is the same at every meal). Some report that the 'right' dose will produce a 'full feeling' after you eat and/or reduce the spike of insulin that tends to happen after meals. If you do not experience this, you may need to increase your dose.

Pramlintide can cause weight loss and usually decreases the

amount of insulin one has to use. Nausea is a common side effect but usually goes away. Other potential side effects include redness at the injection site, stomach pain, tiredness, dizziness, cough, sore throat, and joint pain.

When starting this medication, it's important to work with your doctor on lowering your insulin dose from the start to prevent your blood sugar from going too low.

When starting pramlintide, your insulin doses should be cut in half then adjusted from there to keep your blood sugar from going too low.

Sodium-glucose Cotransporter 2 Inhibitors (SGLT2)

Effectiveness: Intermediate
Chance of causing low blood sugar: Low
Weight change?: Loss
How to take it: oral

Sodium-glucose Cotransporter 2 Inhibitors (SGLT2) and combination products that contain SGLT2 inhibitors include:

- Canagliflozin (Invokana®)
- Dapagliflozin (Farxiga®)
- Empagliflozin (Jardiance®)
- Empagliflozin and linagliptin (Glyxambl®)
- Empagliflozin and metformin (Synjardy®)
- Dapagliflozin and metformin (Xigduo XR®)

These medications are taken by mouth and are FDA-approved to help lower blood sugar in people with type 2 diabetes. SGLT2s can decrease blood sugar, A1C, weight, and blood pressure. Medications in this category have also been shown to decrease the risk of death in patients with type 2 diabetes, especially in those with a history of cardiovascular disease and/or heart failure. They may also decrease the risk of heart attack and stroke. On the downside, one trial showed that they may increase the risk of amputation, increase LDL cholesterol, and increase the risk of bone fractures and certain genital infections.

SGLT2s do not work well in patients with decreased kidney function. Side effects of these medications stem from the fact that these drugs can cause dehydration. As a result they can cause kidney impairment, low blood pressure, fainting and falls. There have also been reports of these medications causing DKA (diabetic ketoacidosis) in patients with type 1 and type 2 diabetes.

It is recommended that people taking one of these medications stop the medication 24 hours before a scheduled surgery and before intense physical activity (like intense sport activities). When taking medications from this class of drugs, one should avoid very low carbohydrate meal plans and avoid drinking too much alcohol. Doing these things while taking a medication from this class of drugs can increase the risk of experiencing dangerously low blood sugar levels.

Thiazolidinediones [TZDs] or "Glitazones"

Effectiveness: High
Chance of causing low blood sugar: No
Weight change?: Gain
How to take them: oral

Examples of thiazolidinediones (TZDs or "glitazones") include:
- Pioglitazone (Actos®)
- Rosiglitazone (Avandia®)
- Rosiglitazone and glimepiride (Avandaryl®)
- Pioglitazone and metformin (ACTOplus Met®)
- Rosiglitazone and metformin (Avandamet®)
- Pioglitazone and glimepiride (Duetact®)

Glitazones have been shown to decrease the risk of future development of diabetes in 60 to 75% of people with prediabetes. They can lower A1C and have a low risk of causing low blood sugar. However, these drugs have been associated with the development of weight gain, water retention, and possible heart failure (especially in people with pre-existing heart dysfunction). There is also an increased risk of bone fractures. For these reasons, many doctors prefer to reserve them for those people who don't respond to other therapies.

Glucagon-like peptide 1 (GLP1) receptor agonists

Effectiveness: High
Chance of causing low blood sugar: No
Weight change?: Loss
How to take them: subcutaneous injection

Examples of these medications include:
- Exenatide (Byetta® and Bydureon®)
- Liraglutide (Victoza® and Saxenda®)
- Lixisenatide (Lyxumia®)
- Albiglutide (Tanzeum®)
- Dulaglutide (Trulicity®)
- Semaglutide (Ozempic®)

These medications are given as a subcutaneous injection (like insulin and pramlintide). They stimulate insulin production and suppress glucagon production. They may be effective in preventing diabetes in people with prediabetes. These drugs have been associated with a decrease in weight, blood lipids, and blood pressure. They have been shown to decrease the risk of kidney problems and death from cardiovascular problems (like heart attack and stroke) in people with type 2 diabetes who have cardiovascular disease.

GLP1 medications should be avoided by those people with a family history of thyroid cancer. Exenatide should not be used in those with very low kidney function. Liraglutide, albiglutide, and dulaglutide may be used in certain people with kidney disease. All of the drugs in this class should be used with caution, if at all in people with a history of pancreatitis as these drugs can aggravate or cause pancreatitis. They also can delay emptying of the stomach and therefore should be used with caution in people with severe gastro-esophageal reflux disease (GERD) and/or gastroparesis (condition where the stomach is slow to move food out of the stomach and into the intestines). These medications have a very low risk of causing blood sugar that is dangerously low. However, there is a lack of long-term safety data with these drugs.

Dipeptidyl peptidase 4 (DPP4) inhibitors (the "gliptins")

Effectiveness: Intermediate
Chance of causing low blood sugar: No
Weight change?: Neutral
How to take them: oral

Examples of peptidyl peptidase 4 (DPP4) inhibitors (AKA the gliptins) include:
- Sitagliptin (Januvia®)
- Saxagliptin (Onglyza®)
- Linagliptin (Tradjenta®)
- Alogliptin (Nesina®)
- Vildagliptin (Galvus®)
- Alogliptin (Nesina®, Vipidia®)
- Metformin and alogliptin (Kazano®)
- Sitagliptin and metformin (Janumet®)

DPP4 inhibitors increase the production of insulin and suppress the production of glucagon in the body. They can lower A1C but do not tend to cause either weight gain or weight loss. Unlike some other diabetes medications, these medications have not been shown to decrease the risk of death from cardiovascular disease.

There is little risk of low blood sugar with DPP4 inhibitors. They should be used with caution in people with kidney disease (a dose adjustment may be necessary) and/or pancreatitis (they can aggravate or cause pancreatitis). Also, saxagliptin and alogliptin have been shown to increase the risk of heart failure.

Alpha-glucosidase Inhibitors

Effectiveness: Intermediate
Chance of causing low blood sugar: no
Weight change?: Loss
How to take: oral

Examples of these medications include:
- Acarbose (Precose®)
- Miglitol (Glyset®)

These medications are taken before meals. They slow down carbohydrate digestion so glucose is absorbed from the food at a slower rate. This lessens the spike in blood sugar that can happen after meals.

It's best to take these medications before meals. Side effects of these medications include: bloating, diarrhea, nausea, stomach pain, and flatulence.

Pancreatic Surgery

There is a surgical procedure available called "Islet transplantation". This type of procedure involves replacing the cells in the pancreas that make insulin so your body can make insulin again. The down side of this procedure is that it requires the patient to be on life-long immunosuppressive medications to prevent their body's immune system from attacking the newly implanted cells.

Which Medications Should I Use?

When it comes to figuring out which medications to use, the ADA makes the following recommendations:[4]

For people with type 1 diabetes:

- Most people with type 1 diabetes should be treated with multiple daily injections of insulin before meals and basal (intermediate or long-acting) insulin or continuous subcutaneous insulin infusion

- Most people with type 1 diabetes should use rapid-acting insulin
- People with type 1 diabetes should learn to take into consideration one's carbohydrate intake, premeal blood sugar levels, and physical activity
- People with type 1 diabetes who have been successfully using continuous subcutaneous insulin infusion should have continued access to this therapy after they turn 65 years of age

People with type 2 diabetes:

- Metformin is the preferred initial medication that should be used for treatment of type 2 diabetes (as long as it is tolerated and not contraindicated (strong recommendation NOT to use)).
- Long-term use of metformin may be associated with biochemical vitamin B12 deficiency. Vitamin B12 levels should be considered in metformin-treated patients, especially in those with anemia or peripheral neuropathy.
- Conmetformin, canagliflozin may be considered to reduce major adverse cardiovascular events.
- Continuous reevaluation of the medication regimen and adjustment is recommended
- For patients with type 2 diabetes who are not achieving their blood sugar goals, drug intensification, including consideration of insulin therapy, should be promptly considered
- Metformin should be continued when used in combination with other medications, including insulin, if not contraindicated and if tolerated.

Treating Low Blood Sugar at Home

People taking insulin are especially prone to having bouts of very low blood sugar. **Make sure you talk to your doctor about having a plan for when your blood sugar is too high, too low, or you feel the symptoms of low blood sugar coming on.** Symptoms of low blood sugar may include shakiness, confusion, fast heart rate, irritability, and hunger. Severely low blood sugar may cause loss of consciousness, coma, or death.

About 15-20 grams of glucose is the preferred treatment for someone who is conscious with a blood sugar less than or equal to 70 mg/dL (3.9 mmol/L).[4] You may need to carry a monitor and a small bag of low-fat candies (like Skittles®) or glucose tablets (available at the drug store) with you for when you have blood sugar that is too low.

Carbohydrates That Can Be Used for Treating Low Blood Sugar

Quick carbohydrates that can be used for treating low blood sugar include (each contains 15-30 grams of carbohydrate):
- 12 gummy bears
- 6 large jelly beans
- 5 Life Savers®
- 15 Skittles®
- 4 Starburst®
- ½ cup of soda (not diet)
- 1 cup fat free milk
- ½ cup of orange juice
- ½ banana
- 1 small apple
- 3 to 4 glucose tablets
- 1 tube of glucose gel

It's important that the candy you carry for this purpose be <u>low fat.</u> Fat slows the absorption of sugar. When treating low blood sugar you need to treat it quickly. Therefore, you don't want any fat in the candy you choose to slow absorption. So candy bars, ice cream, and cookies are NOT a good option.

After you eat the candy to treat your low blood sugar and your blood sugar has returned to normal, a well-balanced snack (preferably containing protein, fat, and carbohydrates) is recommended. If you need help choosing some well-balanced snacks for this purpose, talk to your doctor, pharmacist or RD.

It is recommended that people with diabetes who are prone to bouts of low blood sugar **(less than 54 mg/dL (93 mmol/L))** carry a glucagon pen with them. A glucagon pen can be obtained at your retail pharmacy. Family, friends, and school personnel should be trained on how to use the pen. In the event that your blood sugar dips so low that you become unconscious, someone will be able to use the pen to give you a glucagon injection.

Glucagon is a hormone in the body that caused the liver to release glucose into the blood stream. This raises your blood sugar. It has the opposite action of insulin which lowers blood sugar.

What Types of Things Affect Blood Sugar Levels?

Besides, insulin, many things can affect your blood sugar levels. That's why testing is so important. Things that can affect your blood sugar levels include:

- Activity/ exercise
- Food intake
- Alcohol intake
- Illness

How to Avoid Low Blood Sugar

Check your blood sugar if you have any of these symptoms:

- Weakness
- Dizziness
- Headache
- Sweating
- Anxiety
- Shaking
- Increased heartbeat or heart palpitations

Special Occasions

Here are some circumstances where trying to avoid low blood sugar while dosing your insulin can be tricky.

Eating Out: Sometimes (like in a restaurant) you don't know how long it will take for your food to arrive. Consider not giving your rapid/regular/short-acting insulin dose until you **see** your food. This will avoid any potentially serious dips in blood sugar.

Exercise: Exercise naturally lowers your blood sugar so it's important to dose and time your insulin so your blood sugar doesn't go too low. Always check your blood sugar before you exercise and talk to your doctor about having a plan of what to do if your blood sugar is low, normal or high.

The following is an example 'plan'. **NOTE: this is only one example of how one's plan could look**. Talk to your doctor about tailoring an exercise plan that is right for you.

My Exercise Plan (example)*

Before exercise, check blood sugar (If exercising before a meal, do not take pre-meal insulin yet):

o **If it's critically low (less than 55 mg/dL),** eat at least 30-60 grams of carbohydrates (2-3 servings) to get your blood sugar up. Test again and eat another 15 to 40 grams (1-2 servings) if needed. Then once blood sugar is 100 mg/dL to 120 mg/dL, consider eating a snack that contains at least 30-60 grams of carbohydrates (2-3 servings), some protein and some fat. Consider exercising only after blood sugar is above 150 mg/mL. Don't take any insulin yet. Call an ambulance if feel faint, dizzy, have blurred vision, are confused, feel like fainting, or are extremely weak.

o **If it's 56 mg/dL to 99 mg/dL,** eat at 30-60 grams of carbohydrates (2-3 servings) to get your blood sugar up. Test again and eat another 15 to 40 grams (1-2 servings) if needed. Once blood sugar is between 100 mg/dL to 120 mg/dL, consider eating a snack that contains at least 30-60 grams of carbohydrates (2-3 servings), some protein and some fat. Don't take any insulin yet. Call an ambulance if feel faint, dizzy, have blurred vision, are confused, feel like fainting, or are extremely weak. Consider exercising only after blood sugar is above 150 mg/mL.

o **If it's 100 mg/dL to 120 mg/dL),** Consider eating a snack that contains at least 30-60 grams of carbohydrates (2-3 servings), some protein and some fat. Consider exercising only after blood sugar is above 150 mg/mL. Don't take any insulin yet. Call an ambulance if feel faint, dizzy, have blurred vision, are confused, feel like fainting, or are extremely weak.

o **If it's 150 mg/dL to 199 mg/dL,** can go ahead and exercise or consider having a snack of about 30-60 grams of carbohydrates (1-2 servings) about ½ hour before you exercise but don't take any insulin yet. Unless blood sugar is more than 250 mg/dL.

o **If it's 200 mg/dL to 250 mg/,** do not eat a snack. Do not take insulin yet. Proceed to exercising.

o **If it's very high (251 mg/dL or more),** follow your 'plan'. Talk to your doctor ahead of time about a plan for what to do when your blood sugar is very high. Decide together how much insulin you will take. Seek medical attention if you feel faint, dizzy, have blurred vision, are confused, feel like fainting, or are extremely weak.

Then after you are finished exercising, test your blood sugar again. or are extremely weak. Do not take any meal-time insulin.

*This plan is only a suggestion and may not work for everyone. Talk to your doctor about coming up with a plan that works for you.

In general, it takes about 1 unit of short/rapid insulin to lower blood sugar by 45 mg/dL, however this ratio may very from person to person. After you get a feel for how your blood sugar will react to exercise, you will be able to adjust your pre-exercise insulin dose going forward; but proceed cautiously. The amount of carbs you eat before exercise on how strenuous your workout will be. *When in doubt, error on the side of giving LESS insulin because the more insulin you give, the higher the chance you could overshoot your goal and end up with dangerously low blood sugar*. Blood sugar that is too low poses more of an immediate danger than blood sugar that is a little too high.

Bringing it All Together

Learning to manage your diabetes is crucial to your success. Unlike many other conditions where your doctor tells you to 'take one of these pills every day', diabetes often requires you to constantly reassess your own condition and adjust your treatment accordingly. This is especially true if you find yourself taking insulin. For this reason, it is important that you find a doctor who is willing to work closely with you and refer you to the proper educational resources.

REFERENCES

1. Alan J. Garber, MD, PhD, FACE1; Martin J. Abrahamson, MD2; Joshua I. Barzilay, MD, FACE3; Lawrence Blonde, MD, FACP, MACE4 et. al. Consensus statement by the American association of clinical endocrinologists and American college of endocrinology (AACE/ACE) on the comprehensive type 2 diabetes management algorithm-2018 executive summary, Endocrine Practice Vol 24 No. 1 January 2018.

2. Centers for Disease Control and Prevention. National diabetes statistics report, 2017. Centers for Disease Control and Prevention website. https://www.cdc.gov/features/diabetes-statistic-report/index.html. Updated July 18, 2017. Accessed April 30, 2018.

3. ADA website:
http://www.diabetes.org/living-with-diabetes/treatment-and-care/blood-glucose-control/checking-for-ketones.html

4. 2018 ADA guidelines. Standards of medical care in diabetes. Diabetes Care. January 1, 2018; volume 41 issue Supplement. Accessed at:
http://care.diabetesjournals.org/content/41/Supplement_1

5. Alzheimer's Association website available at: https://www.alz.org/alzheimers-dementia/what-is-dementia

6. Johns Hopkins University website available at: https://www.hopkinsmedicine.org/health/healthy_aging/healthy_body/hip-fractures-five-powerful-steps-to-prevention

7. Schifano F,

8. Bhansali A

9. Diabetes mellitus and risk of dementia: a meta-analysis of prospective observational studies. J Diabetes Investig 2013;**4**:640–650

10. Toobert DJ, Glasgow RE, Strycker LA, Barrera M, Jr, Radcliffe JL, Wander RC, et al. Biologic and quality-of-life outcomes from the Mediterranean lifestyle program: a randomized clinical trial. Diabetes Care (2003) 26:2288–93.10.2337/diacare.26.8.2288

11. Estruch R, Martínez-González MA, Corella D, Salas-Salvadó J, Ruiz-Gutiérrez V, Covas MI, et al. Effects of a Mediterranean style diet on cardiovascular risk factors: a randomized trial. Ann Intern Med (2006) 145:1–11.10.7326/0003-4819-145-1-200607040-00004

12. Shai I, Schwarzfuchs D, Henkin Y, Shahar DR, Witkow S, Greenberg I, et al. Weight-loss with a low carbohydrate Mediterranean, or low-fat diet. N Engl J Med (2008) 359:229–41.10.1056/NEJMoa0708681

13. Esposito K, Maiorino MI, Di Palo C, Giugliano D. Campanian postprandial hyperglycemia study group. Adherence to a Mediterranean diet and glycemic control in type 2 diabetes mellitus. Diabet Med (2009) 26:900–7.10.1111/j.1464-5491.2009.02798.x

14. Elhayany A, Lustman A, Abel A, Attal-Singer J, Vinker S. A low carbohydrate Mediterranean diet improves cardiovascular risk factors and diabetes control among overweight patients with type 2 diabetes mellitus. A one-year prospective randomized intervention study. Diabetes Obes Metab (2010) 12(3):204–9.10.1111/j.1463-1326.2009.01151.x

15. Itsiopoulos C, Brazionis L, Kaimakamis M, Cameron M, Best JD, O'Dea K, et al. Can the Mediterranean diet lower HbA1c in type 2 diabetes? Results from a randomized cross-over study. Nutr Metab Cardiovasc Dis (2011) 21(9):740–7.10.1016/j.numecd.2010.03.005

16. Fexofenadine hydrochloride: Adverse effects. (2015). In Micromedex (Columbia Basin College Library ed.) [Electronic

17. version].Greenwood Village, CO: Truven Health Analytics. Retrieved October 18, 2015, from

http://www.micromedexsolutions.com

18. American Diabetes Association DiabetesPRo. Accessed online at: https://professional.diabetes.org/diapro/glucose_calc.

19. Dietary Guidelines Advisory Committee. Dietary Guidelines for Americans 2015-2020. Washington, DC: US Department of Agriculture; 2015.

CHAPTER 5

OSTEOPOROSIS

The Empowered Medicine Guide to Osteoporosis

How to Use This Chapter

Welcome to the Empowered Medicine Guide to osteoporosis. This chapter is arranged in a step-by-step fashion. First, we will go over the basics of osteoporosis such as what it is and why treating it is important. Then we will follow a step-by-step process for figuring out what your treatment goals should be. Feel free to write your own information in the blanks provided to aid in your calculations. Finally, we will look what medications may work best for you.

If you wish, use Appendix VI in the back to log your own information for easy calculations and sharing with your doctor. Finally, at the end of this chapter you will find a section called 'The Bottom Line'. This box sums up the main points of the chapter.

The Basics

There are about 10 million (yes, million) men and women in the U.S. at this very moment who have osteoporosis.[2] To give you another idea of how common it is, osteoporosis-related fractures affect approximately one in two white women and one

in five white men in their lifetime.[9] Osteoporosis is a condition where bone density deteriorates. The work 'osteoporosis' actually means 'spongy bones'. When your bones are not as dense, you are at more risk for bone fractures. Hip and spine fractures, especially in the elderly, can be debilitating and can significantly decrease the length and quality of one's life. In order to decrease the risk of fractures, we need to increase the strength of the bones.

Screening for Osteoporosis

The U.S. Preventive Services Task Force (USPSTF) recommends screening for osteoporosis with bone measurement testing to prevent osteoporotic fractures in women 65 years and older.[7, 9]

For postmenopausal women younger than 65 years who have at least 1 risk factor, a reasonable approach to determine who should be screened with bone measurement testing is to use a clinical risk assessment tool. Several tools are available to assess osteoporosis risk, such as OST, ORAI, OSIRIS, SCORE, and FRAX (see below for more information on these tools).

STEP 1: Check all of the risk factors that apply:

Table 1: **Risk Factors for Osteoporosis Fractures**[9]

☐	**Parental history of hip fracture**
☐	**Smoking**
☐	**Excess alcohol consumption (> 4 drinks per day for men or > 2 drinks per day for women**
☐	**Caffeine intake (> 2.5 cups of coffee per day)**
☐	**Low body weight**
☐	**Woman who is post-menopausal**
☐	**Gonadal hormone deficiency** (gonad hormones help with breast development in women, testicular development in men, and pubic hair growth)
☐	**Inadequate activity**
☐	**Increased age**
☐	**Low body weight (< 58 kg (128 lb)**
☐	**Low calcium or vitamin D intake**
☐	**History of fracture**
☐	**White or Asian race**

STEP 2: Next you'll figure out if you need to complete a risk assessment or talk to your doctor about a bone scan. Check the box that applies to you:

☐	I am a woman age 65 or older	Ask your doctor to schedule a bone scan to see if you have osteopenia or osteoporosis
☐	I am a woman younger than 65 and have at least 1 risk factor listed in Table 1	Complete one of the screening tools listed in Table 2. Write your OST score in the box provided
☐	I am a woman younger than 65 and do **NOT** have any of the risk factors listed above	Congratulations! You do not need to have a bone scan at this time
☐	I am a man **over** the age of 70	Consider using the screening tool for men in Table 2
☐	I am a man **under** the age of 70	Congratulations! You do not need to have a bone scan at this time unless your doctor thinks it would be helpful

Screening Tools for Osteoporosis

There are several tools available that you can use to see if you are at risk for osteoporosis. These tools include:
- OST - Osteoporosis self-assessment tool
- ORAI - osteoporosis risk assessment instrument
- OSIRIS - osteoporosis index of risk
- SCORE - simple calculated osteoporosis risk estimation
- FRAX - fracture risk assessment tool

Any of these tools may be used to see if you are at risk for osteoporosis. However, FRAX, ORAI, SCORE and OSIRIS are a little more complex. The USPSTF recommends dual-energy X-ray absorptiometry (DXA) scans for younger women who have an increased fracture risk as determined by the World Health Organization's FRAX Fracture Risk Assessment Tool. The problem is this tool needs to be downloaded to a desktop and is not readily available online. Studies have shown that the more complex tools may not be any better at predicting osteoporosis fractures than the simpler tools.[8] Therefore, for the sake of simplicity in this chapter, we will use the OST for women and OST for men.

STEP 3: If in Step 2 it was recommended that you complete a risk assessment, use one of the assessments below to see if you are at high risk for osteoporosis.

Table 2: **Calculators Used to See if One is at Risk for Osteoporosis**

Tool	Where to Find It
OST for women	https://reference.medscape.com/calculator/osteoporosis-self-assessment-women
OST for men (optional)	https://reference.medscape.com/calculator/osteoporosis-self-assessment-men

My OST score is:	☐	**Low (No DXA scan needed at this time)**	☐	**Medium (No DXA scan needed at this time)**	☐	**High (talk to your doctor about getting a DXA scan)**

Most guidelines mention that screening is not necessary for men under the age of 70, but think it may be beneficial to screen men over the age of 70.[9]

So, now you should have a pretty good idea whether you should have a DXA bone scan. Let's take a closer look at the DXA bone scan and what the results mean.

Diagnosis of Osteopenia and Osteoporosis

Unfortunately, there is no way to visualize the inside of the bone without actually taking a piece of it via a biopsy. Likewise, there is no good way to measure bone strength. Since a biopsy of the bone is a very impractical way to diagnose osteoporosis, physicians rely on bone scans to determine bone density and diagnose osteoporosis. By measuring bone mineral density (BMD) via a DXA bone scan, we can measure bone mass, which may account for approximately 70% of bone strength.[3]

Peak BMD is reached in the first twenty to thirty years of life.[4] BMD is usually measured at the hip and spine with the DXA scan. A BMD reading provides two different scores. The first score, called the 'T score', shows us how our bone mass compares to that of a young, healthy adult of the same sex. The second score, the 'Z score', shows us how our bone mass compares to a healthy individual of the same sex and age.[5] These readings are used to diagnosis and categorize osteoporosis in individuals.

When it comes to T scores, the more negative the number, the closer one is to a diagnosis of osteoporosis. A normal T score reading is considered anything above or equal to –1. Anything less than –1 but greater than –2.5 is considered osteopenia. Osteopenia indicates a decrease in bone mass that is not yet severe enough to be classified as osteoporosis. However, there is still a high risk of fracture with osteopenia,. In fact, data suggests the majority of bone fractures occur in those with osteopenia rather than in those with osteoporosis.[5] Osteopenia is considered to be a precursor to osteoporosis. A T score less than or equal to –2.5 indicates osteoporosis. With Z scores, a reading of greater than –2 means the individual is within the expected range for that age. A Z score of –2 or less is defined as "below the expected range for age" and does not necessarily warrant a diagnosis of osteoporosis.

Table 3: **Diagnosis of Osteopenia and Osteoporosis based on T Scores from BMD[9]**

Category	T Score from DXA Scan
Normal	T score greater than or equal to -1.0
Osteopenia	T score between -1.0 and -2.5
Osteoporosis	T score less than or equal to -2.5
Severe osteoporosis	T score less than or equal to -2.5 with one or more fractures

The criteria in Table 3 should not be applied to men younger than 50 years old, children or premenopausal women. These groups of people should use the Z score. NOTE: the presence of osteoporosis in mean younger than 50 cannot be diagnosed based on BMD alone. These men should talk to their doctor.

Table 4: **Diagnosis of Low Bone Density Based on Z Scores from BMD[9]**

Category	Z Score from DXA Scan
Normal	Z score greater than or equal to -2.0
Suggestive of low bone density	Z score less than -2.0

Guidelines are not really clear on re-testing women who have normal bone mineral density on initial screening, intervals of at least 4 years appear safe according to the USPSTF.

STEP 4: After you get your DXA scan at the doctor's office, check the box below that applies to you based on your T or Z score. Do you have osteoporosis?

Check one:	Category	T Score from DXA Scan
Women 65 or older, a woman younger than 65 and have at least 1 risk factor listed in Table 1, or man older than 70		
☐	Normal	T score greater than or equal to -1.0
☐	Osteopenia	T score between -1.0 and -2.5
☐	Osteoporosis	T score less than or equal to -2.5
☐	Severe osteoporosis	T score less than or equal to -2.5 with one or more fractures
OR: men younger than 50 years old, children or premenopausal women		
	Category	**Z Score from DXA Scan**
☐	Normal	Z score greater than or equal to -2.0
☐	Suggestive of low bone density	Z score less than -2.0
Do I have osteoporosis, severe osteoporosis or low bone density?		☐ Yes ☐ No

If you answered "Yes" to the question above, read on to see what you can do to treat osteoporosis and other measures you can take to keep it from getting worse. If it was determined that you have 'low bone density' due to your Z score, talk to your doctor to see if he/she thinks you would benefit from osteoporosis therapy.

Other Tests to Find a Cause

It's recommended that patients who are newly-diagnosed with osteoporosis have other tests done to see if the cause for osteoporosis can be found. These tests may include[9]:

- serum 25-hydroxyvitamin D
- calcium
- creatinine
- thyroid-stimulating hormone

STEP 5: Check the box below once you have talked with your doctor about screening to see if a secondary cause of osteoporosis can be found

☐	**Yes, I have spoken with my doctor about screening for secondary causes of osteoporosis.**

In additions to the risk factors listed in Table 1, there are medications that you may be taking that can contribute to the development of osteoporosis.

Table 5: **Medications That Can Contribute to Osteoporosis**

- Heparin
- Anticonvulsants
- Cyclosporine A
- Tacrolimus
- Barbituates
- Lithium
- Depo-medroxyprogesterone
- Chemotherapy
- Intravenous nutrition
- Glucocorticoids

STEP 6: Check the box below if you are on any of the medications listed in Table 5.

☐	**Yes, I am currently taking medications that may be contributing to osteoporosis. These medications include:** _____ _____ _____

NOTE: Do **NOT** stop taking any the medications listed in Table 5 without talking to your doctor first. Some medications need to be tapered off of slowly. It is also positive that the benefit of using that medications outweighs the risk of osteoporosis.

Non-medication Therapy to Decrease the Risk of Fractures

Prevention is key with osteoporosis. Once you have osteoporosis, it is difficult to get rid of it. Although there are medications available, they are not necessarily a cure. The main class of medications used to treat osteoporosis, called 'bisphosphonates', help lay down a matrix within the bone to help strengthen it. Medications such as these have been shown to decrease the risk of fracture; however, they cannot get rid of the risk completely, and therefore prevention is key. By modifying the risk factors talked about earlier in this chapter, you can decrease your chances of osteoporosis. Stopping smoking, increasing physical activity, and taking actions to prevent falls are just a few examples of things that can be done.

Remember, all of the medications mentioned below are meant to be used in conjunction with other measures, like fall prevention, smoking cessation, decreased caffeine intake, exercise, vitamin D intake, and moderation of alcohol.

Table 6: **Non-medication Therapy to Decrease the Risk of Fractures**[9]

• Alcohol and caffeine in moderation
• Less than or equal to 4 alcoholic drinks per day for men or 2 drinks per day for women
• Less than or equal to 2.5 cups of coffee or 5 cups of tea per day
• Smoking cessation
• Consider exercise and strength training
• Calcium and Vitamin D supplementation (consider more exposure to sunlight)
• Fall prevention measures

Avoidance of Smoking, Excessive Alcohol, and Excessive Caffeine

The National Osteoporosis Foundation (NOF) recognizes smoking and excessive alcohol intake as possible contributors to the development of osteoporosis. For this reason, the NOF strongly recommends that patients avoid tobacco products and excessive alcohol intake. Alcohol in excess of 3 drinks per day for men or 2 drinks per day for women, puts one at a higher risk of falls and may be harmful to bone health.[9]

The NOF also recommend one limit their caffeine intake to Less than or equal to 2.5 cups of coffee or 5 cups of tea per day. These recommendations are not only important for maintaining strong bones, but also for overall health.

Exercise

There are many things you can do to prevent osteoporosis and the risk of fractures. First, we need to get adequate exercise. Proper exercise can be beneficial when it comes to getting and keeping bone and muscle mass.

Muscle-strengthening and weight-bearing exercises are recognized by the NOF as being helpful in preventing falls and fractures.[9] Muscle-strengthening exercises, like weight training, are those that make the muscles stronger. Weight-bearing exercises are those that work against gravity while the feet and legs bear the weight of the body. Examples of weight-bearing exercises include walking, jogging, and tai chi.

Regularly performed, these types of exercise can help keep one agile and strong. This can help decrease the risk of falls. In addition, these types of exercises can help increase and maintain bone mass. When the bones are slightly stressed, as they are when performing these types of exercises, they are forced to build themselves up. The body does this in anticipation of further bone stress. It's recommended that people plan to make such exercise a life-long endeavor. The benefits of these exercises are quickly lost after exercise is stopped for a period of time. Before starting a new exercise program, make sure to talk to your doctor to make sure it won't aggravate any existing conditions you may have.

Calcium and Vitamin D

When it comes to preventing osteoporosis, it is imperative that we get enough calcium and vitamin D. Calcium is not only needed by the body to create bone, but it is also needed for muscle contraction and nerve function. The body stores 99% of its calcium in bones.[16] When we do not take in adequate amounts of calcium, our body pulls it from our bones.

Vitamin D is needed to absorb the calcium we take into our bodies. Taking adequate calcium and vitamin D have been shown to slow bone loss over time.[15] Getting calcium from your diet is preferable because this type of calcium is more easily absorbed than the calcium found in pills. However, many people find it difficult to get the recommended daily intake of calcium from diet alone. For this reason, for many people, a calcium supplement is recommended.

Several dietary sources of calcium are listed below. Although vitamin D can be obtained from diet, sunlight is another way to obtain vitamin D. Going out into the sun actually triggers our body to make its own vitamin D.

Table 7: **Good Natural Sources of Calcium**[16]

- Dairy products
- Beans
- Dark green, leafy vegetables (i.e., spinach, kale)
- Fortified orange juice
- Almonds
- Tofu
- Soy

Table 8: **Good Sources of Vitamin D**

- Fortified milk
- Egg yolks
- Salt water fish
- Liver
- Sunlight (30 minutes, 5 days per week)[9]

How Much Calcium and Vitamin D Do I Need?

So how much calcium do we need each day? It is important to note that our calcium requirements depend on factors such as age and lactation status. It is important to note that increasing calcium intake beyond these recommendations may put you at risk for kidney stones or cardiovascular disease.[17]

Table 9: **Recommended Daily Allowances for Dietary Calcium**[16]

Age	Male	Female
0-6 months	200 mg	200 mg
7-12 months	260 mg	260 mg
1-3 years	700 mg	700 mg
4-8 years	1000 mg	1000 mg
9-13 years	1300 mg	1300 mg
14-18 years	1300 mg	1300 mg
19-50 years	1000 mg	1000 mg
51-70 years	1000 mg	1200 mg
71+ years	1200 mg	1200 mg

Notice that the table tells us how much *elemental* calcium is needed. It is important to read labels carefully and realize that many times the milligrams indicated on the front of the bottle note the milligrams of *whole* calcium complex in the product. It is important to look instead at the 'Drug Facts' label on the back of the bottle to get the real story. Here you will find the amount of *elemental calcium* in the product.

For example, a bottle of calcium carbonate may say 'calcium carbonate 1500mg' on the front. However, if you look on the 'Drug Facts' label on the back, it will tell you that even though the formula contains 1500mg of calcium carbonate, it only contains 600mg of *elemental* calcium per serving. In other words, elemental calcium refers to the amount of actual calcium in the formula (i.e., calcium carbonate, minus the carbonate).

When taking a calcium supplement, it is also important to decide which kind to take. There are two main choices on the market: calcium carbonate and calcium citrate. Calcium carbonate should be taken with food as it needs the stomach acid produced when we eat to be absorbed. Calcium carbonate is usually not a good choice in the elderly. This is because we produce much less stomach acid as we age. Calcium carbonate is also not a good choice if you are taking certain medications that decrease your stomach acid like Zantac®, Pepcid® or Prevacid®. If this applies to you, you may consider calcium citrate. Calcium citrate can be taken on an empty stomach.

It is usually best to get a supplement that includes vitamin D as well. It is recommended that most adults over fifty years old get 1000 to 1200 IU of vitamin D per day.[16] It is necessary to break up your calcium supplementation throughout the day. This is because our bodies can only absorb about 500–600 mg at one time. For example, let's say your daily elemental calcium requirement is 1200 mg of elemental calcium. Your calcium carbonate supplement contains 600 mg of elemental calcium per tablet. You could take one tablet with breakfast and one tablet with lunch or dinner.

Fall Prevention

According to the NOF, each year about one-third of all people over age 65 will fall.[13] They have a really nice page on their website that goes over things you can do every day to prevent falls located at: https://www.nof.org/patients/fracturesfall-prevention.

Here is an abbreviated list of things you can do when you go out, or even around the house, to help reduce the risk of falls. Please see the NOF's website for a comprehensive list.

Table 10: **Safety Tips to Prevent Falls**

- Use a cane, walker, or other assistive device
- If using a cane in an icy region, consider using ice tips at the end to get better grip
- When using a cane or walker, consider suing rubber tips at the tips to get better grip
- Consider using a long-handled gripping device to reach things on the ground
- Avoid walking on slippery surfaces
- Use hand rails when available
- Install handles and rails in the bathroom around the toilet and bath tub
- Consider a plastic shower chair in the shower
- Keep floors inside and outside free of clutter and in good repair
- Be careful when stepping on or off of curbs
- Keep surroundings well-lit. You may consider carrying a small flashlight for times when you might find yourself in dimly-lit areas while away from home
- Wear comfortable, low-heeled footwear
- Consider carrying a bag or using a fannypack/backpack to keep your hands free
- Find out which grocery stores and pharmacies in your community deliver to your home
- Consider getting a personal emergency response system to wear in case you fall when you are alone
- For those that are prone to falls, wearing undergarments with hip pad protectors may also help prevent hip fractures.

There are many types of assistive devices including:

- Cane
- Offset cane (a cane with a crook in the neck)
- Quadripod cane (a cane with 4 feet at the bottom)
- Forearm (Lofstrand) crutches
- Standard walker
- Front-wheeled walker
- Four-wheeled walker (also called a rollator)

You'll need to talk to your doctor about which assistive device may be right for you. Your doctor can write you a prescription for these items so they can be covered by Medicare and/or possibly your private insurance. However, to be covered, they need to be covered by a Medicare-certified durable medical equipment provider.

It's extremely important to make sure that you are using a cane or walker that's the right size for you. Using one that's not the right size can cause serious injuries. To find a **cane** that's the right size for you, stand up straight and measure from the crease of your wrist to the floor. This should be level with the top of the cane.

To measure for a **walker or rollator**, stand up straight with your arms relaxed at your sides. Now gently bend your elbows at a 15-30 degree angle as if you were gripping the handles of a walker or rollator. This is where you will want the handles of the walker or rollator to be.[14]

Medication for the Treatment of Osteoporosis

Remember in STEP 4 earlier in this chapter, we discussed how the NOF recommends starting medication treatment only in the following groups:

Table 11: **People Who Should Consider Medication Treatment for Osteoporosis[9]**

Women 65 or older, women younger than 65 and have at least 1 risk factor listed in Table 1, or men older than 70 with:
T score less than or equal to -2.5
OR: men younger than 50 years old, children, or premenopausal women with:
Z score less than -2.0

The World Health Organization (WHO) only recommends that people with or at risk of osteoporosis should be considered for treatment.[15]

Trials that have examined the treatment of osteoporosis have shown that only two groups of people appear to experience a reduction in fractures while being treated[12]:

1. People with a T-score of less than -2.5

2. People who have already had a fracture of the hip or vertebrae

There are many medications available to treat osteoporosis. However, a class of mediations called 'bisphosphonates' appear to be the work horses of these. Let's look at bisphosphonates and the other medications available.

Bisphosphonates

Examples of these medications include alendronate (Fosamax®), ibandronate (Boniva®), risedronate (Actonel®), zoledronic acid (Reclast®, Zometa®). Bisphosphonates are given by mouth except for zoledronic acid which is given by injection.

Although bisphosphonates are generally considered to be the treatment of choice for osteoporosis, there are currently no head to head studies that show one bisphosphonate is better than another. Many studies may quote data such as, 'drug x has been shown to decrease fractures by 50%'. Meanwhile another drug study may show that 'drug y decreases fractures by 40%'. It is important to note that due to differences in study methods, these two results should not be directly compared. In other words, it cannot be concluded that drug x is better than drug y. Until there are head to head studies that compare bisphosphonates, we will have to assume that all are equally effective. If you and your doctor chose to go with a bisphosphonate factors like dosing, cost and general preference will probably determine which one you use.

Take your bisphosphonate first thing in the morning, at least 30 minutes before you eat or drink anything or take any other medicine. If you take it only once per week, take it on the same day each week and always first thing in the morning.

Take it with a full glass (6 to 8 ounces) of plain water. Do **not** use coffee, tea, soda, juice, or mineral water. Do **not** eat or drink anything other than plain water.

Do not take your bisphosphonate if you cannot sit upright or stand for at least 30 minutes after taking the medicine. You should not take a bisphosphonate if you have problems with your esophagus, or low levels of calcium in your blood.

Common side effects may include:

- heartburn, indigestion
- stomach pain
- diarrhea
- back pain
- joint pain
- muscle pain
- flu-like symptoms

Bisphosphonates can cause serious problems in the stomach or esophagus. Stop using your bisphosphonate and call your doctor at once if you have chest pain, new or worsening heartburn, or pain when swallowing.

Also call your doctor if you have muscle spasms, numbness or tingling (in hands and feet or around the mouth), new or unusual hip pain, or severe pain in your joints, bones, or muscles.

In rare cases, this medicine may cause bone loss (osteonecrosis) in the jaw. Symptoms include jaw pain or numbness, red or swollen gums, loose teeth, or slow healing after dental work. The longer you use your bisphosphonate, the more likely you are to develop this condition.

Osteonecrosis of the jaw may be more likely if you have cancer or received chemotherapy, radiation, or steroids. Other risk factors include blood clotting disorders, anemia (low red blood cells), and a pre-existing dental problem.

You should not take a bisphosphonate if you are allergic to it, or if you have:

- low levels of calcium in your blood (hypocalcemia); or
- problems with the muscles in your esophagus (the tube that connects your mouth and stomach).

Stop using your bisphosphonate and call your doctor at once if you have:

- chest pain, new or worsening heartburn
- difficulty or pain when swallowing
- pain or burning under the ribs or in the back
- severe heartburn, burning pain in your upper stomach, or coughing up blood
- new or unusual pain in your thigh or hip
- jaw pain, numbness, or swelling
- severe joint, bone, or muscle pain
- low calcium levels, muscle spasms or contractions, numbness or tingly feeling (around your mouth, or in your fingers and toes)

For zoledronic acid: drink at least 2 glasses of water within a few hours before your injection to keep from getting dehydrated. Zoledronic acid can cause serious kidney problems, especially if you are dehydrated, if you take diuretic medicine, or if you already have kidney disease. Call your doctor if you urinate less than usual, if you have swelling in your feet or ankles, or if you feel tired or short of breath.

Pay special attention to your dental hygiene while using zoledronic acid. Brush and floss your teeth regularly. If you need to have any dental work (especially surgery), tell the dentist ahead of time that you are using zoledronic acid.

Common side effects of zoledronic acid specifically may include:

- nausea, vomiting, diarrhea, constipation
- bone pain, muscle or joint pain
- fever or other flu symptoms
- pain in your arms or legs
- red or puffy eyes
- headache, tiredness
- trouble breathing
- muscle spasms, numbness or tingling (in hands and feet or around the mouth)
- new or unusual thigh or hip pain
- severe pain in your joints, bones, or muscles

Call your doctor at once if you have:

- new or unusual pain in your thigh or hip
- jaw pain, numbness, or swelling
- kidney problems--little or no urination, swelling in your feet or ankles, feeling tired or short of breath
- severe joint, bone, or muscle pain
- low calcium levels--muscle spasms or contractions, numbness or tingly feeling (around your mouth, or in your fingers and toes)
- As with any medication, get emergency medical help if you have signs of an allergic reaction like rash, hives, trouble breathing, swelling of your face, lips, tongue, or throat.

Serious side effects on the kidneys may be more likely in older adults. In rare cases, this medicine may cause bone loss (osteonecrosis) in the jaw. Symptoms include jaw pain or numbness, red or swollen gums, loose teeth, or slow healing after dental work. The longer you use zoledronic acid, the more likely you are to develop this condition.

To make sure a bisphosphonate is safe for you, tell your doctor if you have ever had:

- kidney disease
- hypocalcemia
- thyroid or parathyroid surgery
- surgery to remove part of your intestine
- asthma caused by taking aspirin
- any condition that makes it hard for your body to absorb nutrients from food (malabsorption); or
- a dental problem (you may need a dental exam before you receive zoledronic acid)

It's recommended that doctors consider discontinuing bisphosphonate therapy after five years in women without a history of vertebral fractures.[9]

Selective Estrogen Receptor Modulators (SERMs)

Selective estrogen receptor modulators (SERMs) combat osteoporosis by acting like estrogen in the body. This increases bone density. There are several SERMS, however, raloxifene (Evista®) is the SERM that's used for the treatment osteoporosis.

Common side effects may include:

- flu symptoms
- increased sweating
- hot flashes
- leg cramps
- swelling in your hands, feet, or ankles
- joint pain

Taking a SERM can increase your risk of blood clots. These clots most commonly happen in one's leg, lung, or eye. If the clot happens in your brain, it can cause a stroke. This can be fatal. If you already have a history of blood clots, you should not take this medication. Your risk for developing a blood clot while taking a SERM goes up if you have coronary heart disease, diabetes, smoking, high blood pressure, high cholesterol, menopause, or hysterectomy.[18]

Before you take a SERM, tell your doctor if you have:

- coronary artery disease or heart disease
- high blood pressure
- history of stroke
- liver or kidney disease
- high cholesterol (especially high triglycerides)
- if you have not gone through menopause
- if you have had breast cancer
- if you take a blood thinner
- if you take estrogen hormone replacement therapy

If you need to have any type of surgery or will be on bed rest, you will need to stop taking your SERM for at least 72 hours before your surgery or before you plan to be immobile. This is because while you are recovering, there is a lack of blood flow that occurs while you are immobile. This lack of blood flow puts you at a higher risk for blood clots especially if you are taking a SERM.

Stop using your SERM and call your doctor at once if you have:

- lumps or other changes in the breast;
- signs of a stroke (these may include weakness, severe headache, slurred speech, vision problems)
- signs of a blood clot in the lung (these may include chest pain, shortness of breath, cough, rapid breathing, rapid heart rate)
- signs of a blood clot in your leg (these may include pain, swelling, warmth, tightness or redness in one or both legs

- As with any medication, get emergency medical help if you have signs of an allergic reaction like rash, hives, trouble breathing, swelling of your face, lips, tongue, or throat.

Teriparatide (Forteo®)

Teriparatide (Forteo®) is a man-made form of parathyroid hormone; a hormone that exists naturally in the body. Teriparatide is considered an anabolic ('bone growing') drug. It increases bone mineral density and bone strength, which may prevent fractures.

Teriparatide is given as an injection once a day. Teriparatide should be clear. If the medicine is a different color, is cloudy, or has particles in it, do not use it. Call your pharmacist to see if you can get new medication.

Rotate injection sites. In other words, do not inject into the same place two times in a row.

Your teriparatide injection pen should be stored in the refrigerator when not in use. After you use it, make sure to remove the needle, recap the pen, and put it back into the refrigerator. However, take care not to freeze teriparatide. Throw away the medicine if it becomes frozen.

Potential side effects may include:
- nausea
- joint pain
- pain anywhere in your body
- dizziness

Teriparatide can cause you to feel dizzy or like you might faint. Make sure you have a place to sit or lie down for a while after giving your injection.

Teriparatide has caused bone cancer in animals but it is not known whether it can cause it in people using this medicine. While using teriparatide, you will likely be asked to provide your name to a patient registry. This is to collect information so any possible risk of bone cancer associated with this medication can be assessed.

While taking teriparatide, call your doctor if you:

• feel like you might pass out (especially within 4 hours after injection)

• experience pounding heartbeats or heart palpitations after using an injection

• have high levels of calcium in your blood (possible symptoms of low calcium in the blood include nausea, vomiting, constipation, muscle weakness, and feeling very tired)

• As with any medication, get emergency medical help if you have signs of an allergic reaction like rash, hives, trouble breathing, swelling of your face, lips, tongue, or throat.

Teriparatide is not for use in children or young adults. This is because their bones are still growing and they might be negatively impacted by the medication.

Before you start teriparatide, tell your doctor if you have ever had:

• Paget's disease or another bone disease other than osteoporosis

• high levels of calcium in the blood

• overactive parathyroid glands

• history of bone cancer or radiation treatment involving your bones

• kidney stones

Each prefilled injection pen contains 28 separate teriparatide injections. After the 28th injection, throw the pen away, even if there is still medicine left inside.

Use only the injection pen provided with teriparatide. Do not transfer the medicine to a syringe. Use a new disposable needle for each dose. Follow your state or local laws about throwing away used needles. Always use a puncture-proof disposal container, preferably a "sharps" container (ask your pharmacist where to get one and how to throw it away). Keep this container out of the reach of children and pets.

Talk to your doctor about how long you should take this medicine. Teriparatide is often given for only 2 years.

Denosumab (Prolia®)

Denosumab is a monoclonal antibody. This means it is made to target and destroy certain cells in the body. Denosumab's job is to seek and destroy the proteins that break down bone.

Denosumab is injected every 6 months. It is injected under the skin. Typical places to inject include the stomach, upper thigh, or upper arm. You receive this injection at your doctor's office.

Store denosumab in the original container in the refrigerator. Protect from light and take care not to freeze. After you have taken it out of the refrigerator, you may keep it at room temperature for up to 14 days.

You may take the medicine out of the refrigerator and allow it to reach room temperature before the injection is given, but do NOT heat the medicine before using.

Do NOT shake the prefilled syringe or you may ruin the medicine. Do not use the medicine if it looks cloudy or has particles in it. Call your pharmacist for a new prescription.

Each prefilled syringe of this medicine is for one dose only. Throw away after one use, even if there is still some medicine left in it after injecting your dose.

Follow any state or local laws about throwing away used needles and syringes. Use a puncture-proof "sharps" disposal container (ask your pharmacist where to get one and how to throw it away). Keep this container out of the reach of children and pets.

Do not share this medicine with another person, even if they have the same symptoms you have.

Potential side effects may include:

- Bladder infection
- Back pain
- Pain in your arms or legs
- Bone loss in the jaw. Call your doctor if you have signs of this like:

- Jaw pain or numbness
- Red or swollen gums
- Loose teeth
- Gum infection
- Slow healing after dental work
- Serious infections. Call your doctor if you have signs of infection like:
  o Fever
  o Chills
  o Night sweats
  o Swelling, pain, tenderness, warmth, or redness anywhere on your body
  o Pain or burning when you urinate
  o Increased or urgent need to urinate
  Ssevere stomach pain
  o Cough, feeling short of breath

When taking denosumab, call your doctor if you have:
- New pain in your thigh, hip, jaw, or groin
- New bone, joint, or muscle pain
- Skin problems (including excessive dryness, redness, itching, blisters, drainage
- Low calcium levels--muscle spasms or contractions, numbness or tingly feeling (around your mouth, or in your fingers and toes)

As with any medication, get emergency medical help if you have signs of an allergic reaction like rash, hives, trouble breathing, swelling of your face, lips, tongue, or throat.

If you already have low levels of calcium in your blood, you should not use denosumab.

Before starting denosumab, tell your doctor if you have:
- Kidney disease
- A weak immune system

- A history of parathyroid disease or thyroid surgery
- Problems absorbing nutrients from food
- If you are allergic to latex
- If you need to have dental work done (especially surgery)

Make sure to take good care of your teeth while taking denosumab. You should brush and floss every day. It may be a good idea to have a dental exam before starting denosumab if you are concerned you might need some work done.

Let's review the medications that can be used for the treatment of osteoporosis.

Table 12: **Medications for the Prevention and Treatment of Osteoporosis**

Class of Medications	Examples of Medications in this Class	Approved for Prevention or Treatment	Fracture Type	How to Take it
Bisphosphonates	Alendronate (Fosamax®)	Prevention Treatment	Hip, vertebral*, nonvertebral**	Oral once daily or weekly
	Alendronate with cholecalciferol (Fosamax plus D®)	Treatment	Hip, vertebral, nonvertebral	Oral once daily or weekly
	Ibandronate (Boniva®)	Prevention Treatment	Vertebral only	Oral once a month
	Risedronate (Actonel®, Atelvia®)	Prevention Treatment	Hip, vertebral, nonvertebral	Different options: Once per day, once per week, once per month,

Class of Medications	Examples of Medications in this Class	Approved for Prevention or Treatment	Fracture Type	How to Take it
				or for 2 days in a row once per month
	Risedronate with calcium (Actonel with calcium®)	Prevention Treatment	Hip, vertebral, nonvertebral	Different options: Once per day, once per week, once per month, or for 2 days in a row once per month
	Zoledronic acid (Reclast®, Zometa®)	Prevention Treatment	Hip, vertebral, nonvertebral	Injection once every 1-2 years
Selective estrogen receptor modulators (SERMs)	Raloxifene (Evista®)	Prevention Treatment	Vertebral only	Oral daily
Anabolic Drug	Teriparatide (Forteo®)	Treatment	Vertebral, nonvertebral	Injection once daily
	Denosumab (Prolia®)	Treatment	Hip, vertebral, nonvertebral	Injection every 6 months

*Vertebral: means involving the vertebrae (bones that make up the spine)
**Nonvertebral: means NOT involving the vertebrae (bones that make up the spine)

First line treatment for osteoporosis is to start bisphosphonate therapy. However, people who can't take bisphosphonates or don't

respond to them might consider other medications like raloxifene, teriparatide, and denosumab.

Remember, all of these medications are meant to be used in conjunction with other measures like fall prevention, smoking cessation, decreased caffeine intake, exercise, vitamin D intake, and moderation of alcohol.

The Bottom Line

Osteoporosis is a condition where bone density deteriorates. The work 'osteoporosis' actually means 'spongy bones'. When your bones are not as dense, you are at more risk for bone fractures. Hip and spine fractures, especially in the elderly, can be debilitating and can significantly decrease the length and quality of one's life. In order to decrease the risk of fractures, we need to increase the strength of the bones.

The U.S. Preventive Services Task Force (USPSTF) recommends screening for osteoporosis with bone measurement testing to prevent osteoporotic fractures in women 65 years and older.[7, 9]

For postmenopausal women younger than 65 years who have at least 1 risk factor, a reasonable approach to determine who should be screened with bone measurement testing is to use a clinical risk assessment tool. Several tools are available to assess osteoporosis risk, such as OST, ORAI, OSIRIS, SCORE, and FRAX

STEP 1: Check all of the risk factors that apply:

Risk Factors for Osteoporosis Fractures[9]

- ☐ **Parental history of hip fracture**
- ☐ **Smoking**
- ☐ **Excess alcohol consumption (> 4 drinks per day for men or > 2 drinks per day for women**
- ☐ **Caffeine intake (> 2.5 cups of coffee per day)**
- ☐ **Low body weight**
- ☐ **Woman who is post-menopausal**
- ☐ **Gonadal hormone deficiency**
  (gonad hormones help with breast development in women, testicular development in men, and pubic hair growth)

☐	**Inadequate activity**
☐	**Increased age**
☐	**Low body weight (< 58 kg (128 lb))**
☐	**Low calcium or vitamin D intake**
☐	**History of fracture**
☐	**White or Asian race**

STEP 2: Next you'll figure out if you may need to talk to your doctor about a bone scan or maybe need to complete a risk assessment. Check the box that applies to you:

☐	I am a woman age 65 or older	Ask your doctor to schedule a bone scan to see if you have osteopenia or osteoporosis
☐	I am a woman younger than 65 and have at least 1 risk factor listed in Table 1	Complete one of the screening tools listed in Table 2. Write your OST score in the box provided
☐	I am a woman younger than 65 and do **NOT** have any of the risk factors listed above	Congratulations! You do not need to have a bone scan at this time
☐	I am a man **over** the age of 70	Consider using the screening tool for men in Table 2
☐	I am a man **under** the age of 70	Congratulations! You do not need to have a bone scan at this time unless your doctor thinks it would be helpful

STEP 3: If in Table 2 it was recommended that you complete a risk assessment, use one of the assessments below to see if you are at high risk for osteoporosis.

Calculators Used to See if One is at Risk for Osteoporosis

Tool	Where to Find It
OST for women	https://reference.medscape.com/calculator/osteoporosis-self-assessment-women
OST for men (optional)	https://reference.medscape.com/calculator/osteoporosis-self-assessment-men

Mark the box that describes you:

My OST score is:	☐ Low (No DXA scan needed at this time)	☐ Medium (No DXA scan needed at this time)	☐ High (Talk to your doctor about getting a DXA scan)

Most guidelines mention that screening is not necessary for men under the age of 70, but think it may be beneficial to screen men over the age of 70.[9]

So, now you should have a pretty good idea if you should have a DXA bone scan. Let's take a closer look at the DXA bone scan and what the results mean.

STEP 4: After you get your DXA scan at the doctor's office, check the box below that applies to you based on your T or Z score below. Do you have osteoporosis?

Check the box that applies to you:

Check one:	Category	T Score from DXA Scan
Women 65 or older, women younger than 65 and have at least 1 risk factor listed in Table 1, or men older than 70		
☐	Normal	T score greater than or equal to -1.0
☐	Osteopenia	T score between -1.0 and -2.5
☐	Osteoporosis	T score less than or equal to -2.5
☐	Severe osteoporosis	T score less than or equal to -2.5 with one or more fractures
OR: men younger than 50 years old, children, or premenopausal women		
	Category	**Z Score from DXA Scan**
☐	Normal	Z score greater than or equal to -2.0
☐	Suggestive of low bone density	Z score less than -2.0

Based on your score above, mark the box that describes you:

Do I have Osteoporosis?	☐ Yes	☐ No

If you answered "Yes" to the question above, read on to see what you can do to treat osteoporosis and other measures you can take to keep it from getting worse.

Other Tests

It's recommended that patients who are newly diagnosed with osteoporosis have other tests done to see if the cause for osteoporosis can be found. These tests include[9]:

- serum 25-hydroxyvitamin D
- calcium
- creatinine
- thyroid-stimulating hormone

In additions to the risk factors listed in Table 1, there are medications that you may be taking that can contribute to the development of osteoporosis.

Medications That Can Contribute to Osteoporosis

- Heparin
- Anticonvulsants
- Cyclosporine A
- Tacrolimus
- Barbituates
- Lithium
- Depo-medroxyprogesterone
- Chemotherapy
- Intravenous nutrition
- Glucocorticoids

Non-medication Therapy to Decrease the Risk of Fractures

Remember, all of the medications mentioned below are meant to be used in conjunction with other measures like fall prevention, smoking cessation, decreased caffeine intake, exercise, vitamin D intake, and moderation of alcohol.

Non-medication Therapy to Decrease the Risk of Fractures[9]

- Alcohol and caffeine in moderation
- Less than or equal to 4 drinks per day for men or 2 drinks per day for women
- Less than or equal to 2.5 cups of coffee or 5 cups of tea per day
- Smoking cessation
- Consider exercise and strength training
- Calcium and Vitamin D supplementation (consider more exposure to sunlight)
- Fall prevention measures

How Much Calcium and Vitamin D Do I Need?

So how much calcium do we need each day? It is important to note that our calcium requirements depend on factors such as age and lactation status. It is important to note that increasing calcium intake beyond these recommendations may put you at risk for kidney stones or cardiovascular disease.[17]

Recommended Daily Allowances for Dietary Calcium[16]

Age	Male	Female
0-6 months	200 mg	200 mg
7-12 months	260 mg	260 mg
1-3 years	700 mg	700 mg
4-8 years	1000 mg	1000 mg
9-13 years	1300 mg	1300 mg
14-18 years	1300 mg	1300 mg
19-50 years	1000 mg	1000 mg
51-70 years	1000 mg	1200 mg
71+ years	1200 mg	1200 mg

Here are some tips on how you can help prevent falls. Falls put you at a higher risk of bone fracture.

Safety Tips to Prevent Falls

- Use a cane, walker or other assistive device
- If using a cane in an icy region, consider using ice tips at the end to get better grip
- When using a cane or walker, consider suing rubber tips at the tips to get better grip
- Consider using a long-handled gripping device to reach things on the ground
- Avoid walking on slippery surfaces
- Use hand rails when available
- Install handles and rails in the bathroom around the toilet and bath tub
- Consider a plastic shower chair in the shower
- Keep floors inside and outside free of clutter and in good repair
- Be careful when stepping on or off of curbs
- Keep surroundings well-lit. You may consider carrying a small flashlight for times when you might find yourself in dimly-lit areas

while away from home
- Wear comfortable, low-heeled footwear
- Consider carrying a bag or using a fannypack/backpack to keep your hands free
- Find out which grocery stores and pharmacies in your community deliver to your home
- Consider getting a personal emergency response system to wear in case you fall when you are alone
- For those that are prone to falls, wearing undergarments with hip pad protectors may also help prevent hip fractures.

If you have trouble walking, there are many types of assistive devices available including:
- Cane
- Offset cane (a cane with a crook in the neck)
- Quadripod cane (a cane with 4 feet at the bottom)
- Forearm (Lofstrand) crutches
- Standard walker
- Front-wheeled walker
- Four-wheeled walker (also called a rollator)

You'll need to talk to your doctor about which assistive device may be right for you

Medication for the Treatment of Osteoporosis

Remember in STEP 4 earlier in this chapter, we discussed how the NOF recommends starting medication treatment only in the following groups:

People Who Should Consider Medication Treatment for Osteoporosis[9]

Women 65 or older, women younger than 65 and have at least 1 risk factor listed in Table 1, or men older than 70 with:
T score less than or equal to -2.5
OR: men younger than 50 years old, children, or premenopausal women with:
Z score less than -2.0

Here is a summary of the medications used to treat or prevent osteoporosis.

Medications for the Prevention and Treatment of Osteoporosis

Class of Medications	Examples of Medications in this Class	Approved for Prevention or Treatment	Fracture Type	How to Take it
Bisphosphonates	Alendronate (Fosamax®)	Prevention Treatment	Hip, vertebral*, nonvertebral**	Oral once daily or weekly
	Alendronate with cholecalciferol (Fosamax plus D®)	Treatment	Hip, vertebral, nonvertebral	Oral once daily or weekly
	Ibandronate (Boniva®)	Prevention Treatment	Vertebral only	Oral once a month
	Risedronate (Actonel®, Atelvia®)	Prevention Treatment	Hip, vertebral, nonvertebral	Different options: Once per day, once per week, once per month, or for 2 days in a row once per month
	Risedronate with calcium (Actonel with calcium®)	Prevention Treatment	Hip, vertebral, nonvertebral	Different options: Once per day, once per week, once per month, or for 2 days in a row once

				per month
	Zoledronic acid (Reclast®, Zometa®)	Prevention Treatment	Hip, vertebral, nonvertebral	Injection once every 1-2 years
Selective estrogen receptor modulators (SERMs)	Raloxifene (Evista®)	Prevention Treatment	Vertebral only	Oral daily
Anabolic Drug	Teriparatide (Forteo®)	Treatment	Vertebral, nonvertebral	Injection once daily
	Denosumab (Prolia®)	Treatment	Hip, vertebral, nonvertebral	Injection every 6 months

*Vertebral: means involving the vertebrae (bones that make up the spine)
**Nonvertebral: means NOT involving the vertebrae (bones that make up the spine)

First line treatment for osteoporosis is to start bisphosphonate therapy. However, people who can't take bisphosphonates or don't respond to them might consider other medications like raloxifene, teriparatide, and denosumab.

Remember, all of these medications are meant to be used in conjunction with other measures like fall prevention, smoking cessation, decreased caffeine intake, exercise, vitamin D intake, and moderation of alcohol.

Bringing It All Together

If you do not have osteoporosis, remember that prevention is key and the risk of osteoporosis should be reevaluated on an ongoing basis. If you have osteoporosis, treatment goals and the effects of medications should be reevaluated on an ongoing basis. The NOF recommends re-testing, using a bone scan, every 1 to 2 years after starting therapy and then every 2 years thereafter.[5] Taking a wholistic approach and treating osteoporosis with medication and non-medication options will help optimize your treatment.

REFERENCES

1. Kristie N. Tu, PharmD, BCPS, CGP, Janette D. Lie, PharmD, BCACP, Chew King Victoria Wan, PharmD Candidate, et. al. Osteoporosis: A Review of Treatment Options. P T. 2018 Feb; 43(2): 92–104.

2. Wright N, Looker A, Saag K, et al. The recent prevalence of osteoporosis and low bone mass in the United States based on bone mineral density at the femoral neck or lumbar spine. J Bone Miner Res. 2014;29(11):2520–2526. [PMC free article] [PubMed]

3. Optimal Calcium Intake: NIH Consensus Statement, 1994. Bethesda, MD. National Institutes of Health, 1994;12(4):1–31.

4. National Osteoporosis Foundation. Clinician's Guide to Prevention and Treatment of Osteoporosis (2014 update).

5. Pauline M. Camacho, MD, FACE; Steven M. Petak, MD, MACE, FACP, FCLM, JD; Neil Binkley, MD, et. al. American Association of Clinical Endocrinologists and American College of Endocrinology Clinical Practice Guidelines for the Diagnosis and Treatment of Postmenopausal Osteoporosis-2016. Endocrine Practice. Vol 22 (Suppl 4) September 2016.

6. Osteoporosis to Prevent Fractures: Recommendation Statement. *Am Fam Physician.* 2018 Nov 15;98(10): online at https://www.aafp.org/afp/2018/1115/od1.html.

7. Katrine Hass Rubin a,b,, Bo Abrahamsen a,c, Teresa Friis-Holmberg, et. al. Comparison of different screening tools (FRAX®, OST, ORAI, OSIRIS, SCORE and age alone) to identify women with increased risk of fracture. A population-based prospective study. Bone 56 (2013) 16–22.

8. Michael P. Jeremiah, MD; Brian K. Unwin, MD, and Mark H. Greenwald, MD. Diagnosis and Management of Osteoporosis. *Am Fam Physician.* 2015 Aug 15;92(4):261-268.

9. World Health Organization. Prevention and management of osteoporosis: report of a WHO Scientific Group. Geneva, Switzerland; 2003. http://whqlibdoc.who.int/trs/WHO_TRS_921.pdf. Accessed September 6, 2014

10. F. Cosman, S. J. de Beur, M. S. LeBoff, et. al. Clinician's Guide to Prevention and Treatment of Osteoporosis. Osteoporos Int. 2014; 25(10): 2359–2381.

11. Crandall CJ, Newberry SJ, Diamant A, et al. Comparative effectiveness of pharmacologic treatments to prevent fractures: an updated systematic review. *Ann Intern Med.* 2014;161(10):711-723.

12. Accessed 2018, December 5. *Fractures/Fall Prevention.* Retrieved from https://www.nof.org/patients/fracturesfall-prevention.

13. Kumar R, Roe MC, Scremin OU. Methods for estimating the proper length of a cane. *Arch Phys Med Rehabil.* 1995;76(12):1173–1175.

14. Optimal Calcium Intake: NIH Consensus Statement, 1994. Bethesda, MD. National Institutes of Health, 1994;12(4):1–31.

15. Committee to Review Dietary Reference Intakes for Vitamin D and Calcium, Food and Nutrition Board, Institute of Medicine. Dietary Reference Intakes for Calcium and Vitamin D. Washington, DC: National Academy Press, 2010

16. Jian-Ping Peng, PhD and Hang Zheng, PhD. Kidney stones may increase the risk of coronary heart disease and stroke; A PRISMA-Compliant meta-analysis. Medicine (Baltimore). 2017 Aug; 96(34): e7898.

17. Micromedex (2018). In Micromedex (Columbia Basin College Library ed.) [Electronic version].Greenwood Village, CO: Truven Health Analytics. Retrieved October 18, 2015, from http://www.micromedexsolutions.com

CHAPTER 6

STROKE

The Empowered Medicine Guide to Stroke

How to Use This Chapter

Welcome to the Empowered Medicine Guide to stroke. First, we will go over the basics of stroke such as what it is and why treating it is important. Then you will be able to plug your own information into the tools provided to see if you should consider medication to protect against stroke. Finally, we will look at what medications may work best for you.

Please refer to Appendices I, II and VII in the back of this book to log your own information for easy calculations and sharing with your doctor. All 3 of these Appendices will be used in this chapter. Also, at the end of this chapter you will find a section called 'The Bottom Line'. This box sums up the main points of the chapter.

Stroke: The Basics

A stroke is when damage to the brain happens as a result of a lack of blood flow to the brain. Another term for stroke the medical community uses is cerebrovascular accident (CVA). For the sake of this chapter, we will use the term stroke.

There are 2 main types of stroke:

1. **Ischemic stroke** – this type of stroke happens when blood clots become trapped in the blood vessels of the brain. These clots can originate in the brain or can form elsewhere in the body and

travel to the brain. Similar to a heart attack, this causes an interruption in the blood flow to the brain. This can result in damage to the brain.

2. **Hemorrhagic stroke** – this type of stroke happens when a blood vessel in the brain bursts. This can also cause an interruption in the blood flow to the brain.

A transient ischemic attack (TIA) is sometimes referred to as a 'mini stroke'. This happens when an artery is only partially and temporarily blocked. It can cause a temporary lack of blood flow to the brain and may produce symptoms that are temporary.

In this chapter we will be focusing on ischemic stroke as it is responsible for the majority of strokes. Stroke is the 5th leading cause of death in the United States. Unfortunately, someone has a stroke every 40 seconds. This results in 1 out of every 20 deaths in the United States being the result of a stroke.[1-4]

What are the Symptoms of Stroke?

It's important to recognize the symptoms of a stroke so that you can seek emergency help right away. Every second your brain is without oxygen can result in more brain cells being damaged, sometimes permanently. This can lead to problems with movement, speech, thinking, and more.

Table 1: **Symptoms of Stroke**

- Severe headache
- Numbness or weakness on one side of the body (for example: face, arm, leg)
  - Loss or disturbance in vision in one or both eyes
  - Problems talking
  - Problems understanding what other people are saying
  - Loss of balance or problems walking

To make things easier to remember, the American Heart Association (AHA) has developed the F.A.S.T. campaign. This is designed to help people recognize the symptoms of a stroke fast.

Table 2: **F.A.S.T Symptoms of Stroke**

F – Facial droop – Does one side of the face droop? Ask the person to smile. **A – Arm weakness** – Ask the person to raise both arms. One may stay down or is numb. **S – Speech difficulty** – Person may be hard to understand or unable to speak. **T – Time to call 9-1-1** – Call immediately, even if the symptoms go away.

Ischemic Stroke

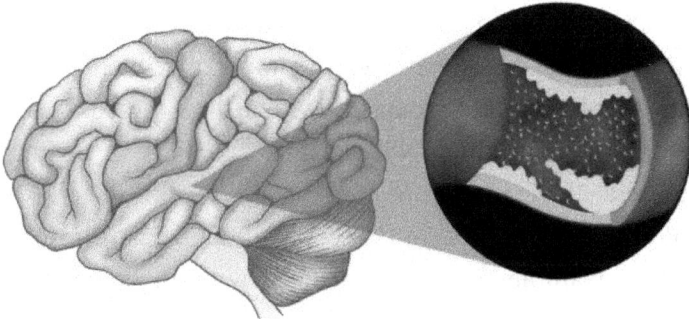

If you or someone you know experiences any of the symptoms listed above in Table 1 or 2, call emergency services immediately (9-1-1). Wait for the ambulance. Do **NOT** drive or have someone drive you to the hospital. People who use an ambulance get to the hospital faster and receive treatment faster.

What Happens Next?

Let's say you have called 9-1-1 and an ambulance has transported you to the hospital. What happens next? The guidelines urge hospitals to get an image of your brain within 20 minutes of arrival.[5] This usually involves using a CT scan. If you have a stroke caused by a clot, depending on which criteria you meet, the guidelines suggest you receive one of two therapies:[5]

1. **Alteplase** – This medication is able to help dissolve the clot causing the stroke and possibly restore blood flow to the brain. The guidelines urge hospitals to give (patients who qualify) alteplase therapy within 60 minutes from the time they arrive at the hospital, when at all possible. They call this "door to needle (DTN) time". Hospitals should strive to achieve this in at least 50% of their stroke patients. [5] This is because this medication works better the sooner it is given.

The guidelines also say that selected people should receive alteplase within 3 hours of the last known normal and that certain people can receive up to 4.5 hours after the last known normal.[5]

One study showed that each 15-minute reduction in time to receiving alteplase was associated with a 4% increase in odds of walking at discharge and a 4% decrease in odds of death prior to discharge.[6]

You might NOT be able to receive alteplase if you meet certain criteria. For example, if have a history of brain hemorrhage, have blood pressure greater than 185/110, are taking blood thinners, or have had a gastrointestinal bleed within the past 21 days.[5]

2. **Thrombectomy (mechanical clot removal)** – If the patient is a candidate and the necessary tools are available, the clot may be mechanically removed by inserting a tool into the vein and physically removing the clot. This therapy is generally for people who have a clot in one of the large veins of the brain. This treatment

strategy needs to be used within 24 hours of the last time the patient was known to be well and symptom-free.[5]

Key to Success

If you have symptoms of a stroke, do NOT attempt to drive yourself to the hospital or have someone drive you to the hospital. Call Emergency Services (9-1-1) for an ambulance. People who use an ambulance get to the hospital faster and receive treatment faster.

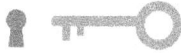

Sometimes the hospital you are brought to will want to start therapy and then transport you to a facility that has a higher level of care. For example, they might want to transport you to a hospital that has more tools to treat your stroke (perhaps they have the equipment needed to perform a thrombectomy). The medical community sometimes calls this "drip and ship".

Other Medications for Stroke

As we will see in a moment, there are other medications that may be used if you are diagnosed with an ischemic stroke. For example, once you leave the hospital (after your initial emergency treatment for a stroke caused by a clot), your doctor may prescribe you medications to help make sure the clot that caused the stroke is gone. Some medications (like alteplase mentioned above), help dissolve the clot. Other medications help prevent more clots from forming while your body gets rid of the clot. Aspirin plus clopidogrel, starting within 24 hours of a minor stroke and continued for 21 days, has been shown to be beneficial.[5] In addition, most patients who have had a stroke will receive long term medication to prevent another stroke from happening again. The type of medication you receive will depend on what other health conditions you have.

Preventing Stroke

Although you cannot completely get rid of your risk for stroke, there are things you can do to minimize your risk.

A surgical option to prevent stroke is angioplasty. Angioplasty is a procedure where a small balloon is inserted into a carotid artery and expanded to open up the vessel to help blood move more freely through it. There is a carotid artery on either side of your neck. These supply the brain with oxygen. Sometimes these can get clogged with fatty deposits. Angioplasty may be used with the placement of stents (tubular devices placed into the carotid arteries that expand to let blood flow through easier).

You can also modify some of your risk factors. There are two types of risk factors; 1) those you can improve, and 2) those you cannot. You can decrease your risk of stroke by treating the risk factors that you can improve.

Table 3: Risk Factors for Stroke[15]

Risk Factors You Can Treat	
High blood pressure	Smoking
Diabetes	High cholesterol
Physical inactivity	Obesity
Illegal drug use	Sleep apnea
Carotid artery disease	Transient ischemic attacks (TIAs)
Excessive alcohol intake	Atrial fibrillation
Risk Factor You Can NOT Control	
Prior stroke	Sickle cell anemia
Increasing age	Gender
Heredity	Race

According to the American Heart Association and American Stroke Association, knowing about the ones you can't control might motivate you to treat the risk factors you can control.

For example, high blood pressure is a risk factor for stroke that can be treated. In other words, if you have high blood pressure, treating it (using medications and/or lifestyle changes) so that your blood pressure becomes closer to normal can greatly decrease your risk of stroke.

Avoiding excess sodium and making sure you get adequate amounts of potassium in your diet can also help decrease blood pressure. Finally, regular, vigorous aerobic activity for 40 minutes per day, at least 3 to 4 days per week is recommended.[5] This can help decrease blood pressure and lower your risk of stroke. See the "High Blood Pressure" chapter in this book for more tips on how to improve your blood pressure.

Diabetes is a risk factor for stroke that might be avoidable for some people. If you take care to watch your weight and stay physically active, you will decrease your risk of type 2 diabetes, which can also decrease your risk of stroke. For more information on how to manage diabetes, see the "Diabetes" chapter in this book.

Having high cholesterol is also a risk factor that can be treated to decrease your risk of stroke. It is thought that having high levels of certain types of cholesterol in the blood can increase the risk of clots that can cause a heart attack or stroke. To learn more about how to treat high cholesterol, see the "high cholesterol" chapter of this book.

Besides those risk factors listed above, there are other health conditions that can put you at a higher risk for stroke. These include having artificial heart valves, atrial fibrillation (a. fib.), heart attack, angina, heart stents, and peripheral artery disease.

Reducing Your Risk of Heart Attack and Stroke after a Stroke

Simply having a stroke can put you at a greater risk for having another one. For patients who have had a stroke where the clot did not form in the heart, the use of antiplatelet drugs is recommended to reduce the risk of recurrent stroke or heart attack.[15] Platelets are special cells found in the blood stream whose job it is to stick together and form a clot when needed. This is to prevent excessive bleeding. Antiplatelet drugs work by decreasing the ability of the body's platelets to stick together and form a clot.

According to the guidelines, options for initial therapy after an ischemic stroke to prevent a second stroke include aspirin, clopidogrel (Plavix®) or a combination of aspirin and extended-release dipyridamole (Aggrenox®)[15] Other medications like ticagrelor (Brilinta®), ticlopidine (Ticlid®), and vorapaxar (Zontivity®) are reserved as possible alternatives to the recommended first line medications. Some of these second line drugs have not been shown in recent trials to have a definite benefit so they are not listed as first line agents in the guidelines.

You can learn more about these medications in the "Medications for the Prevention of Stroke" section toward the end of this chapter.

Reducing Your Risk of Heart Attack and Stroke with Mechanical Heart Valves

People who have had a mechanical heart valve implanted to replace a faulty heart valve are at a higher risk of blood clots. This is because the synthetic materials that make up the mechanical valve provide an ideal place for clots to form. These clots can travel from the heart, where they are formed, to the brain and cause a stroke. But there is a way people with mechanical heart valves can reduce their risk of stroke. The guidelines recommend that patients with artificial heart valves be given oral aspirin or warfarin (Coumadin®) to help prevent a stroke.[7] This is not usually necessary if the heart valves are bioprosthetic. Bioprosthetic valves are often made of animal tissue. Clots are not likely to form on this bioprosthetic surface.

Dipyridamole is also approved to prevent blood clots after heart valve replacement surgery when added to warfarin therapy.

Reducing Your Risk of Heart Attack and Stroke by Taking Statins

Basically strokes caused by a clot should be thought of like a heart attack; both are due to a blood clot that impedes the flow of blood to the brain (in the case of a stroke) or to the heart (in the case of a heart attack). Statins are a type of medication used to treat high cholesterol. High cholesterol is thought to increase the risk of heart attack and stroke.

The *2013 ACC/AHA Guidelines on the Treatment of Blood Cholesterol to Reduce Atherosclerotic cardiovascular Risk in Adults AND the 2017 AACE/ACE Guidelines for Managing Dyslipidemia and Prevention of CVD*, have taken data from the latest scientific trials and created tools to help predict your risk of having a first heart attack or stroke in the next 10 years.

Both guidelines have agreed that statin therapy is the most effective option for treating high cholesterol and thereby decreasing the risk of stroke. However, each guideline goes about determining all of this slightly differently. You will find these risk tools in Appendix I and II at the end of this book. *To see if you should consider taking a statin, turn to Appendix I and II and plug in your numbers. Then share your results with your doctor.*

The 2013 guidelines tell us that there are 4 groups of people who should be taking a statin.

Table 4: **4 Groups of People Who Should Take a Statin According to 2013 ACC/AHA Lipid Guidelines[8]**

1	**I have been diagnosed with cardiovascular disease, including angina, previous heart attack or stroke.**
2	My LDL-C is 190 mg/dL or above.
3	I have type 2 diabetes **AND** am between 40 and 75 years old **AND** my LDL-C 70-189 mg/dL **AND** I do **NOT** have cardiovascular disease.
4	I do **NOT** have cardiovascular disease or diabetes **AND** I am 40 to 75 years old **AND** my 10-year risk of heart attack or stroke greater than 7.5% (according to the 2013 risk calculator explained below).

The 2013 guidelines provide a risk calculator to see if you fit into line 4 above. The risk calculator looks at your age, history of diabetes, if you are male or female, what race you are and if you smoke or not. These guidelines suggest that people with a score of 7.5% or higher should consider a statin.

The authors of the 2013 ACC/AHA guidelines tell us (based on their research) that to get a true reduction in the number of cardiovascular events, moderate or high doses of statin drugs must be used. But at higher doses, side effects may be more common. They also suggest that instead of trying to dose your statin to reach a certain cholesterol goal, you should take the maximum dose of a moderate or high intensity statin that is tolerated and stick with it as tolerated.

The 2017 guidelines also have you calculate your risk, but they recommend you use one of a handful of online risk calculators they recommend. They also have you determine how many risk factors you have, but have a slightly different list of risk factors.

In contrast to the 2013 guidelines which recommend you take the maximum statin dose that is tolerated, the 2017 guidelines have you determine what your cholesterol treatment goals should be. Then they suggest using the statin dose that allows you to reach that goal.

Table 5: **Risk Categories and Lipid Goals**

Your Risk Level	**This is What your LDL-C goal should be**
Low Risk	**LDL-C goal is < 130 mg/dL**
Moderate Risk	**LDL-C goal is < 100 mg/dL**
High Risk	**LDL-C goal is < 100 mg/dL**
Very High Risk	**LDL-C goal is < 70 mg/dL**
Extreme Risk	**LDL-C goal is < 55 mg/dL**

Remember, to discover if you should consider a statin or not (and which statin you should consider) turn the Appendix I and II at the end of this book and plug in your numbers.

Let's look at which statins are available on the market today.

Table 6: **Low, Moderate and High-intensity Statin Drug**[8]

Low-intensity Statins	Moderate-intensity Statins	High-intensity Statins
Lowers LDL-C by less than 30%	**Lowers LDL-C by 30-50%**	**Lowers LDL-C by more than 50%**
Simvastatin 10 mg	Atorvastatin 10-20 mg	Atorvastatin 40-80 mg
Pravastatin 10-20 mg	Rosuvastatin 5-10 mg	Rosuvastatin 20-40 mg
Lovastatin 20 mg	Simvastatin 20-40 mg	
Fluvastatin 20-40 mg	Pravastatin 40-80 mg	
Pitavastatin 1 mg	Lovastatin 40 mg	
	Fluvastatin XL 80 mg	
	Fluvastatin 40 mg twice daily	
	Pitavastatin 2-4 mg	

When deciding if you should take a statin or not, the authors of the 2013 guidelines mention that you and your doctor should consider adverse effects, drug-drug interactions, and patient preferences as well.

You and your doctor might want to think about other factors too. Consider using information from the risk assessment combined with items such as LDL-P, non-HDL-C, Apo B level, cardiovascular health, weight, and family history to determine if a moderate to high dose statin is for you. Statins are capable of certain side effects including muscle and liver damage, neurological damage and increased risk of type 2 diabetes. So, the decision to take a statin should not be taken lightly.

To learn more about statins, check out the section toward the end of this chapter titled, "Medications for the Prevention of Stroke".

Reducing Your Risk of Stroke When You're Already taking a Statin

Alirocumab (Praluent®) and evolocumab (Repatha®)[5] are drugs used in addition to a statin in an effort to meet cholesterol goals. Both of these medications are available as an injection. You take it every two weeks OR once a month.

Alirocumab and evolocumab work by changing how the liver deals with fat in the blood stream. As a result, they may help lower cholesterol.

People who have had an ischemic stroke who are already taking the optimal amount of statin, may be a candidate for these types of injections.[5] After you start either of these medications, it's recommended you measure LDL-C in 4 to 8 weeks.

To learn more about alirocumab and evolocumab, turn to the "Medications for the Prevention of Stroke" section of this chapter.

Reducing Your Risk of Stroke if You Have Atrial Fibrillations (a. fib)

A condition called atrial fibrillation (a. fib.) has been associated with an increased risk of stroke. When one has a. fib., their heart beats irregularly. This is due to disorganized electrical signals in the chambers of the heart. This can cause you to feel a fast and/or fluttery heartbeat. Sometimes, this allows blood to pool in the chambers of the heart, allowing tiny clots to form. These clots can travel to the brain through the arteries and cause a stroke.

If you have a. fib., you can reduce your risk of stroke. If you meet the criteria, you may be a candidate for aspirin or oral anticoagulation therapy. Like aspirin, anticoagulation medications are drugs that help keep your blood from clotting.

Table 7 below is for people who have a. fib. Points are awarded depending on which risk factors you have. The number of points you have will let you and your doctor know if you should consider aspirin or an anticoagulation drug to decrease your risk of stroke. If you'd like, fill use Appendix VII for easy calculation and sharing with your doctor.

Table 7: **Stroke Risk Assessment for Atrial Fibrillation**[7]

	Criteria		Points	
C	Congestive Heart Failure	☐ ☐	Yes No	1 0
H	**H**igh blood pressure (> 140/90 mmHg on at least 2 occasions or current blood pressure treatment)	☐ ☐	Yes No	1 0
A	**A**ge 75 years or older	☐ ☐	Yes No	2 0
D	**D**iabetes mellitus (fasting glucose > 125 mg/dL or treatment with an oral hypoglycemic agent or insulin)	☐ ☐	Yes No	1 0
S	**S**troke or transient ischemic attack (TIA)- both of these involve a loss of blood flow to the brain	☐ ☐	Yes No	2 0

V	Vascular disease (Prior heart attack, peripheral arterial disease or aortic plaque)	☐	Yes	1
		☐	No	0
A	Age 65 to 74 years old	☐	Yes	1
		☐	No	0
SC	Sex Category female	☐	Yes	1
		☐	No	0
			Total Points:	

STEP 2: Add up the points you earned. Write the answer in the space labeled "Total points" above.

STEP 3: Check to box below that corresponds with how many "Total points" you have. Note what medications are recommended for you.

Table 8: **A. fib. Stroke Risk Score**

	Score	Risk
☐	0	Low risk. May not require anticoagulation
☐	1	Low-moderate risk. Should consider anticoagulation

In general, those with a score of 1 should consider full oral anticoagulation. This means aspirin is probably not potent enough for you and you should choose another medication from Table 3. The one exception, however, is in patients who have a score of 1 due to gender alone. In these patients (female < 65 years old without other risk factors), antithrombotic therapy should NOT be given.

If your score indicates you might be a candidate for anticoagulation, you will have the following medications to choose from:

Table 9: **Types of Anticoagulation Used to Treat Atrial Fibrillation**

- **Aspirin**
- **Warfarin (Coumadin®)**
- **Apixaban (Eliquis®)**
- **Dabigatran (Pradaxa®)**
- **Rivaroxaban (Xarelto®)**
- **Edoxaban (Savaysa®)**

Warfarin requires a lab called an (International Normalized Ration) INR to be monitored while you are taking it. The drug is dosed to achieve an INR of 2 to 3. This is because data shows that this is the optimal range for the INR to be to successfully prevent clots. However, it may take several days to achieve goal INR. This is why sometimes when warfarin is started for other health conditions besides a. fib., it is first overlapped with heparin, enoxaparin (Lovenox®) or fondaparinux (Arixtra®) until the goal INR is reached. However, this overlapping of therapies is not recommended for treating a. fib. and may do more harm than good. It could possibly lead to unwanted bleeding. For this reason, warfarin is generally used by itself when treating a. fib.

There is another option for people with a. fib to decrease the risk of stroke. The Watchman is a small device that looks kind of like a net. It is implanted in the heart. It can keep clots that form from traveling to the brain and causing a stroke. The procedure takes no more than an hour and typically involves staying the hospital one day.

Reducing Your Risk of Heart Attack and Stroke if You Have a History of Heart Attack or Angina

People who have had a heart attack or who have angina (chest pain caused by the heart not getting enough oxygen) are at a higher risk of heart attack and stroke. However, there are medications these people can take to decrease this risk.

Aspirin is commonly prescribed after a heart attack to prevent a second heart attack or stroke. In patients who can't take aspirin, clopidogrel is recommended. The combination of aspirin plus clopidogrel has not been shown to offer any more protection and may be associated with a higher risk of bleeding.

Ticagrelor (Brilinta®) and vorapaxar (Zontivity®) are other antiplatelet medications approved to prevent heart attacks and strokes in patients who have had a heart attack or who have angina (chest pain caused by a lack of oxygen to the heart). Warfarin (Coumadin®) are also indicated to prevent stroke in people who have had a heart attack.

Reducing Your Risk of Heart Attack and Stroke if You Have Had a Heart Stent Placed or Have Peripheral Artery Disease

Sometimes after a heart attack, the doctor may place one or many stents into the blood vessels of the heart. These stents are small tubes that expand after they are placed in the vessel to help keep the vessel open so blood can move freely through it. The down side of stents is that they are prone to having platelets in the blood stick to them. This can form clots that travel to the heart to cause a heart attack or to the brain and cause a stroke.

Aspirin plus clopidogrel (Plavix®), ticagrelor (Brilinta®), prasugrel (Efient®), or ticlopidine (Ticlid®) are often used after stent placement to reduce the risk of clots. However, prasugrel should NOT be used in people who have had a stroke due to an increased risk of bleeding that was shown during trials. These antiplatelet drugs help keep the platelets in the blood from sticking to each other. The combination of two antiplatelet drugs is referred to as "Dual antiplatelet Therapy (DAPT)".

Peripheral artery disease (PAD) is a condition where the blood vessels in the legs narrow, usually due to plaques that build up due to high cholesterol. This decreases the amount of blood that can flow through the vessels of the leg. This condition can make the arteries of the legs prone to clots.

There are many medications that can be used to help decrease the formation of clots in the legs with PAD. Aspirin, aspirin plus dipyridamole (Aggrenox®), clopidogrel (Plavis®), ticagrelor (Brilinta®), cilostazol (Pletal®), and Vorapaxar (Zontivity®) are often used.

Angioplasty is sometimes used to treat PAD. During this procedure, a small balloon is inserted and inflated in the narrowed vessel to widen it. A stent may also be placed to help keep these arteries open. Bypass surgery is also an option. During this procedure a vessel is grafted to the narrowed vessel offering an alternative route for blood to flow through.

Reducing Your Risk of Heart Attack and Stroke if You Have Blood Pressure

High blood pressure is strongly associated with a higher risk of stroke. It's important to work closely with your doctor to manage your blood pressure. Here we will look at a list of different blood pressure medications. For more information on blood pressure medications, please refer to the "high blood pressure" chapter in this book.

Table 9: **4 Main Drug Classes Recommended for the Initial Treatment of High Blood Pressure**

Class of Medications	Examples Recommended by Panel
Thiazide diuretics	Chlorthalidone (Thalitone®), Hydrochlorothiazide (Microzide®, Hydrodiuril®), Indapamide (Lozol®)
ACEI (angiotensin converting enzyme inhibitors)	Captopril (Capoten®), Enalapril (Vasotec®), Lisinopril (Prinivil®, Zestril®, Qbrelis®)
ARB (angiotensin receptor blocker)	Eprosartan (Teveten®), Candesartan (Atacad®), Losartan (Cozaar®), Valsartan (Diovan®), Irbesartan (Avapro®)
CCB (calcium channel blocker)	Amlodipine (Norvasc®), Diltiazem extended release, Verapamil

Remember, these 4 classes of drugs are those recommended for the *initial* treatment of high blood pressure. In other words, when one is first diagnosed with high blood pressure, it is recommended the doctor prescribe a drug from one of these categories. However, many people may require a combination of drugs from these 4 groups or even the addition of drugs outside of these 4 groups, to control their high blood pressure.

Table 10: **Other Medications that are Less Commonly Used for High Blood Pressure**

Class of Medications	Examples
Loop Diuretics	Bumetanide (Bumex®), Furosemide (Lasix®) and Torsemide (Demadex®).
Potassium-sparing diuretics	Amiloride (Midamor®) and Triamterene. Eplerenone (Inspra®) and Spironolactone (Aldactone®)
β-blockers (or 'beta blockers')	• Atenolol (Tenormin®) Betaxolol (Kerlone®) • Bisoprolol (Zebeta®)

	• Metoprolol (Lopressor®, Toprol-XL®) • Nebivolol (Bystolic®) • Adolfo (Corgard®) • Propranolol (Inderal®) • Acebutolol (Sectral®) • Penbutolol (Levatol®) • Pindolol (Visken®) • Carvedilol (Coreg®) • Labetalol (Normodyne®, Trandate®)
Alpha Blockers	Doxazosin (Cardura®), Prazosin (Minipress®), Terazosin (Hytrin®)
Centrally-acting Drugs	Clonidine (Catapress®), Methyldopa (Aldomet®), Guanfacine (Tenex®)
Vasodilators	Hydralazine (Apresoline®), Minoxidil (Loniten®)
Renin Inhibitor	Aliskiren (Tekturna® and Rasilez®)

Remember, for more information on blood pressure medications, please refer to the "high blood pressure" chapter in this book.

Reducing Your Risk of Heart Attack and Stroke If You Have an Irregular Heart Rate or Rhythm

If your stroke was due to an irregular heart rhythm, your doctor may have you take a medication that helps slow down your heart rate and/or helps your heart beat at a more regular rhythm. Here is a list of drugs commonly prescribed for one or both of these purposes. You can read more about each drug in the "Medications for the Prevention of Stroke" section toward the end of this chapter.

Table 11: **Drugs for Heart Rate and/or Rhythm**

Class of Medication	Examples
Drugs for Heart Rate	
Calcium channel blockers	Verapamil (Calan SR®, Verelean®)
	Diltiazem (Cardizem CD®, Dilacor XR®)
Beta blockers	Acebutolol (Sectral®)
	Atenolol (Tenormin®)
	Betaxolol (Kerlone®)
	Labetalol (Trandate®)
	Bisoprolol (Zebeta®)
	Carvedilol (Coreg®)
	Metoprolol tartrate (Lopressor®)
	Metoprolol succinate (Toprol XL®)
	Nebivolol (Bystolic®)
	Penbutolol (Levatol®)
	Propranolol (Inderal®)
	Sotalol (Betapace®)
	Nadolol (Corgard®)
	Pindolol (Visken®)
Digitalis drugs	Digoxin
Drugs for Heart Rhythm	
Sodium Channel Blockers	Disopyramide (Norpace®)
	Flecainide (Tambocor®)
	Mexiletine (Mexitil®)
	Quinidine
	Procainamide
	Propafenone (Rythmol®)
Class III Antiarrhythmic	Amiodarone (Cordarone®, Pacerone®)

Reducing Your Risk of Heart Attack and Stroke If You Have Diabetes

Diabetes is associated with a higher risk of stroke. Here is a list of diabetes medications. For more information on diabetes and the medications that treat it, turn to the "Diabetes" chapter in this book.

Metformin

- Metformin (Glucophage®, Glumetza®, Riomet®, Fortamet®)
- Repaglinide and metformin (Prandimet®)
- Metformin and glipizide (Metaglip®)
- Metformin and pioglitazone (ACTOplus Met®)
- Metformin and glyburide (Glucovance®)
- Metformin and rosiglitazone (Avandamet®)
- Metformin and sitagliptin (Janumet®)

Sulfonylureas

- Glimepiride (Amaryl®)
- Glyburide (DiaBeta®, Micronase®)
- Glipizide (Glucotrol®)
- Chlorpropamide
- Tolazamide (Tolinase®)
- Tolbutamide
- Glipizide and metformin (Metaglip®)
- Glimepiride and rosiglitazone (Avandaryl®)
- Glyburide and metformin (Glucovance®)
- Glimepiride and pioglitazone (Euetact®)

Glinides

- Nateglinide (Starlix®)
- Repaglinide (Prandin®)
- Repaglinide and metformin (Prandimet®)

Pramlintide (Symlin®, SymlinPen®)

Thiazolidinediones [TZDs] or "Glitazones"

- Pioglitazone (Actos®)
- Rosiglitazone (Avandia®)
- Rosiglitazone with glimepiride (Avandaryl®)

- Pioglitazone and metformin (ACTOplus Met®)
- Rosiglitazone and metformin (Avandamet®)
- Pioglitazone and glimepiride (Duetact®)

Glucagon-like peptide 1 (GLP1) receptor agonists

- Exenatide (Byetta® and Bydureon®)
- Liraglutide (Victoza® and Saxenda®)
- Lixisenatide (Lyxumia®)
- Albiglutide (Tanzeum®)
- Dulaglutide (Trulicity®)
- Semaglutide (Ozempic®)

Dipeptidyl Peptidase 4 (DPP4) Inhibitors (the "gliptins")

- Sitagliptin (Januvia®)
- Saxagliptin (Onglyza®)
- Linagliptin (Tradjenta®)
- Alogliptin (Nesina®)
- Vildagliptin (Galvus®)
- Alogliptin (Nesina®, Vipidia®)
- Metformin and alogliptin (Kazano®)
- Sitagliptin and metformin (Janumet®)

Alpha-glucosidase Inhibitors

- Acarbose (Precose®)
- Miglitol (Glyset®)

Medications for the Prevention of Stroke

We have just gone over many of the health conditions that can put you at a higher risk of stroke. It's important to make sure you are treating these conditions properly so you can lower your risk of stroke.

Aside from the medications that we use to treat other health conditions to lower our risk of stroke (like diabetes and high blood pressure), we looked at two main categories of drugs used to prevent stroke: anticoagulants and antiplatelet drugs. Both of these types of medications are sometimes referred to as "blood thinners". Neither of these classes of drugs dissolve blood clots. They actually just keep the blood from clotting more so your body can take care of the existing blood clot. Let's look at the drugs included in each of these groups then we will look at them separately.

Antiplatelet drugs

First we will look at the antiplatelet drugs used for the prevention of a stroke.

Table 12: **Antiplatelet Drugs for Prevention of a Stroke**

First line
Aspirin
Clopidogrel (Plavix®)
Cilostazol (Pletal®)-used mostly with PAD
Aspirin plus extended-release dipyridamole (Aggrenox®)
Second line
Ticagrelor (Brilinta®)
Ticlopidine (Ticlid®)
Vorapaxar (Zontivity®)

As we just learned, these medications are used to prevent stroke in a variety of situations including after an initial stroke, after a cardiac stent, after cardiac valves, after a heart attack and with peripheral artery disease (PAD).

Let's take a look at each of these drugs in more detail.

Aspirin

Aspirin is a nonsteroidal anti-inflammatory drug. It is also an antiplatelet drug. It works by reducing substances in the body that cause pain, fever, and inflammation. It also helps keep the platelets in the blood from sticking together. Aspirin is used to treat pain, fever and inflammation. Aspirin is sometimes used to treat or prevent heart attacks, strokes, and angina (chest pain).

Before starting aspirin therapy, ask your doctor. This way he or she can make sure it's safe for you to take aspirin. For example, you should avoid aspirin if you have a bleeding disorder such as hemophilia, a history of stomach, or intestinal bleeding or it you are allergic to NSAIDS. If you are planning surgery (including dental procedures), make sure your surgeon/dentist knows. Aspirin may need to be stopped before surgery and restarted after.

Aspirin is the most widely used antiplatelet agent. It reduces the risk of recurrent stroke by 15%.[13] Aspirin is the mainstay therapy for prevention of second ischemic stroke.

You can take aspirin with food if it upsets your stomach. Do not crush or chew enteric-coated or delayed-release pills. Swallow them whole. The chewable aspirin must be chewed though. Be sure to follow the instructions on the bottle for the type of aspirin you will be using.

Make sure to discard aspirin after its expiration date printed on the bottle. If you smell a vinegar-like odor from the bottle, do not take it. It has probably gone bad.

Aspirin should not be given to a child or teenager with flu symptoms or fever, or those with chicken pox. This is because aspirin can cause a serious condition in these people called Reye syndrome. This condition causes swelling of the liver and brain and can be fatal.

Aspirin should be used with caution in people with the following conditions:

- asthma or seasonal allergies
- stomach ulcers
- kidney disease
- a bleeding or blood clotting disorder
- gout
- high blood pressure
- hemorrhagic stroke
- congestive heart failure

What are the possible side effects of aspirin?

- Asthma
- Stomach ulcers
- Kidney disease
- Confusion
- Seizure
- Nausea, vomiting, stomach pain
- Bleeding
- Hemorrhagic stroke
- If you have high blood pressure, taking aspirin can increase your risk of having a hemorrhagic stroke.
- Aspirin can aggravate gout because aspirin can increase uric acid levels.
- Aspirin can worsen congestive heart failure.
- Aspirin can cause or worsen ringing in the ears

Let your doctor know right away if you have any symptoms of abnormal bleeding like blood in your urine, coughing up blood or coffee ground-like vomit, have bright red blood in your stools or black, tarry stools. If you experience any symptoms of stroke (drooping of one side of the face, weakness on one side of the body or difficulty talking) or if you experience any symptoms of an allergic reaction (trouble breathing, swelling of the throat or tongue), call emergency help immediately.

If you are planning surgery (including dental procedures), make sure your surgeon/dentist knows. Aspirin may need to be stopped before surgery and restarted after. But do not stop taking it without first letting your doctor know, even if you have signs of bleeding because stopping it can put you at risk for stroke.

Clopidogrel (Plavix®)

Clopidogrel is an antiplatelet drug that helps keep platelets in your blood from sticking together to form a blood clot that could block blood flow. It is sometimes taken with aspirin, depending on what health condition is being treated. Clopidogrel can be taken with or without food.

Before taking clopidogrel, let your doctor know if you have a history of:
- abnormal bleeding
- stomach ulcers or intestinal bleeding
- bleeding in the brain
- bleeding or clotting disorder

Potential side effects of clopidogrel may include:
- liver toxicity/jaundice
- abnormal bleeding
- systemic Inflammatory Response Syndrome (SIRS)
- kidney dysfunction
- seizure

Let your doctor know right away if you have:
- abnormal bleeding like: nose bleeds, pink urine, coughing up blood or coffee ground-like vomit, have bright red blood in your stools or black, tarry stools
- unusual bruising, red or purple spots under your skin
- symptoms of stroke (drooping of one side of the face, weakness on one side of the body or difficulty talking)
- jaundice (yellowing of skin or eyes)

- fever
- fast heart beat
- decreased urine output
- seizure

If you experience any symptoms of an allergic reaction (trouble breathing, swelling of the throat or tongue), call emergency help immediately.

If you are planning surgery (including dental procedures), make sure your surgeon/dentist knows. Clopidogrel may need to be stopped before surgery and restarted after. But do not stop taking it without first letting your doctor know, even if you have signs of bleeding because stopping it can put you at risk for stroke.

Ticagrelor (Brilinta®)

Ticagrelor is an antiplatelet drug that helps keep platelets in the blood from sticking together to form a clot. It is used to prevent blood clots after a heart attack. It's also sometimes used to prevent clots in people with peripheral artery disease (PAD). It is typically used in combination with aspirin. It is indicated by the Food and Drug Administration (FDA) to prevent a stroke after an initial stroke, but is not listed in the guidelines as a first line drug for this purpose because recent trials have not shown a definite benefit.

Take ticagrelor with or without food. If you can't swallow it whole, you may crush it up and mix it with water.

Before taking ticagrelor, let your doctor know if you have a history of:

- abnormal bleeding
- stomach ulcers or intestinal bleeding
- bleeding in the brain
- bleeding or clotting disorder
- heart problems
- liver disease/jaundice

Potential side effects of ticagrelor may include:

- abnormal bleeding
- liver toxicity/jaundice
- heart block
- possible lung issues or worsening asthma

Let your doctor know right away if you have:

- abnormal bleeding like nose bleeds, pink urine, coughing up blood or coffee ground-like vomit, have bright red blood in your stools, or black, tarry stools
- unusual bruising, red or purple spots under your skin
- symptoms of stroke (drooping of one side of the face, weakness on one side of the body or difficulty talking)
- jaundice (yellowing of skin or eyes)
- slow heartbeat
- shortness of breath

If you experience any symptoms of an allergic reaction (trouble breathing, swelling of the throat or tongue), call emergency help immediately.

If you are planning surgery (including dental procedures), make sure your surgeon/dentist knows. Ticagrelor may need to be stopped before surgery and restarted after. But do not stop taking it without first letting your doctor know, even if you have signs of bleeding because stopping it can put you at risk for stroke.

Ticlopidine (Ticlid®)

Ticlopidine helps to prevent platelets in your blood from sticking together and forming a blood clot. Ticlopidine is used to prevent blood clots after heart attack or stroke. It also may be used in people who have had a stent placed.

Ticlopidine has been shown to be more effective than aspirin in preventing stroke in people who have already had a stroke, but it has more side effects. For this reason it is reserved for those who cannot tolerate aspirin when trying to prevent a second stroke.[17]

Take ticlopidine exactly as your doctor instructs. Taking too much can put you at a higher risk for bleeding. Taking too little can put you at risk for a stroke. You can take it with food if it upsets your stomach.

Before taking ticlopidine, let your doctor know if you have a history of:
- abnormal bleeding
- stomach ulcers or intestinal bleeding
- bleeding in the brain
- bleeding or clotting disorder
- low platelets
- anemia
- liver disease/jaundice
- kidney impairment
- immune disorder that affects your body's ability to fight infection
- high cholesterol

Potential side effects of ticlopidine may include:
- liver toxicity/jaundice
- abnormal bleeding
- kidney dysfunction
- seizure
- low white blood cells (signs of illness including fever, chills, sore throat
- low platelet count and possible thrombotic thrombocytopenic purpura (TTP), a sometimes-fatal condition
- diarrhea, nausea, vomiting
- upset stomach
- rash

While taking ticlopidine, you will frequently be asked to get bloodwork done at the lab, especially in the first 3 months of therapy.

This is because ticlopidine can cause a life-threatening decrease in white blood cells (WBCs) and/or platelets.

Let your doctor know right away if you have:

• abnormal bleeding like: nose bleeds, pink urine, coughing up blood or coffee ground-like vomit, have bright red blood in your stools, or black, tarry stools

• unusual bruising, red or purple spots under your skin

• symptoms of stroke (drooping of one side of the face, weakness on one side of the body or difficulty talking)

• jaundice (yellowing of skin or eyes)

• seizures

• symptoms of illness like fever, chills, sore throat

• excessive bleeding or bruising, decreased urine output, red or purple spots under the skin or fever all can be signs of a condition called thrombotic thrombocytopenic purpura (TTP), a sometimes-fatal condition

If you experience any symptoms of an allergic reaction (trouble breathing, swelling of the throat or tongue), call emergency help immediately.

If you are planning surgery (including dental procedures), make sure your surgeon/dentist knows. Ticlopidine may need to be stopped before surgery and restarted after. But do not stop taking it without first letting your doctor know, even if you have signs of bleeding because stopping it can put you at risk for stroke

Dipyridamole (Persantine®)

Dipyridamole is an antiplatelet drug that helps keep platelets in your blood from sticking together and causing a clot. It also helps dilate or open up the blood vessels to let blood flow more freely. It is sometimes used in combination with aspirin, depending on what health condition is being treated. By itself, it is used to keep blood clots from forming after mechanical valve placement. The combination of dipyridamole and aspirin (Aggrenox®) is used to prevent blood clots in people with peripheral arterial disease (PAD) and to prevent another stroke in people who have had a stroke.

Follow the directions for taking dipyridamole precisely. Do not take more or less than is prescribed to you. Do not stop taking dipyridamole without talking to your doctor first. Doing so will put you at a higher risk of stroke.

Before taking dipyridamole, let your doctor know if you have a history of:

- abnormal bleeding
- stomach ulcers or intestinal bleeding
- bleeding in the brain
- bleeding or clotting disorder
- severe heart disease
- liver disease
- low blood pressure

Potential side effects of dipyridamole may include:

- liver toxicity/jaundice
- abnormal bleeding
- low blood pressure
- heart problems in people with severe heart disease
- dizziness or feeling like you might pass out
- chest pain
- nausea
- stomach pain

Let your doctor know right away if you have:

- abnormal bleeding like: nose bleeds, pink urine, coughing up blood or coffee ground-like vomit, have bright red blood in your stools, or black, tarry stools
- unusual bruising
- symptoms of stroke (drooping of one side of the face, weakness on one side of the body or difficulty talking)
- jaundice (yellowing of skin or eyes)

- Signs of blood pressure that is too low (dizziness, fainting)

If you experience any symptoms of an allergic reaction (trouble breathing, swelling of the throat or tongue), call emergency help immediately.

If you are planning surgery (including dental procedures), make sure your surgeon/dentist knows. Dipyridamole may need to be stopped before surgery and restarted after. But do not stop taking it without first letting your doctor know, even if you have signs of bleeding because stopping it can put you at risk for stroke.

Aspirin plus Dipyridamole (Aggrenox®)

As we just learned, the combination of dipyridamole and aspirin (Aggrenox®) is used to prevent blood clots in people with peripheral arterial disease (PAD) and to prevent another stroke in people who have had a stroke.

To learn more about the combination of aspirin and dipyridamole, please refer to the "Aspirin" and "Dipyridamole" sections of this chapter.

Anticoagulants

Anticoagulants are typically used in people with atrial fibrillation (a. fib) to help prevent clots from forming that can cause a stroke.

Table 13: **Types of Anticoagulants Used to Treat Atrial Fibrillation**

- **Aspirin**
- **Warfarin (Coumadin®)**
- **Apixaban (Eliquis®)**
- **Dabigatran (Pradaxa®)**
- **Rivaroxaban (Xarelto®)**
- **Edoxaban (Savaysa®)**

Aspirin

Aspirin is considered an "Antiplatelet drug" and an "Anticoagulant". To read more about aspirin, please refer to the "Aspirin" section of this chapter.

Warfarin (Coumadin®)

Warfarin is an anticoagulant. Vitamin K is needed for the blood to make a clot. Warfarin works by inhibiting vitamin K dependent clotting factors. This helps keep the blood from clotting.

Warfarin can be used to prevent stroke in people who have atrial fibrillation (a. fib.), have an artificial heart valve and in those who have had a heart attack.

While taking warfarin, you must have frequent blood tests to determine your International Normalized Ration (INR). The INR gives your doctor an idea of how fast your blood is clotting. The INR can be obtained by a finger prick using a small, hand held device or by a blood draw. The ideal INR goal range is 2 to 3. However, people taking warfarin for a mechanical heart valve usually have an INR goal of 2.5 to 3.5. The dose of warfarin is adjusted to keep the INR at goal. The INR will be monitored more frequently in the beginning (possibly once or twice a week) but can be spaced out more when the INR becomes stable.

Because warfarin works with vitamin K, the food you eat can affect how warfarin works and affect your INR. ***Vitamin K rich foods decrease the INR, making you more prone to developing a clot.*** Vitamin K rich foods include:

- Greens
- Broccoli
- Brussel sprouts
- Beef liver
- Pork chops
- Chicken

- Green beans
- Prunes
- Kiwi
- Cheese
- Avocado
- Peas

You don't necessarily need to avoid these foods. You should, however, aim to keep your consumption of them consistent. For example, if you like to have a green salad with your dinner 4 times a week, then eat it 4 times per week consistently.

Warfarin also has many more drug interactions than the other anticoagulants. This is because it affects enzymes in the liver that are responsible for eliminating other drugs in the body. Drugs that frequently interact with warfarin are listed below. All of the drugs listed below increase the INR so the dose of warfarin will have to be decreased while taking these other drugs:

- Antibiotics
- Antifungals
- NSAIDS like aspirin, ibuprofen, naproxen
- Acetaminophen
- Some heart rhythm drugs (amiodarone)

There are many supplements that interact with warfarin too including:

Table 14: **Supplements That Interact with Warfarin**

Decreases INR, increasing the risk of clotting
Coenzyme Q10
St. John's wort
Ginseng
Green tea (contains vitamin K)
Increases INR, increasing the risk of bleeding
Ginkgo biloba
Garlic

This is just a small portion of the list of drugs that can interact with warfarin.

Before taking warfarin, let your doctor know if you have a history of:

- abnormal bleeding
- stomach ulcers or intestinal bleeding
- bleeding in the brain
- bleeding or clotting disorder
- liver disease
- high blood pressure
- Recent spinal anesthesia or spinal tap

Potential side effects of dipyridamole may include:

- abnormal bleeding
- headache

Let your doctor know right away if you have:

- abnormal bleeding like: nose bleeds, pink urine, coughing up blood or coffee ground-like vomit, have bright red blood in your stools or black, tarry stools
- unusual bruising
- symptoms of stroke (drooping of one side of the face, weakness on one side of the body or difficulty talking)

If you experience any symptoms of an allergic reaction (trouble breathing, swelling of the throat or tongue) call emergency help immediately.

If you are planning surgery (including dental procedures), make sure your surgeon/dentist knows. Warfarin may need to be stopped before surgery and restarted after. But do not stop taking it without first letting your doctor know, even if you have signs of bleeding because stopping it can put you at risk for stroke.

Statins

As mentioned earlier, examples of statins include Atorvastatin (Lipitor®), Fluvastatin (Lescol®), Lovastatin (Mevacor®, Altocor®), Pitavastatin (Livalo®), Pravastatin (Pravachol®), Simvastatin (Zocor®) and Rosuvastatin (Crestor®).

Table 15: **Low, Moderate and High-intensity Statin Drugs**

Low-intensity Statins	Moderate-intensity Statins	High-intensity Statins
Lowers LDL-C by less than 30%	Lowers LDL-C by 30-50%	Lowers LDL-C by more than 50%
Simvastatin 10 mg	Atorvastatin 10-20 mg	Atorvastatin 40-80 mg
Pravastatin 10-20 mg	Rosuvastatin 5-10 mg	Rosuvastatin 20-40 mg
Lovastatin 20 mg	Simvastatin 20-40 mg	
Fluvastatin 20-40	Pravastatin 40-80 mg	
mg	Lovastatin 40 mg	
Pitavastatin 1 mg	Fluvastatin XL 80 mg	
	Fluvastatin 40 mg twice daily	
	Pitavastatin 2-4 mg	

Statins are a class of medications (also called HMG-CoA reductase Inhibitors). Statin drugs are recommended by the 2013 ACC/AHA and 2017 AACE/ACE guidelines as the primary medications that should be used to treat dyslipidemia.[20, 21]. They can lower LDL-C by 21 to 55%. They can decrease triglycerides by anywhere from 6 to 30%. They also may increase HDL-C by 2 to 10%.[20]

Before taking warfarin, let your doctor know if you have a history of:

- liver disease
- kidney disease
- diabetes

Potential side effects of statins include:

- Liver problems, nerve problems and muscle pain.
  - It is a good idea to get a baseline measurement of your liver enzymes so that your liver function can be monitored if you begin having symptoms of liver toxicity (fatigue, weakness, loss of appetite, dark-colored urine, yellowing of the skin or eyes).

- Raised blood sugar levels and type 2 diabetes
    - Although they appear to be less frequent with pravastatin or pitavastatin.
    - The risk of developing increased blood sugar and type 2 diabetes by using statins does not outweigh the benefits of using a statin according to the guidelines.
    - People taking statins should be screened for new-onset diabetes according to the newest diabetes guidelines. If diabetes develops, they encourage one to continue to statin therapy and focus on adhering to a heart healthy diet and increase physical activity. One is also encouraged to maintain a healthy body weight and avoid tobacco.
- Rhabdomyolysis
    - A rare, serious condition called rhabdomyolysis can occur. This is where muscle fibers break down releasing proteins into the blood that can damage the kidneys.
    - Report any muscle pain to your doctor while you are taking a statin.
    - Your doctor may want to measure your creatine kinase (CK) level.[6] This can tell him/her if the pain is due to rhabdomyolysis.
    - The 2013 authors also advise stopping the statin following symptoms of rhabdomyolysis such as extreme fatigue or muscle pain.
- Finally, if confusion or memory loss develops while taking a statin, the patient should be evaluated for a variety of causes including statin use.

While taking a statin, let your doctor know right away if you have:
- New muscle pain
- Raised blood sugar
- liver toxicity/jaundice

Medications if You are Already on Statins

Alirocumab (Praluent®) and evolocumab (Repatha®)[5] are part of a new class of drugs called PCSK9 inhibitors . They are used in addition to a statin in an effort to meet lipid goals. Both of these medications are available as an injection you take every two weeks OR once a month.

Alirocumab and evolocumab work by changing how the liver deals with fat in the blood stream. As a result, they may help lower cholesterol.

Patients and caregivers should be trained on how to prepare and administer either alirocumab or evolocumab.

Table 16: **How to Administer Alirocumab** (Praluent®)

• **To administer the 300 mg dose, give two 150 mg alirocumab injections consecutively at two different injection sites.**
• **Store alirocumab in the refrigerator. Allow alirocumab to warm to room temperature for 30 to 40 minutes prior to use. If needed, it may be kept at room temperature up to 77°F (25°C) for a maximum of 30 days in original carton to protect from light. Do not store above 77°F (25°C). After removal from the refrigerator, alirocumab must be used within 30 days or discarded.**
• **Before administration, alirocumab should be inspected visually for particulate matter and discoloration prior to administration. If the solution is discolored or contains visible particulate matter, do not use it**
• **Follow** aseptic **injection technique every time alirocumab is administered.**
• **Administer alirocumab by subcutaneous injection into the thigh, abdomen, or upper arm using a single-dose pre-filled pen or single-dose pre-filled syringe.**
• **Rotate the injection site with each injection.**
• **Do NOT inject alirocumab into areas of active skin disease or injury such as sunburns, skin rashes, inflammation, or skin infections.**
• **Do NOT co-administer alirocumab with other injectable drugs at the same injection site.**

Table 17: **How to Administer Evolocumab (Repatha®)**

The 420 mg dose of evolocumab can be administered 2 ways:

1. Over 9 minutes by using the single use on-the-body infusor that has a prefilled cartridge OR
2. By giving 3 injections consecutively within 30 minutes using the single-use prefilled autoinjector or single use prefilled syringe.

- Evolocumab should be kept in the refrigerator. Right before use, it should be removed from the refrigerator and allowed to come to room temperature for at least 30 minutes (for the single use prefilled autoinjector or single use prefilled syringe) or at least 45 minutes (for the single use on-the-body infusor with prefilled cartridge.

- Once it has been brought to room temperature it should be used within 30 days. Do not put in the microwave or attempt to heat it on the stove, as this may damage the drug.

- Before you inject evolocumab

- Inspect it for particles and make sure the solution in clear to opalescent or pale yellow. If the solution is cloudy, another color or has particles in it, do not use it.

- Administer evolocumab into the abdomen, thigh or upper arm.

- Do not give other injectable drugs at the same sight, at the same time.

- Rotate injection sites so you are not using the same injection site for evolocumab, every day.

Before taking alirocumab or evolocumab, let your doctor know if you have a history of:
- abnormal bleeding
- liver dysfunction
- if you are pregnant

Side effects of alirocumab and evolocumab may include:
- bleeding, pain or bruising at the injection site
- liver dysfunction
- back pain

- cold or flu-like symptoms like stuffy nose, sore throat, sneezing
- bronchitis
- sinusitis
- muscle pain
- muscle spasm
- urinary tract infection
- cough
- dizziness
- stomach ache
- diarrhea
- confusion
- memory impairment
- extremely low LDL-C levels

Let your doctor know right away if you have:

- liver toxicity/jaundice

There have been reports of the body producing antibodies against the drug resulting in injection site reaction and allergic reactions requiring hospitalization. Get emergency medical help if you have signs of an allergic reaction: hives; difficult breathing; swelling of your face, lips, tongue, or throat.

These medications are still relatively new on the market. There is little data showing that they are effective in decreasing heart attack and stroke. We are learning more about them as reports come in from people who use them.

Blood pressure medications

High blood pressure is strongly associated with a higher risk of stroke. It's important to work closely with your doctor to manage your blood pressure. Here we will look at a list of different blood pressure medications. For more information on blood pressure medications, please refer to the "high blood pressure" chapter in this book.

Table 18: **4 Main Drug Classes Recommended for the Initial Treatment of High Blood Pressure**

Class of Medications	Examples Recommended by Panel
Thiazide diuretics	Chlorthalidone (Thalitone®), Hydrochlorothiazide (Microzide®, Hydrodiuril®), Indapamide (Lozol®)
ACEI (angiotensin converting enzyme inhibitors)	Captopril (Capoten®), Enalapril (Vasotec®), Lisinopril (Prinivil®, Zestril®, Qbrelis®)
ARB (angiotensin receptor blocker)	Eprosartan (Teveten®), Candesartan (Atacad®), Losartan (Cozaar®), Valsartan (Diovan®), Irbesartan (Avapro®)
CCB (calcium channel blocker)	Amlodipine (Norvasc®), Diltiazem extended release, Verapamil

Remember, these 4 classes of drugs are those recommended for the *initial* treatment of high blood pressure. In other words when one is first diagnosed with high blood pressure, it is recommended the doctor prescribe a drug from one of these categories. However, many people may require a combination of drugs from these 4 groups or even the addition of drugs outside of these 4 groups, to control their high blood pressure.

Table 19: **Other Medications that are Less Commonly Used for High Blood Pressure**

Class of Medications	Examples
Loop Diuretics	Bumetanide (Bumex®), Furosemide (Lasix®) and Torsemide (Demadex®).
Potassium-sparing diuretics	Amiloride (Midamor®) and Triamterene. Eplerenone (Inspra®) and Spironolactone (Aldactone®)

β-blockers (or 'beta blockers')	• Atenolol (Tenormin®) Betaxolol (Kerlone®) • Bisoprolol (Zebeta®) • Metoprolol (Lopressor®, Toprol-XL®) • Nebivolol (Bystolic®) • Nadolol (Corgard®) • Propranolol (Inderal®) • Acebutolol (Sectral®) • Penbutolol (Levatol®) • Pindolol (Visken®) • Carvedilol (Coreg®) • Labetalol (Normodyne®, Trandate®)
Alpha Blockers	Doxazosin (Cardura®), Prazosin (Minipress®), Terazosin (Hytrin®)
Centrally-acting Drugs	Clonidine (Catapress®), Methyldopa (Aldomet®), Guanfacine (Tenex®)
Vasodilators	Hydralazine (Apresoline®), Minoxidil (Loniten®)
Renin Inhibitors	Aliskiren (Tekturna® and Rasilez®)

Remember, for more information on blood pressure medications, please refer to the "high blood pressure" chapter in this book.

Heart rate and Rhythm drugs

If your stroke was due to an irregular heart rhythm, your doctor may have you take a medication that helps slow down your heart rate and/or helps your heart beat at a more regular rhythm. Here is a list of drugs commonly prescribed for one or both of these purposes.

Table 20: Drugs for Heart Rate and/or Rhythm

Class of Medication	Examples
Drugs for Heart Rate	
Calcium channel blockers	Verapamil (Calan SR®, Verelean®)
	Diltiazem (Cardizem CD®, Dilacor XR®)
Beta blockers	Acebutolol (Sectral®)
	Atenolol (Tenormin®)
	Betaxolol (Kerlone®)
	Labetalol (Trandate®)
	Bisoprolol (Zebeta®)
	Carvedilol (Coreg®)
	Metoprolol tartrate (Lopressor®)
	Metoprolol succinate (Toprol XL®)
	Nebivolol (Bystolic®)
	Penbutolol (Levatol®)
	Propranolol (Inderal®)
	Sotalol (Betapace®)
	Nadolol (Corgard®)
	Pindolol (Visken®)
Digitalis drugs	Digoxin
Drugs for Heart Rhythm	
Sodium Channel Blockers	Disopyramide (Norpace®)
	Flecainide (Tambocor®)
	Mexiletine (Mexitil®)
	Quinidine
	Procainamide
	Propafenone (Rythmol®)
Class III Antiarrhythmic	Amiodarone (Cordarone®, Pacerone®)

Here is a rundown of the main classes of heart rate and arrhythmia drugs.

Calcium Channel Blockers

Calcium channel blockers work by blocking some of the calcium that enters the muscles of the heart. This has an effect of slowing down the force at which the heart beats. It also dilates (widens) the blood vessels a bit so blood can move freely through them. They are used to treat many health conditions including high blood pressure, chest pain and heart arrhythmias.

Verapamil and diltiazem differ from amlodipine (another calcium channel blocker) a bit. Verapamil and diltiazem reduce the strength of the heart's contractions. Amlodipine does not affect the strength of the heart's contraction much. It is not used to treat abnormal heart rhythms.

Side Effects of Calcium Channel Blockers May Include:
- Headache
- Constipation
- Rash
- Nausea
- Edema
- Flushing
- Drowsiness
- Low blood pressure
- Dizziness
- Sexual dysfunction
- Liver dysfunction
- Overgrowth of gums

Let your doctor know right away if you have:
- liver toxicity/jaundice
- dizziness or feel like you're going to faint

Get emergency medical help if you have signs of an allergic reaction: hives; difficult breathing; swelling of your face, lips, tongue, or throat.

Beta blockers

Beta blockers work by blocking the effects of the hormone epinephrine (AKA adrenaline). Adrenaline is the 'fight or flight' hormone produced by the body when it senses a threat to its survival. Among other actions, adrenaline shunts blood away from the digestive tract, sex organs and skin and sends it to the heart, muscles and lungs to prepare the body to fight or run.

By blocking the actions of adrenaline, beta blockers cause your heart to beat slower and with less force. This lowers your blood pressure and decreases the work for your heart. Some beta blockers also help keep your blood vessels dilated so that blood can move through them easier.

Let's look at some examples of beta blockers now.

Table 21: **Examples of Beta-blockers**

Type of beta-blocker	Details
Beta-blockers that target the heart • Atenolol (Tenormin®) Betaxolol (Kerlone®) • Bisoprolol (Zebeta®) • Metoprolol (Lopressor®, Toprol-XL®)	□ □These drugs focus on the heart □ □These drugs are preferred in people who have asthma, chronic obstructive pulmonary disease (COPD) and emphysema •
Beta blockers that target the heart and also help widen blood vessels • Nebivolol (Bystolic®)	• These drugs focus on the heart but also help relax the blood vessels (widen the blood vessels so blood can flow easier)
More beta blockers that target the heart and also help relax blood vessels • Carvedilol (Coreg®) • Labetalol (Normodyne®, Trandate®)	• These drugs, like nebivolol, focus on the heart and also help relax blood vessels. They work in a slightly different way than nebivolol • Carvedilol is preferred in people with heart failure
Beta-blockers that don't just target the heart (they affect the lungs too) • Nadolol (Corgard®) • Propranolol (Inderal®)	• These are generally not prescribed for patients with asthma, chronic obstructive pulmonary disease (COPD) and emphysema because these drugs can affect the lungs as well as the heart

Type of beta-blocker	Details
Beta-blockers that block the effects of adrenaline but can also stimulate the heart • Acebutolol (Sectral®) • Penbutolol (Levatol®) • Pindolol (Visken®)	• These are usually avoided for the treatment of high blood pressure, especially in people with cardiovascular disease or heart failure.

Side Effects of Beta Blockers May Include:
- Cold hands and feet
- Stomach cramps
- Dizziness
- Slow heart beat
- Low blood pressure
- Tiredness and sleep disturbances
- Increases in blood sugar
- Masking of symptoms of low blood sugar (so may have low blood sugar and not realize it)

Let your doctor know right away if you have:
- Dizziness or feel like you're going to faint
- Very slow heart beat
- Very low blood pressure

Get emergency medical help if you have signs of an allergic reaction: hives; difficult breathing; swelling of your face, lips, tongue, or throat.

Digoxin

Digoxin is made from the leaves of the digitalis plant. It's used to treat health conditions like heart failure and atrial fibrillation (a. fib.). A. fib., in particular, is known to put one at a higher risk of stroke.

Your digoxin levels will need to be measured periodically using a blood test. This is to ensure the amount of digoxin in your body is within the target range. This helps make sure you are getting enough digoxin so you will see the potential benefits. It's also to make sure you're not getting too much digoxin. Digoxin levels that are too high can lead to a higher incidence of side effects and abnormal heart rhythms.

Before taking digoxin, let your doctor know if you have a history of:

- Sick sinus syndrome or AV block
- History of heart attack
- Wolff-Parkinson-White syndrome
- Thyroid disorder
- Are taking a diuretic ("water pill")
- Abnormal electrolyte levels (like potassium, calcium, magnesium)
- Kidney disease

Side Effects of Digoxin May Include:

- Nausea, vomiting
- Irregular heart beat
- Vision disturbances
- Confusion, hallucinations
- Weakness
- Dizziness
- Headache
- Enlarged breasts in men
- rash

Let your doctor know right away if you have:

- Dizziness or feel like you're going to faint
- Very slow heart beat

Get emergency medical help if you have signs of an allergic reaction: hives; difficult breathing; swelling of your face, lips, tongue, or throat.

Sodium Channel Blockers

Sodium channel blockers are a class of anti-arrhythmia drugs that work by slowing the rate and strength of the electrical impulses within the heart. This can 'calm down' erratic heart rhythms.

Side Effects of Sodium Channel Blockers May Include:

- Very fast heart rate
- Dry mouth
- Urinary retention
- Blurred vision
- Constipation
- Diarrhea
- Nausea
- Headache
- Dizziness

Quinidine can cause a potentially fatal condition called torsades de pointes in certain people. Disopyramide should not be used in certain people with heart failure.

Let your doctor know right away if you have:

- Very fast or very slow heart rate
- Dizziness like you're going to faint

Get emergency medical help if you have signs of an allergic reaction: hives; difficult breathing; swelling of your face, lips, tongue, or throat.

Amiodarone

Amiodarone helps the heart maintain a normal rhythm.

Before taking amiodarone, let your doctor know if you have a history of:

- Lung disease
- Thyroid disease

- A neurological disorder
- Liver disease

Side effects of Amiodarone may include:

- Wheezing or other lung problems
- Heart arrhythmia (abnormal heart rhythms)
- Dizziness
- Blurred vision
- liver toxicity/jaundice
- Thyroid toxicity-problems like weight loss, thinning hair, feeling hot, jitteriness, tremors, goiter (swelling in the neck)
- Loss of coordination
- Muscle weakness
- Nausea, vomiting
- constipation

Let your doctor know right away if you have:

- Wheezing or other lung problems
- Very fast or slow or force full heart beat
- Dizziness like you're going to faint
- Blurred vision
- liver toxicity/jaundice
- Signs of thyroid problems like weight loss, thinning hair, feeling hot, jitteriness, tremors, goiter (swelling in the neck)
- Loss of coordination
- Muscle weakness

Diabetes medications

Diabetes is associated with a higher risk of stroke. Here is a list of diabetes medications. For more information on diabetes and the medications that treat it, turn to the "Diabetes" chapter in this book.

Metformin

- Metformin (Glucophage®, Glumetza®, Riomet®, Fortamet®)
- Repaglinide with metformin (Prandimet®)
- Metformin with glipizide (Metaglip®)
- Metformin and pioglitazone (ACTOplus Met®)
- Metformin and glyburide (Glucovance®)
- Metformin with rosiglitazone (Avandamet®)
- Metformin with sitagliptin (Janumet®)

Sulfonylureas

- Glimepiride (Amaryl®)
- Glyburide (DiaBeta®, Micronase®)
- Glipizide (Glucotrol®)
- Chlorpropamide
- Tolazamide (Tolinase®)
- Tolbutamide
- Glipizide with metformin (Metaglip®)
- Glimepiride and rosiglitazone (Avandaryl®)
- Glyburide with metformin (Glucovance®)
- Glimepiride with pioglitazone (Euetact®)

Glinides

- Nateglinide (Starlix®)
- Repaglinide (Prandin®)
- Repaglinide with metformin (Prandimet®)

Pramlintide (Symlin®, SymlinPen®)

Thiazolidinediones [TZDs] or "Glitazones"

- Pioglitazone (Actos®)
- Rosiglitazone (Avandia®)
- Rosiglitazone with glimepiride (Avandaryl®)

- Pioglitazone and metformin (ACTOplus Met®)
- Rosiglitazone and metformin (Avandamet®)
- Pioglitazone and glimepiride (Duetact®)

Glucagon-like peptide 1 (GLP1) receptor agonists

- Exenatide (Byetta® and Bydureon®)
- Liraglutide (Victoza® and Saxenda®)
- Lixisenatide (Lyxumia®)
- Albiglutide (Tanzeum®)
- Dulaglutide (Trulicity®)
- Semaglutide (Ozempic®)

Dipeptidyl peptidase 4 (DPP4) inhibitors (the "gliptins")

- Sitagliptin (Januvia®)
- Saxagliptin (Onglyza®)
- Linagliptin (Tradjenta®)
- Alogliptin (Nesina®)
- Vildagliptin (Galvus®)
- Alogliptin (Nesina®, Vipidia®)
- Metformin with alogliptin (Kazano®)
- Sitagliptin with metformin (Janumet®)

Alpha-glucosidase Inhibitors

- Acarbose (Precose®)
- Miglitol (Glyset®)

For more information on these medications refer to the "Diabetes" chapter of this book.

The Bottom Line

A stroke is when damage to the brain happens as a result of a lack of blood flow to the brain. Another term for stroke the medical community uses is cerebrovascular accident (CVA). For the sake of this chapter, we will use the term stroke.

There are 2 main types of stroke:

1. **Ischemic stroke**-this type of stroke happens when blood clots or fatty deposits become trapped in the blood vessels of the brain. These clots/deposits can originate in the brain or can form elsewhere in the body and travel to the brain. Similar to a heart attack, this causes an interruption in the blood flow to the brain. This can result in damage to the brain.

2. **Hemorrhagic stroke** – this type of stroke happens when a blood vessel in the brain bursts. This can also cause an interruption in the blood flow to the brain.

A transient ischemic attack (TIA) is sometimes referred to as a 'mini stroke'. This happens when an artery is only partially and temporarily blocked. It can cause a temporary lack of blood flow to the brain and may produce symptoms that are temporary.

F.A.S.T Symptoms of Stroke

F – Facial droop – Does one side of the face droop? Ask the person to smile.

A – Arm weakness – Ask the person to raise both arms. One may stay down or is numb.

S – Speech difficulty – Person may be hard to understand or unable to speak.

T – Time to call 9-1-1 – Call immediately, even if the symptoms go away.

If you or someone you know experiences any of the symptoms listed above in Table 1 or 2, call emergency services immediately (9-1-1). Wait for the ambulance. Do **NOT** drive or have someone drive you to the hospital. People who use an ambulance get to the hospital faster and receive treatment faster.

If you have a stroke caused by a clot, depending on which criteria you meet, the guidelines suggest you receive one of two therapies:[5]

1. **Alteplase**-This medication is able to help dissolve the clot causing the stroke and possibly restore blood flow to the brain. The guidelines urge hospitals to give (patients who qualify) alteplase therapy within 60 minutes from the time they arrive at the hospital, when at all possible. They call this "door to needle (DTN) time". Hospitals should strive to achieve this in at least 50% of their stroke patients. [5] This is because this medication works better, the sooner it is given.

The guidelines also say that all people eligible to receive alteplase should receive it within 3 hours of the last known normal and that certain people can receive up to 4.5 hours after the last known normal.[5]

One study showed that each 15-minute reduction in time to receiving alteplase was associated with a 4% increase in odds of walking at discharge and a 4% decrease in odds of death prior to discharge.[6]

You may NOT be able to receive alteplase if you meet certain criteria. For example, if have a history of brain hemorrhage, have blood pressure greater than 185/110, are taking blood thinners or have had a gastrointestinal bleed within the past 21 days.[5]

2. **Thrombectomy (mechanical clot removal)** – If the patient is a candidate and the necessary tools are available, the clot may be mechanically removed by inserting a tool into the vein and physically removing the clot. This therapy is generally for people who have a clot in one of the large veins of the brain. This treatment strategy needs to be used within 24 hours of the last time the patient was known to be well and symptom-free.[5]

Another surgical option to treat stroke is angioplasty. Angioplasty is a procedure where a small balloon is inserted into the blocked blood vessel and expanded to open up the vessel to help blood move more freely through it. Angioplasty may be used with the placement of stents (tubular devices placed into the blood vessels of the brain that expand to let blood flow through easier).

Other Medications for stroke

There are other medications that may be used if you are diagnosed with an ischemic stroke. For example, once you leave the hospital (after your initial emergency treatment for a stroke caused by a clot), your doctor may prescribe you medications to help make sure the clot that caused the stroke is gone. Some medications (like alteplase mentioned above), help dissolve the clot. Other medications help prevent more clots from forming while your body gets rid of the clot. Aspirin plus clopidogrel, starting within 24 hours of a minor stroke and continued for 21 days, has been shown to be beneficial.[5] In addition, most patients who have had a stroke will receive long term medication to prevent another stroke from happening.

Preventing Stroke

Although you cannot completely get rid of your risk for stroke, there are things you can do to minimize your risk. There are two types of risk factors; 1.) those you can improve and 2.) those you cannot. You can decrease your risk of stroke by treating the risk factors that you can improve.

Risk Factors for Stroke[15]

Risk Factors You Can Treat	
High blood pressure	Smoking
Diabetes	High cholesterol
Physical inactivity	Obesity
Illegal drug use	Sleep apnea
Carotid artery disease	Transient ischemic attacks (TIAs)
Excessive alcohol intake	Atrial fibrillation
Risk Factor You Can NOT Control	
Prior stroke	Sickle cell anemia
Increasing age	Gender
Heredity	Race

According to the American Heart Association and American Stroke Association, knowing about the ones you can't control might motivate you to treat the risk factors you can control.

Besides those risk factors listed above, there are other health conditions that can put you at a higher risk for stroke. These include artificial heart valves, atrial fibrillation, heart attack, angina, heart stents and peripheral artery disease.

Reducing Your Risk of Heart Attack and Stroke after a Stroke

For patients who have had a stroke where the clot did not form in the heart, the use of antiplatelet drugs is recommended to reduce the risk of recurrent stroke or heart attack.[15] Antiplatelet drugs work by decreasing the ability of the body's platelets to stick together and form a clot.

According to the guidelines, options for initial therapy after an ischemic stroke to prevent a second stroke include aspirin, clopidogrel (Plavix®) or a combination of aspirin and extended-release dipyridamole (Aggrenox®)[15] Other medications like ticagrelor (Brilinta®), ticlopidine (Ticlid®), and vorapaxar (Zontivity®) are reserved as possible alternatives to the recommended first line medications.

Reducing Your Risk of Heart Attack and Stroke with Mechanical Heart Valves

People who have had a mechanical heart valve implanted to replace a faulty heart valve are at a higher risk of blood clots. This is because the synthetic materials that make up the mechanical valve provide a good place for clots to form. The guidelines recommend that patients with artificial heart valves be given oral aspirin or warfarin (Coumadin®) to help prevent a stroke.[7] This is not usually necessary if the heart valves are bioprosthetic. Bioprosthetic valves which are often made of animal tissue. Clots are not likely to form on this bioprosthetic surface.

Dipyridamole is also approved to prevent blood clots after heart valve replacement surgery when added to warfarin therapy.

Reducing Your Risk of Heart Attack and Stroke by Taking Statins

Statins are a type of medication used to treat high cholesterol. It is possible for some people to lower their risk of stroke by taking a statin. Basically, an ischemic stroke is considered to be an atherosclerotic cardiovascular disease (ASCVD) event, like a heart attack. This means

341

that strokes caused by a clot should be thought of like a heart attack; both are due to a blood clot that impedes the flow of blood to the brain (in the case of a stroke) or to the heart (in the case of a heart attack).

The *2013 ACC/AHA Guidelines on the Treatment of Blood Cholesterol to Reduce Atherosclerotic cardiovascular Risk in Adults AND the 2017 AACE/ACE Guidelines for Managing Dyslipidemia and Prevention of CVD*, have taken data from the latest scientific trials and created tools to help predict your risk of having a first heart attack or stroke in the next 10 years. They both have agreed that statin therapy is the most effective option when treating high cholesterol and thereby decreasing the risk of stroke. However, each guideline goes about determining all of this slightly differently. You will find these risk tools in Appendix I and II at the end of this book. ***To see if you should consider taking a statin, turn to Appendix I and II and plug in your numbers. Then share your results with your doctor.***

Reducing Your Risk of Stroke When You're Already taking a Statin

Alirocumab (Praluent®) and evolocumab (Repatha®)[5] are drugs used by themselves or in addition to a statin in an effort to meet lipid goals. Both of these medications are available as an injection you take every two weeks OR once a month.

Reducing Your Risk of Stroke if You Have Atrial Fibrillations (a. fib)

A condition called atrial fibrillation (a. fib.) has been associated with an increased risk of stroke. When one has a. fib., their heart beats irregularly. This is due to disorganized electrical signals in the chambers of the heart. This can cause you feel a fast and/or fluttery heartbeat. Sometimes, this allows blood to pool in the chambers of the heart, allowing tiny clots to form. These clots can travel to the brain through the arteries and cause a stroke.

If you have a. fib., you can reduce your risk of stroke. If you meet the criteria, you may be a candidate for aspirin or oral anticoagulation. Anticoagulation medications are drugs that help keep your blood from clotting. They are sometimes called "blood thinners".

You will find these risk tools in Appendix VII at the end of this book. *To see if you should consider anticoagulation for you're a. fib., turn to Appendix I and II and plug in your numbers. Then share your results with your doctor.*

Types of Anticoagulation Used to Treat Atrial Fibrillation

- **Aspirin**
- **Warfarin (Coumadin®)**
- **Apixaban (Eliquis®)**
- **Dabigatran (Pradaxa®)**
- **Rivaroxaban (Xarelto®)**
- **Edoxaban (Savaysa®)**

Reducing Your Risk of Heart Attack and Stroke if You Have a History of Heart Attack or Angina

People who have had a heart attack or who have angina (chest pain caused by the heart not getting enough oxygen) are at a higher risk of heart attack and stroke. However, there are medications these people can take to decrease this risk.

Aspirin is commonly prescribed after a heart attack to prevent a second heart attack or stroke. In patients who can't take aspirin, clopidogrel is recommended. The combination of aspirin plus clopidogrel has not been shown to offer any more protection and may be associated with a higher risk of bleeding.

Ticagrelor (Brilinta®) and vorapaxar (Zontivity®) are other antiplatelet medications approved to prevent heart attacks and strokes in patients who have had a heart attack or who have angina (chest pain caused by a lack of oxygen to the heart). Warfarin (Coumadin®) are also indicated to prevent stroke in people who have had a heart attack.

Reducing Your Risk of Heart Attack and Stroke if You Have Had a Heart Stent Placed or Have Peripheral Artery Disease

Sometimes after a heart attack, the doctor may place one or many stents into the blood vessels of the heart. These stents are small tubes that expand after they are placed in the vessel to help keep the vessel open so blood can move freely through it. The down side of stents is that they are prone to having platelets in the blood stick to them. This can form clots that travel to the heart to cause a heart attack or to the brain and cause a stroke.

Aspirin plus clopidogrel (Plavix®), ticagrelor (Brilinta®), prasugrel (Efient®) or ticlopidine (Ticlid®) are often used after stent placement to reduce the risk of clots. However, prasugrel should NOT be used in people who have had a stroke due to an increased risk of bleeding that was shown during trials. These antiplatelet drugs help keep the platelets in the blood from sticking to each other. The combination of two antiplatelet drugs is referred to as "Dual antiplatelet Therapy (DAPT)".

Peripheral artery disease (PAD) is a condition where the blood vessels in the legs narrow, usually due to plaques that build up due to high cholesterol. This decreases the amount of blood that can flow through the vessels of the leg. This condition can make the arteries of the legs prone to clots.

There are many medications that can be used to help decrease the formation of clots in the legs with PAD. Aspirin, aspirin plus dipyridamole (Aggrenox®), clopidogrel (Plavis®), ticagrelor (Brilinta®), cilostazol (Pletal®) and vorapaxar (Zontivity®) are often used.

Angioplasty is sometimes used to treat PAD. During this procedure, a small balloon is inserted and inflated in the narrowed vessel to widen it. A stent may also be placed to help keep these arteries open. Bypass surgery is also an option. During this procedure a vessel is grafted to the narrowed vessel offering an alternative route for blood to flow through.

Reducing Your Risk of Heart Attack and Stroke if You Have High Blood Pressure

High blood pressure is strongly associated with a higher risk of stroke. It's important to work closely with your doctor to manage your blood pressure. Here we will look at a list of different blood pressure medications. For more information on blood pressure medications, please refer to the "high blood pressure" chapter in this book.

4 Main Drug Classes Recommended for the Initial Treatment of High Blood Pressure	
Class of Medications	**Examples Recommended by Panel**
Thiazide diuretics	Chlorthalidone (Thalitone®), Hydrochlorothiazide (Microzide®, Hydrodiuril®), Indapamide (Lozol®)
ACEI (angiotensin converting enzyme inhibitors)	Captopril (Capoten®), Enalapril (Vasotec®), Lisinopril (Prinivil®, Zestril®, Qbrelis®)
ARB (angiotensin receptor blocker)	Eprosartan (Teveten®), Candesartan (Atacad®), Losartan (Cozaar®), Valsartan (Diovan®), Irbesartan (Avapro®)
CCB (calcium channel blocker)	Amlodipine (Norvasc®), Diltiazem extended release, Verapamil

Remember, these 4 classes of drugs are those recommended for the *initial* treatment of high blood pressure. However, many people may require a combination of drugs from these 4 groups or even the addition of drugs outside of these 4 groups, to control their high blood pressure.

Other Medications that are Less Commonly Used for High Blood Pressure

Class of Medications	**Examples**
Loop Diuretics	Bumetanide (Bumex®), Furosemide (Lasix®), Torsemide (Demadex®).
Potassium-sparing diuretics	Amiloride (Midamor®), Triamterene (Dyrenium), Eplerenone (Inspra®), Spironolactone (Aldactone®)
β-blockers (or 'beta blockers')	Atenolol (Tenormin®)Betaxolol (Kerlone®) Bisoprolol (Zebeta®) Metoprolol (Lopressor®, Toprol-XL®) Nebivolol (Bystolic®)

	Nadolol (Corgard®)
	Propranolol (Inderal®)
	Acebutolol (Sectral®)
	Penbutolol (Levatol®)
	Pindolol-(Visken®)
	Carvedilol (Coreg®)
	Labetalol (Normodyne®, Trandate®)
Alpha Blockers	Doxazosin (Cardura®), Prazosin (Minipress®), Terazosin (Hytrin®)
Centrally-acting Drugs	Clonidine (Catapress®), Methyldopa (Aldomet®), Guanfacine (Tenex®)
Vasodilators	Hydralazine (Apresoline®), Minoxidil (Loniten®)
Renin Inhibitors	Aliskiren (Tekturna® and Rasilez®)

Remember, for more information on blood pressure medications, please refer to the "high blood pressure" chapter in this book.

Reducing Your Risk of Heart Attack and Stroke if You Have an Irregular Heart Rate or Rhythm

If your stroke was due to an irregular heart rhythm, your doctor may have you take a medication that helps slow down your heart rate and/or helps your heart beat at a more regular rhythm. Here are a list of drugs commonly prescribed for one or both of these purposes.

Drugs for Heart Rate and/or Rhythm

Class of Medication	Examples
Drugs for Heart Rate	
Calcium channel blockers	Verapamil (Calan SR®, Verelean®) Diltiazem (Cardizem CD®, Dilacor XR®)

Beta blockers	Acebutolol (Sectral®)
	Atenolol (Tenormin®)
	Betaxolol (Kerlone®)
	Labetalol (Trandate®)
	Bisoprolol (Zebeta®)
	Carvedilol (Coreg®)
	Metoprolol tartrate (Lopressor®)
	Metoprolol succinate (Toprol XL®)
	Nebivolol (Bystolic®)
	Penbutolol (Levatol®)
	Propranolol (Inderal®)
	Sotalol (Betapace®)
	Nadolol (Corgard®)
	Pindolol (Visken®)
Digitalis drugs	Digoxin
Drugs for Heart Rhythm	
Sodium Channel Blockers	Disopyramide (Norpace®)
	Flecainide (Tambocor®)
	Mexiletine (Mexitil®)
	Quinidine
	Procainamide
	Propafenone (Rythmol®)
Class III Antiarrhythmic	Amiodarone (Cordarone®, Pacerone®)

Reducing Your Risk of Heart Attack and Stroke if You Have Diabetes

Diabetes is associated with a higher risk of stroke. Here is a list of diabetes medications. For more information on diabetes and the medications that treat it, turn to the "Diabetes" chapter in this book.

Metformin
- Metformin (Glucophage®, Glumetza®, Riomet®, Fortamet®)
- Repaglinide and metformin (Prandimet®)
- Metformin and glipizide (Metaglip®)

- Metformin and pioglitazone (ACTOplus Met®)
- Metformin and glyburide (Glucovance®)
- Metformin and rosiglitazone (Avandamet®)
- Metformin and sitagliptin (Janumet®)

Sulfonylureas
- Glimepiride (Amaryl®)
- Glyburide (DiaBeta®, Micronase®)
- Glipizide (Glucotrol®)
- Chlorpropamide
- Tolazamide (Tolinase®)
- Tolbutamide
- Glipizide and metformin (Metaglip®)
- Glimepiride and rosiglitazone (Avandaryl®)
- Glyburide and metformin (Glucovance®)
- Glimepiride and pioglitazone (Euetact®)

Glinides
- Nateglinide (Starlix®)
- Repaglinide (Prandin®)
- Repaglinide and metformin (Prandimet®)

Pramlintide (Symlin®, SymlinPen®)

Thiazolidinediones [TZDs] or "Glitazones"
- Pioglitazone (Actos®)
- Rosiglitazone (Avandia®)
- Rosiglitazone and glimepiride (Avandaryl®)
- Pioglitazone and metformin (ACTOplus Met®)
- Rosiglitazone and metformin (Avandamet®)
- Pioglitazone and glimepiride (Duetact®)

Glucagon-like peptide 1 (GLP1) receptor agonists
- Exenatide (Byetta® and Bydureon®)
- Liraglutide (Victoza® and Saxenda®)
- Lixisenatide (Lyxumia®)
- Albiglutide (Tanzeum®)
- Dulaglutide (Trulicity®)

- Semaglutide (Ozempic®)

Dipeptidyl peptidase 4 (DPP4) inhibitors (the "gliptins")
- Sitagliptin (Januvia®)
- Saxagliptin (Onglyza®)
- Linagliptin (Tradjenta®)
- Alogliptin (Nesina®)
- Vildagliptin (Galvus®)
- Alogliptin (Nesina®, Vipidia®)
- Metformin and alogliptin (Kazano®)
- Sitagliptin and metformin (Janumet®)

Alpha-glucosidase Inhibitors
- Acarbose (Precose®)
- Miglitol (Glyset®)

The Good News

The good news is that the new guidelines make recommendations that will allow more people to receive potentially life-saving interventions for stroke.

As far as stroke treatment goes, the new stroke guidelines from 2018 make recommendations that will allow more patients to be treated for stroke using clot removing procedures. This is because the window of time that people could be treated using these procedures has been broadened from 6 hours to up to 24 hours (for certain people).[5]

Another update to the stroke guidelines is that newer anticoagulants can now be used, offering people more options than just warfarin (Coumadin®). Newer drugs don't require as many lab tests but may be more expensive depending on your insurance.

A group of cholesterol medications called 'statins' are highly recommended by the new guidelines. They urge prescribers to consider using them to reduce the risk of stroke.

We not have more tools in our tool box to prevent stroke and to treat stroke so we can help give more people their lives back after a stroke.

REFERENCES

1. Sidney S, Rosamond WD, Howard VJ, Luepker RV; National Forum for Heart Disease and Stroke Prevention. The "heart disease and stroke statistics-2013 update" and the need for a national cardiovascular surveillance system. *Circulation.* 2013;127(1):21-23.

2. American Heart Association, American Stroke Association. Stroke webinar 7: acute stroke therapy. https://learn.heart.org/Activity/2699791/Detail.aspx#lnk2699791.

3. Mozaffarian D, Benjamin EJ, Go AS, et al. Heart disease and stroke statistics-2015 update: a report from the American Heart Association. *Circulation.* 2015;131(4):e29-e322.

4. Vaartjes I, O'Flaherty M, Capewell S, Kappelle J, Bots M. Remarkable decline in ischemic stroke mortality is not matched by changes in incidence. *Stroke.* 2013;44(3):591-597.

5. William J. Powers, MD, FAHA, Chair; Alejandro A. Rabinstein, MD, FAHA, Vice Chair; Teri Ackerson, BSN, RN; 2018 Guidelines for the Early Management of Patients With Acute Ischemic Stroke. A Guideline for Healthcare Professionals From the American Heart Association/American Stroke Association. Stroke 2018;49:e46-e110.

6. Emberson et al. Effect of treatment delay, age, and stroke severity on the effects of intravenous thrombolysis with alteplase for acute ischemic stroke: a meta-analysis of individual patient data from randomised trials. Lancet 2014;384(9958):1929 Saver et al. JAMA 2013;309(23):2480.

7. Gregory Y. H. Lip, MD; Amitava Banerjee, MD, DPhil; Giuseppe Boriani, MD, PhD et. al. Antithrombotic Therapy for Atrial Fibrillation. CHEST Guideline and Expert Panel ReportCHEST 2018; 154(5):1121-1201

8. Goff et al. 2013 ACC/AHA Cardiovascular Risk Assessment Guideline. JACC Vol. 63, No. 25, 2014.

9. Anderson KM, Castelli WP, Levy D. Cholesterol and mortality. 30 years of follow-up from the Framingham study. JAMA 1987 Apr 24;257 (16):2176-80.

10. Robert DuBroff and Michel de Lorgeril. Cholesterol confusion and statin controversy. World J Cardiol. 2015. Jul 26; 7(7): 404-409.

11. Al-Mallah, MH, Hatahet H, Cavalcante JL, Khanal S. Low admission LDL-cholesterol is associated with increased 3-year all-cause mortality in patients with non ST segment elevation myocardial infarction. Cardiol J 2009;16:227-33.

12. Krumholz HM et al. Lack of association between cholesterol and coronary heart disease mortality and morbidity and all-cause mortality in persons older than 70 years. JAMA.272, 1335-40, 1994.

13. Gouya G, Arrich J, Wolzt M, et al. Antiplatelet treatment for prevention of cerebrovascular events in patients with vascular diseases: a systematic review and meta-analysis. Stroke. 2014;45:492–503.

14. Furie KL, Kasner SE, Adams RJ, Albers GW, Bush RL, Fagan SC, et al; American Heart Association Stroke Council, Council on Cardiovascular Nursing, Council on Clinical Cardiology, and Interdisciplinary Council on Quality of Care and Outcomes Research. Guidelines for the prevention of stroke in patients with stroke or transient ischemic attack: a guideline for healthcare professionals from the American Heart Association/ American Stroke Association. Stroke. 2011;42:227–276.

15. Kernan WN, Ovbiagele B, et. al. Guidelines for the prevention of stroke in patients with stroke and transient ischemic attack: a guideline for healthcare professionals from the American Heart Association/American Stroke Association. Stroke. 2014 Jul;45(7):2160-236.

16. Malhotra K, Goyal N, et. al. Ticagrelor for stroke prevention in patients with vascular risk factors: A systematic review and meta-analysis. J Neurol Sci. 2018 Jul 15;390:212-218.

17. *Hass WK, Easton JD, Adams HP Jr, Pryse-Phillips W, Molony BA, Anderson S, Kamm B (24 August 1989). "A randomized trial˄ comparing ticlopidine hydrochloride with aspirin for the prevention of stroke in high-risk patients. Ticlopidine Aspirin Stroke Study Group". N Engl J Med. 321: 501–507.*

18. Jellinger PS, Handelsman Y, Rosenblit PD, et al. American Association of Clinical Endocrinologists and American College of Endocrinology guidelines for the management of dyslipidemia and prevention of cardiovascular disease. *Endocr Pract*2017;23:1-87

19. O'Gara P.T., Kushner F.G., Ascheim D.D., et al. (2013) 2013 ACCF/AHA guideline for the management of ST-elevation myocardial infarction: a report of the American College of Cardiology Foundation/American Heart Association Task Force on Practice Guidelines. J Am Coll Cardiol **61**:e78–e140.

20. Jellinger PS, Handelsman Y, Rosenblit PD, et al. American Association of Clinical Endocrinologists and American College of Endocrinology guidelines for the management of dyslipidemia and prevention of cardiovascular disease. *Endocr Pract*2017;23:1-8

Stone NJ, Robinson JG, Lichtenstein AH, Bairey Merz CN, Blum CB, Eckel RH, Goldberg AC, Gordon D, Levy D, Lloyd-Jones DM, et al. 2013 ACC/AHA guideline on the treatment of blood cholesterol to reduce atherosclerotic cardiovascular risk in adults: a report of the American College of Cardiology/American Heart Association Task Force on Practice Guidelines. J Am Coll Cardiol. 2014;63:2889–2934.

CHAPTER 7

ATRIAL FIBRILLATION (a. fib.)

The Empowered Medicine Guide to Atrial Fibrillation

How to Use This Chapter

Welcome to the Empowered Medicine Guide to atrial fibrillation (a. fib). First, we will go over the basics of a. fib such as what it is and why treating it is important. Then, because having a. fib. can put you at a higher risk for stroke, we will follow a step by step process for figuring out if aspirin or anticoagulation is the right move for you. Finally, we will look at medications used to manage a. fib in more detail.

If you wish, use Appendix VII in the back of this book to log your own information. This makes calculations easy and sharing with your doctor even easier. Also, at the end of this chapter you will find a section called 'The Bottom Line'. This box sums up the main points of the chapter.

Atrial Fibrillation (a. fib): The Basics

A. fib. is a condition where the heart beats irregularly. This is due to disorganized electrical signals in the chambers of the heart. When you have a. fib., your heart beat might often feel fluttery and fast.

The heart's job is to pump oxygen rich blood to the rest of the body. But because of this irregular rhythm, blood is not pumped as efficiently as it should be. This can lead to heart failure. Also with a. fib., blood can pool in the chambers of the heart, allowing tiny clots to form. These clots can travel to the brain through the arteries and cause a stroke. A stroke is when there is damage to the brain due to a lack of blood flow.

So as you can see, treating a. fib. and protecting yourself against stroke and heart failure is very important. There are non-surgical and surgical procedures to manage a. fib. When first being diagnosed with a. fib, your doctor may try to get your heart into the right rhythm again by using either medicine, surgery or electrical current. If a. fib. cannot be converted into a normal heart rhythm, medications to keep the blood from clotting are usually used to protect against stroke.

Non-medication Options to Manage Atrial Fibrillation

Pacemakers and Defibrillators

A pacemaker is a small device that is implanted in the chest. It has wires that go into the heart so it can regulate your heart beat. Pacemakers cannot "fix" a. fib. but can be used to stimulate the heart when the heart rate is too slow (which can sometimes happen with a. fib.).

Many pacemakers act as a defibrillator as well. This means, it can sense when your heart goes into a dangerous rhythm and, in an emergency situation, can deliver a burst of electrical current or "shock" to try to reset your heart.

Some devices only have the pacemaker or defibrillator function. Others serve as both a pacemaker and defibrillator. It may depend on how your doctor has programmed your device.

Ablation

Ablation is a procedure that creates scar tissue in the heart. This scar tissue gets rid of any extra electrical activity that may be causing the heart to beat irregularly. There are open-heart ablation procedures and catheter ablation procedures. Catheter ablation is a minimally-invasive procedure. It involves inserting long flexible tubes through blood vessels to map the heart's electrical signals. Then using very hot or cold temperature, the over-active tissue is destroyed. Sometimes ablation involves placing a pacemaker as well.

Open-heart ablation is just like catheter ablation, but instead of accessing the heart through a few small incisions, it involves open heart surgery. This surgery involves breaking the sternum and opening up the rib cage.

Ablation is typically reserved for patients who do not respond to electrical cardioversion or anti-arrhythmic drugs.

Electrical Cardioversion

Electrical cardioversion is a non-surgical procedure where the patient receives an electrical shock to "reset" the heart's electrical system. Note that the patient is sedated and comfortable during this procedure. Generally, people do not remember the procedure when they wake up.

Before the heart's rhythm and rate are reset, it is recommended to take anticoagulation medications (we will discuss anticoagulation shortly) for 3 weeks before and 4 weeks after cardioversion to make sure there are no clots present in the heart that could cause a stroke.[3] If this is not possible, a transesophageal echocardiogram (TEE) can be performed. This is a type of ultrasound that allows the doctor to see if there are any clots present in the chambers of the heart before the electrical cardioversion is done. This is to decrease the risk of having a clot travel from the heart to the brain during the cardioversion procedure. Remember that clots in the brain can cause a lack of oxygen to the brain which can cause a stroke.

If anticoagulation was not started before the TEE, TEE is performed, anticoagulation should start before or with the TEE and be continued for 4 weeks after the TEE.[3]

Using Anti-arrhythmic Medications to Treat Atrial Fibrillation

If you have a. fib., your doctor may have you take a medication that helps slow down your heart rate and/or helps your heart beat at a more regular rhythm. Here are a list of drugs commonly prescribed for one or both of these purposes. Some of these are not used very often for the treatment of a. fib but may be used with other arrhythmias or electrical conduction issues you may be having, so they've been included here. You can read more about these classes of drugs in the "Medications for the Management of Atrial Fibrillation" section toward the end of this chapter.

Table 1: **Drugs for Heart Rate and/or Rhythm**

Class of Medication	Examples
Drugs for Heart Rate	
Calcium channel blockers	Verapamil (Calan SR®, Verelean®) Diltiazem (Cardizem CD®, Dilacor XR®)
Beta blockers	Acebutolol (Sectral®) Atenolol (Tenormin®) Betaxolol (Kerlone®) Labetalol (Trandate®) Bisoprolol (Zebeta®) Carvedilol (Coreg®) Metoprolol tartrate (Lopressor®) Metoprolol succinate (Toprol XL®) Nebivolol (Bystolic®) Penbutolol (Levatol®) Propranolol (Inderal®)
	Sotalol (Betapace®) Nadolol (Corgard®) Pindolol (Visken®)
Digitalis drugs	Digoxin
Drugs for Heart Rhythm	

Sodium Channel Blockers	Disopyramide (Norpace®)
	Flecainide (Tambocor®)
	Mexiletine (Mexitil®)
	Quinidine
	Procainamide
	Propafenone (Rythmol®)
Class III Anti-arrhythmic	Amiodarone (Cordarone®, Pacerone®)

Reducing Your Risk of Stroke with Aspirin and Anticoagulants

If you have a. fib. your doctor may first recommend trying to fix the a. fib. by using one of the procedures or anti-arrhythmic medications we just discussed. If the a. fib. does not go away, it may be recommended that you take an anticoagulant medication to help prevent stroke. Like aspirin, anticoagulation medications are drugs that help keep your blood from clotting.

If you have a. fib, do not have an artificial heart valve and meet the criteria, you may be a candidate for oral anticoagulation. To see if you meet criteria, see Table 2. Points are awarded, depending on which risk factors you have. The number of points you have will let you and your doctor know if you should consider an anticoagulation drug to decrease your risk of stroke.

Note: The stroke risk assessment above is meant for people with "nonvalvular" a. fib. Sometimes you will hear the terms "nonvalvular" and "valvular a. fib". Valvular a. fib. generally refers to a. fib where one of the two scenarios is present:[3]

1. **There is moderate to severe mitral stenosis** (narrowing of the mitral valve opening that blocks blood flow within the heart) **or...**

2. **There is an artificial (mechanical) heart valve** (Note that biosynthetic heart valves, like those from a human donor or those created from animal donors do not usually require anticoagulation).

So by definition, nonvalvular a. fib. is a. fib in the absence of moderate-to-severe mitral stenosis or a mechanical heart valve.

If you have "valvular" a. fib (for example, an artificial heart valve) warfarin is recommended (instead of apixaban, dabigatran, rivaroxaban or edoxaban). You can read more about artificial heart valves in the "Stroke" chapter of this book.

So if you have nonvalvular a. fib., continue on to the a. fib stroke risk assessment below. Fill in the boxes that describe you.

Table 2: **Stroke Risk Assessment for Atrial Fibrillation**[7]

	Criteria		Points	
C	Congestive Heart Failure	☐	Yes	1
		☐	No	0
H	High blood pressure (> 140/90 mmHg on at least 2 occasions or current blood pressure treatment	☐	Yes	1
		☐	No	0
A	Age 75 years or older	☐	Yes	2
		☐	No	0
D	Diabetes mellitus (fasting glucose > 125 mg/dL or treatment with an oral hypoglycemic agent or insulin)	☐	Yes	1
		☐	No	0

S	Stroke or transient ischemic attack (TIA)- both of these involve a loss of blood flow to the brain	☐	Yes	2
		☐	No	0
V	Vascular disease (Prior heart attack, peripheral arterial disease or aortic plaque)	☐	Yes	1
		☐	No	0
A	Age 65 to 74 years old	☐	Yes	1
		☐	No	0
SC	Sex Category female	☐	Yes	1
		☐	No	0
			Total Points:	

STEP 2: Add up the points you earned. Write the answer in the space labeled "Total points" above.

STEP 3: Check to box below that corresponds with how many "Total points" you have. Note what medications are recommended for you.

Table 3: **A. fib. Stroke Risk Score**

	Score	**Risk**
☐	0	Low risk. May not require anticoagulation
☐	1	Low-moderate risk. Should consider anticoagulation

In general, those with a score of 1 should consider full oral anticoagulation. This means aspirin is probably not potent enough for you, and you should choose another medication from Table 3. ***The one exception, however, is in patients who have a score of 1 due to gender alone. In these patients (female < 65 years old without other risk factors), antithrombotic therapy should NOT be given.***

If your score indicates you might be a candidate for blood thinners, you will have the following medications to choose from.

Table 4: **Types of Anticoagulation Used to Treat Atrial Fibrillation**[*3]

• **Warfarin (Coumadin®)**
• **Apixaban (Eliquis®)**
• **Dabigatran (Pradaxa®)**
• **Rivaroxaban (Xarelto®)**
• **Edoxaban (Savaysa®)**

Apixaban, dabigatran, rivaroxaban and edoxaban should be considered before warfarin in people with non-valvular a. fib.

The newest atrial fibrillation guidelines recommend using apixaban, dabigatran, rivaroxaban or edoxaban instead of warfarin when anticoagulation is needed.[3] There are several reasons for this. First of all, studies that have shown there appears to be a reduced risk of intracranial (inside the head) bleeding with apixaban, dabigatran, rivaroxaban, and edoxaban when compared to warfarin. Also, these newer drugs have fewer drug and food interactions. Finally, people taking warfarin must be seen frequently to have labs drawn to make sure the dose of warfarin that is being given does not need to be adjusted.

The 2019 atrial fibrillation guideline update recommends keeping the following in mind when considering anticoagulation therapy[3]:

- Anticoagulation besides warfarin (apixaban, dabigatran, rivaroxaban or edoxaban) are recommended first for patients with nonvalvular a. fib.

- Warfarin is recommended for people with a. fib. who have an artificial heart valve.

- People taking warfarin should have their international normalized ratio (INR) monitored at least weekly during initiation and at least monthly when the INR is stable (we'll talk about INR in the medication section at the end of this chapter).

- Kidney and liver function should be evaluated before starting anticoagulation and then at least yearly.

- After starting anticoagulation therapy, it is recommended that your doctor reevaluate the need for anticoagulation periodically.

- When deciding whether or not to prescribe an anticoagulant, it is recommended your doctor take into consideration the risk of stroke and bleeding as well as patient preferences.

Key to Success

New anticoagulation drugs are thought to have less drug and food interactions than warfarin.

Factors That Put You at a Higher Risk of Bleeding with Atrial Fibrillation

Even if you meet the criteria in Table 2, anticoagulation therapy may not be for you. Because anticoagulation helps prevent your blood from clotting, it can put you at a higher risk for abnormal bleeding. Abnormal bleeding can be especially serious when it's in the brain. Other major bleeding (in the GI tract for example) can be very serious as well. For this reason, before starting anticoagulation therapy, it's important to see if you are at an increased risk for abnormal bleeding. Before prescribing anticoagulation therapy, your doctor will weigh your risk of stroke with your risk of having a major bleeding incident.

One tool your doctor may use to calculate your bleeding risk is called the HAS-BLED score. The tool used to calculate this score was developed to figure out just what your risk of abnormal bleeding is. To calculate this, your doctor will plug in numbers from your most recent tests. One of these tests is called the INR. It is basically a number that your doctor looks at when you are prescribed warfarin (Coumadin®). The INR gives the doctor an idea of how quickly your blood is clotting.

Here is a look at what is taken into consideration with the HAS-BLED test.

Table 5: **Items Taken into Consideration with the HAS-BLED Score[2]**

• **Uncontrolled high blood pressure (SBP > 160 mmHg)** • **Kidney disease** • **Liver disease** • **History of stroke** • **Prior major bleeding or predisposed to bleeding** • **Unstable or high INR values** • **Age > 65 years old** • **Using medications that predispose you to bleeding (NSAIDS, clopidogrel, aspirin)** • **Alcohol use (> 8 drinks per week)**

*SBP = systolic blood pressure

It is suggested that patients who have a HAS-BLED score of 3 or higher be prescribed anticoagulation and that they should be followed frequently by a doctor. In certain patients, especially in those who have survived a bleed in the brain, other options besides oral anticoagulation may be recommended. These options might include procedures like the left atrial appendage occlusion procedure or the Watchman® device (see below).

Non-medication Options to Prevent Stroke

There are non-medication options people with a. fib can use to decrease their risk of stroke. For example, the Watchman® device is a small gadget that looks kind of like a net. It is implanted in the heart. It can keep clots that form from traveling to the brain and causing a stroke. The procedure usually takes no more than an hour and typically involves staying the hospital one day. According to the 2019 update to the guidelines, oral anticoagulation is still the preferred therapy for stroke prevention for most patients with a. fib. and elevated stroke risk. However, the Watchman® may be especially helpful for patients who can't take oral anticoagulation (because of bleeding for example).[3]

It may be helpful to note that The Centers for Medicare & Medicaid Services (CMS) has determined that patients should have a CHADS2 VASC score ≥2 or a CHA2DS2-VASc (see Table 2) score ≥3 to be considered for the device.[3]

Left Atrial Appendage Occlusion

Another non-medication option to help decrease one's risk of stroke with a. fib. is called left atrial appendage (LAA) occlusion. The LAA is a small, ear-shaped sac in the wall of the left atrium of the heart. In people with a. fib, this sac is where blood clots tend to form. The doctor can perform a procedure that seals off this sac. This is thought to eliminate the need for anticoagulation drugs (which we will discuss next!).

Medications Used to Manage Atrial Fibrillation

Until fairly recently in medical history, there were few choices available for the prevention of stroke in people with a. fib. (who don't have heart valves). Now, newer medications are available that require less monitoring and have less drug and food interactions.

Aspirin and Anticoagulants

Aspirin or Anticoagulants (like those in Table 4) can be used in people with atrial fibrillation (and other conditions) to help prevent clots from forming, thereby reducing your risk of stroke.

Aspirin

Aspirin is considered an "Antiplatelet drug". Platelets are tiny disk-shaped cells found in the blood that bond together to form a clot when the body needs to stop bleeding. Aspirin helps keep platelets from sticking together, therefore, preventing the blood from clotting.

Take aspirin exactly as recommended by your doctor. If it smells like vinegar, do not use it because it is probably spoiled.

Possible side effects of aspirin include:

- ringing in the ears
- asthma
- hallucinations
- seizure
- nausea and/or vomiting
- stomach pain
- stomach ulcers
- fever
- swelling
- worsening of heart failure
- worsening of gout
- abnormal bleeding
- worsening of kidney disease

I know some of these side effects seem a little outlandish but drug companies are required to report all possible side effects that happened while people were taking the drug. Most of these side effects are rarely seen with aspirin. However, it's important to know that if you find yourself coughing up blood, or coffee-ground-like vomit, you will need to contact your doctor or get emergency help right away. This may indicate that there is bleeding in the stomach.

Aspirin can also be tough on the stomach lining; sometimes breaking it down and causing ulcers. These ulcers can bleed. This bleeding is especially concerning because the aspirin also inhibits blood clotting. This means it may be difficult to control the bleeding once it starts. Because aspirin can be irritating to the stomach lining, it can be taken with food if needed. This may help keep the aspirin from irritating your stomach.

Aspirin therapy may not be a good choice for people who have a bleeding disorder or have had a recent stomach or intestinal bleed. So before you take aspirin, let your doctor know if you have a history of abnormal bleeding. Also, before you take aspirin, let your doctor know if you have asthma because aspirin may make it worse.

People with kidney disease should also talk to their doctor before taking aspirin. Aspirin may also worsen heart failure, if you already have it. Finally, people with gout should know that aspirin may increase the level of uric acid in the body. This can worsen gout.

Warfarin (Coumadin®)

Warfarin is an anticoagulant. Vitamin K is needed for the blood to make a clot. Warfarin works by inhibiting vitamin K dependent clotting factors. This helps keep the blood from clotting.

Warfarin can be used to prevent stroke in people who have atrial fibrillation (a. fib.), have an artificial heart valve and in those who have had a heart attack.

Warfarin requires a lab test called an International Normalized Ration (INR) to be monitored while you are taking it. This involves having a blood test. The blood can be obtained by a finger prick using a small, hand held device or by a blood draw.

The average person who doesn't take warfarin will have an INR of 1.0. This is normal. However, the ideal INR goal range for people with a. fib. who are taking warfarin is 2 to 3. People taking warfarin for a mechanical heart valve usually have an INR goal of 2.5 to 3.5.

While taking warfarin, the INR is monitored frequently and the dose of warfarin is adjusted to keep the INR at goal. The INR will be monitored more frequently in the beginning (possibly once or twice a week) but can be spaced out more when the INR becomes stable.

It can take several days to achieve a goal INR. This is why sometimes when warfarin is started for other health conditions besides a. fib., it is first overlapped with other 'blood thinning' drugs like heparin, enoxaparin (Lovenox®), or fondaparinux (Arixtra®) until the goal INR is reached. However, this overlapping of therapies is not recommended for treating a. fib. and may do more harm than good. It could possibly lead to unwanted bleeding. For this reason, warfarin is generally started by itself when treating a. fib.

Because warfarin works with vitamin K, the food you eat can affect how warfarin works and affect your INR. ***Vitamin K rich foods decrease the INR, making you more prone to developing a clot.*** Vitamin K rich foods include:

- Greens
- Broccoli
- Brussel sprouts
- Beef liver
- Pork chops
- Chicken
- Green beans
- Prunes
- Kiwi
- Cheese
- Avocado
- Peas

You don't necessarily need to avoid these foods. You should, however, aim to keep your consumption of them consistent. For example, if you like to have a green salad with your dinner 4 times a week, then eat it 4 times per week consistently.

Warfarin also has many more drug interactions than the other anticoagulants. This is because it affects enzymes in the liver that are responsible for eliminating other drugs in the body. Drugs that frequently interact with warfarin are listed below. All of the drugs listed below increase the INR so the dose of warfarin will have to be decreased while taking these other drugs:

- Antibiotics
- Antifungals
- NSAIDS like aspirin, ibuprofen, naproxen
- Acetaminophen
- Some heart rhythm drugs (amiodarone)

There are many supplements that interact with warfarin too including:

Table 6: **Supplements That Interact with Warfarin**

Decreases INR, increasing the risk of clotting
Coenzyme Q10
St. John's Wort
Ginseng
Green tea (contains Vitamin K)
Increases INR, increasing the risk of bleeding
Ginkgo Biloba
Garlic

This is just a small portion of the list of drugs that can interact with warfarin.

Empowered U

True or False:

Warfarin interacts with many over the counter supplements

Answer: true

Before taking warfarin, let your doctor know if you have a history of:
- abnormal bleeding
- stomach ulcers or intestinal bleeding
- bleeding in the brain
- bleeding or clotting disorder
- liver disease
- high blood pressure
- Recent spinal anesthesia or spinal tap

Potential side effects of dipyridamole may include:
- abnormal bleeding
- headache

Let your doctor know right away if you have:
- abnormal bleeding like: nose bleeds, pink urine, coughing up blood or coffee ground-like vomit, have bright red blood in your stools or black, tarry stools
- unusual bruising
- symptoms of stroke (drooping of one side of the face, weakness on one side of the body or difficulty talking)

If you experience any symptoms of an allergic reaction (trouble breathing, swelling of the throat or tongue) call emergency help immediately.

If you are planning surgery (including dental procedures), make sure your surgeon/dentist knows. Warfarin may need to be stopped before surgery and restarted after. But do not stop taking it without first letting your doctor know, even if you have signs of bleeding because stopping it can put you at risk for stroke.

Anticoagulation in Special Circumstances

Sometimes people with a. fib. have other health conditions that may require additional anticoagulation medications. For examples, sometimes people with a. fib. and who have had stents placed in the blood vessels of the heart are prescribed "triple therapy". This triple therapy consists of and oral anticoagulant, aspirin and a $P2Y_{12}$ inhibitor. A $P2Y_{12}$ inhibitor is a drug that help keep blood from clotting from help keeping platelets from sticking together. Examples of $P2Y_{12}$ inhibitors include clopidogrel (Plavis®), prasugrel (Effient®), ticagrelor (Brillinta®), and cangrelor (Kengreal®)

Anti-arrhythmia Medications

As we mentioned before, if you have a. fib. your doctor may prescribe medications that affect the rate and/or rhythm of your heart. Sometimes this can help the heart reorganize its electrical signals and beat with a normal rate and rhythm again. Here is a rundown of the main classes of heart rate and arrhythmia drugs.

Table 7: **Drugs for Heart Rate and/or Rhythm**

Class of Medication	Examples
Drugs for Heart Rate	
Calcium channel blockers	Verapamil (Calan SR®, Verelean®) Diltiazem (Cardizem CD®, Dilacor XR®)
Beta blockers	Acebutolol (Sectral®) Atenolol (Tenormin®) Betaxolol (Kerlone®) Labetalol (Trandate®) Bisoprolol (Zebeta®) Carvedilol (Coreg®) Metoprolol tartrate (Lopressor®) Metoprolol succinate (Toprol XL®) Nebivolol (Bystolic®) Penbutolol (Levatol®) Propranolol (Inderal®) Sotalol (Betapace®) Nadolol (Corgard®) Pindolol (Visken®)
Digitalis drugs	Digoxin
Drugs for Heart Rhythm	
Sodium Channel Blockers	Disopyramide (Norpace®) Flecainide (Tambocor®) Mexiletine (Mexitil®) Quinidine Procainamide Propafenone (Rythmol®)
Class III Anti-arrhythmic	Amiodarone (Cordarone®, Pacerone®)

Calcium Channel Blockers

Calcium channel blockers work by blocking some of the calcium that enters the muscles of the heart. This has an effect of slowing down the force at which the heart beats. It also dilates (widens) the blood vessels a bit so blood can move freely through them. Calcium channel blockers are used to treat many health conditions including high blood pressure, chest pain, and heart arrhythmias.

Verapamil and diltiazem differ from amlodipine (another calcium channel blocker) a bit. Verapamil and diltiazem reduce the strength of the heart's contractions. Amlodipine does not affect the strength of the heart's contraction much. Amlodipine relaxes the blood vessels. It is usually used to treat high blood pressure and NOT to treat abnormal heart rhythms.

Side Effects of Calcium Channel Blockers May Include:

- Headache
- Constipation
- Rash
- Nausea
- Edema
- Flushing
- Drowsiness
- Low blood pressure
- Dizziness
- Sexual dysfunction
- Liver dysfunction
- Overgrowth of gums

Let your doctor know right away if you have:

- liver toxicity/jaundice
- dizziness or feel like you're going to faint

Get emergency medical help if you have signs of an allergic reaction: hives; difficult breathing; swelling of your face, lips, tongue, or throat.

Beta blockers

Beta blockers work by blocking the effects of the hormone epinephrine (AKA adrenaline). Adrenaline is the 'fight or flight' hormone produced by the body when it senses a threat to its survival. Among other actions, adrenaline shunts blood away from the digestive tract, sex organs, and skin and sends it to the heart, muscles and lungs to prepare the body to fight or run.

By blocking the actions of adrenaline, beta blockers cause your heart to beat slower and with less force. This lowers your blood pressure and decreases the work for your heart. Some beta blockers also help keep your blood vessels dilated so that blood can move through them easier.

Let's look at some examples of beta blockers.

Table 8: Examples of Beta-blockers

Type of beta-blocker	Details
Beta-blockers that target the heart • Atenolol (Tenormin®) Betaxolol (Kerlone®) • Bisoprolol (Zebeta®) • Metoprolol (Lopressor®, Toprol-XL®)	• These drugs focus on the heart • These drugs are preferred in people who have asthma, chronic obstructive pulmonary disease (COPD) and emphysema
Beta blockers that target the heart and also help widen blood vessels • Nebivolol (Bystolic®)	• These drugs focus on the heart but also help relax the blood vessels (widen the blood vessels so blood can flow easier)
More beta blockers that target the heart and also help relax blood vessels • Carvedilol (Coreg®)	• These drugs, like nebivolol, focus on the heart and also help relax blood vessels. They work in a slightly different way than

Type of beta-blocker	Details
• Labetalol (Normodyne®, Trandate®)	nebivolol • Carvedilol is preferred in people with heart failure
Beta-blockers that don't just target the heart (they affect the lungs too) • Nadolol (Corgard®) • Propranolol (Inderal®)	• These are generally not prescribed for patients with asthma, chronic obstructive pulmonary disease (COPD) and emphysema because these drugs can affect the lungs as well as the heart
Beta-blockers that block the effects of adrenaline but can also stimulate the heart • Acebutolol (Sectral®) • Penbutolol (Levatol®) • Pindolol (Visken®)	• These are usually avoided for the treatment of high blood pressure, especially in people with cardiovascular disease or heart failure.

Side Effects of Beta Blockers May Include:
- Cold hands and feet
- Stomach cramps
- Dizziness
- Slow heart beat
- Low blood pressure
- Tiredness and sleep disturbances
- Increases in blood sugar
- Masking of symptoms of low blood sugar (so may have low blood sugar and not realize it)

Let your doctor know right away if you have:
- Dizziness or feel like you're going to faint
- Very slow heart beat
- Very low blood pressure

Get emergency medical help if you have signs of an allergic reaction: hives; difficult breathing; swelling of your face, lips, tongue, or throat.

Digoxin

Digoxin is made from the leaves of the digitalis plant. It's used to treat health conditions like heart failure and atrial fibrillation (a. fib.). A. fib., in particular, is known to put one at a higher risk of stroke.

Your digoxin levels will need to be measured periodically using a blood test. This is to ensure the amount of digoxin in your body is within the target range. It's important to make sure you are getting enough digoxin so you will see the potential benefits. It's also important to make sure you're not getting too much digoxin. Digoxin levels that are too high can lead to a higher incidence of side effects and abnormal heart rhythms.

Before taking digoxin, let your doctor know if you have a history of:

- Sick sinus syndrome or AV block
- History of heart attack
- Wolff-Parkinson-White syndrome
- Thyroid disorder
- Are taking a diuretic ("water pill")
- Abnormal electrolyte levels (like potassium, calcium, magnesium)
- Kidney disease

Side Effects of Digoxin May Include:

- Nausea, vomiting
- Irregular heart beat
- Vision disturbances
- Confusion, hallucinations
- Weakness
- Dizziness

- Headache
- Enlarged breasts in men
- Rash

Let your doctor know right away if you have:

- Dizziness or feel like you're going to faint
- Very slow heart beat

Get emergency medical help if you have signs of an allergic reaction: hives; difficult breathing; swelling of your face, lips, tongue, or throat.

Sodium Channel Blockers

Sodium channel blockers are a class of anti-arrhythmia drugs that work by slowing the rate and strength of the electrical impulses within the heart. This can 'calm down' erratic heart rhythms.

As noted in Table 8, sodium channel blockers include:

- Disopyramide (Norpace®)
- Flecainide (Tambocor®)
- Mexiletine (Mexitil®)
- Quinidine
- Procainamide
- Propafenone (Rythmol®)

Side Effects of Sodium Channel Blockers May Include:

- Very fast heart rate
- Dry mouth
- Urinary retention
- Blurred vision
- Constipation
- Diarrhea
- Nausea
- Headache
- Dizziness

Quinidine can cause a potentially fatal condition called torsades de pointes in certain people. It's important to take quinidine exactly as prescribed and to follow up regularly with your doctor while you are taking quinidine.

Also, it's important to note that disopyramide should not be used in certain people with heart failure.

Let your doctor know right away if you have:

- Very fast or very slow heart rate
- Dizziness like you're going to faint

Get emergency medical help if you have signs of an allergic reaction: hives; difficult breathing; swelling of your face, lips, tongue, or throat.

Amiodarone

Amiodarone helps the heart maintain a normal rhythm.

Before taking amiodarone, let your doctor know if you have a history of:

- Lung disease
- Thyroid disease
- A neurological disorder
- Liver disease

Side effects of Amiodarone may include:

- Wheezing or other lung problems
- Heart arrhythmia (abnormal heart rhythms)
- Dizziness
- Blurred vision
- liver toxicity/jaundice
- Thyroid toxicity-problems like weight loss, thinning hair, feeling hot, jitteriness, tremors, goiter (swelling in the neck)
- Loss of coordination
- Muscle weakness
- Nausea, vomiting
- constipation

Let your doctor know right away if you have:

- Wheezing or other lung problems
- Very fast or slow or force full heart beat
- Dizziness like you're going to faint
- Blurred vision
- liver toxicity/jaundice
- Signs of thyroid problems like weight loss, thinning hair, feeling hot, jitteriness, tremors, goiter (swelling in the neck)
- Loss of coordination
- Muscle weakness

How Can I Expect My Treatment to Progress?

For some people, a. fib. may come and go. This is called "Paroxysmal a. fib" For other people, a. fib is constant and may cause them to have bouts of palpitations or periods of time where their heart rate is really high. Sometimes, a. fib. goes away on its own. If you find yourself with a. fib. that won't go away, don't worry. By managing your symptoms with antiarrhythmia medications and anticoagulation, you will find that a. fib. does not have to slow you down or define who you are.

The Bottom Line

A. fib. is a condition where the heart beats irregularly. This is due to disorganized electrical signals in the chambers of the heart. When you have a. fib., your heart beat might often feel fluttery and fast.

With a. fib., the irregular rhythm can cause blood to pool in the chambers of the heart. This can allow tiny clots to form. These clots can travel to the brain through the arteries and cause a stroke. A stroke is when there is damage to the brain due to a lack of blood flow.

So as you can see, treating a. fib. and protecting yourself against stroke and heart failure is very important. There are non-surgical and surgical procedures used to manage a. fib. When first being diagnosed with a. fib, your doctor may try to get your heart into the right rhythm again by using either medicine, surgery or electrical current. If a. fib.

cannot be converted into a normal heart rhythm, medications to keep the blood from clotting are usually used to protect against stroke.

Some procedures used to manage a. fib include:

- **Pacemakers and Defibrillators**
  - A pacemaker is a small device that is implanted in the chest. It has wires that go into the heart so it can regulate your heart beat. Pacemakers cannot "fix" a. fib. but can be used to stimulate the heart when the heart rate is too slow (which can sometimes happen with a. fib.).

- **Ablation**
  - Ablation is a procedure that creates scar tissue in the heart by using very hot or cold temperatures. This scar tissue gets rid of any extra electrical activity that may be causing the heart to beat irregularly. Ablation is typically reserved for patients who do not respond to electrical cardioversion or anti-arrhythmic drugs.

- **Electrical Cardioversion**
  - Electrical cardioversion is a non-surgical procedure where the patient receives an electrical shock to "reset" the heart's electrical system. Note that the patient is sedated and comfortable during this procedure. Generally, people do not remember the procedure when they wake up. Before the heart's rhythm and rate are reset, it is recommended to take anticoagulation medications (we will discuss anticoagulation shortly) for 3 weeks before and 4 weeks after cardioversion to make sure there are no clots present in the heart that could cause a stroke.[3] If this is not possible, a transesophageal echocardiogram (TEE) can be performed.

If you have a. fib., your doctor may have you take a medication that helps slow down your heart rate and/or helps your heart beat at a more regular rhythm. Here are a list of drugs commonly prescribed for one or both of these purposes. Some of these are not used very often for the treatment of a. fib but may be used with other arrhythmias or electrical conduction issues you may be having, so they've been included here. You can read more about these classes of drugs in the "Medications for the Management of Atrial Fibrillation" section toward the end of this chapter.

If you have a. fib., your doctor may have you take a medication that helps slow down your heart rate and/or helps your heart beat at a more regular rhythm. Here are a list of drugs commonly prescribed for one or both of these purposes. Some of these are not used very often for the treatment of a. fib but may be used with other arrhythmias or electrical conduction issues you may be having, so they've been included here. You can read more about these classes of drugs in the "Medications for the Management of Atrial Fibrillation" section toward the end of this chapter.

Drugs for Heart Rate and/or Rhythm

Class of Medication	Examples
Drugs for Heart Rate	
Calcium channel blockers	Verapamil (Calan SR®, Verelean®) Diltiazem (Cardizem CD®, Dilacor XR®)
Beta blockers	Acebutolol (Sectral®) Atenolol (Tenormin®) Betaxolol (Kerlone®) Labetalol (Trandate®) Bisoprolol (Zebeta®) Carvedilol (Coreg®) Metoprolol tartrate (Lopressor®) Metoprolol succinate (Toprol XL®) Nebivolol (Bystolic®) Penbutolol (Levatol®) Propranolol (Inderal®) Sotalol (Betapace®) Nadolol (Corgard®) Pindolol (Visken®)
Digitalis drugs	Digoxin
Drugs for Heart Rhythm	

Sodium Channel Blockers	Disopyramide (Norpace®)
	Flecainide (Tambocor®)
	Mexiletine (Mexitil®)
	Quinidine
	Procainamide
	Propafenone (Rythmol®)
Class III Anti-arrhythmic	Amiodarone (Cordarone®, Pacerone®)

If you have a. fib. your doctor may first recommend trying to fix the a. fib. by using one of the procedures or anti-arrhythmic medications we just discussed. If the a. fib. does not go away, it may be recommended that you take an anticoagulant medication to help prevent stroke. Like aspirin, anticoagulation medications are drugs that help keep your blood from clotting.

If you have a. fib, do not have an artificial heart valve and meet the criteria, you may be a candidate for oral anticoagulation. See if you meet criteria in the table below. Points are awarded, depending on which risk factors you have. The number of points you have will let you and your doctor know if you should consider an anticoagulation drug to decrease your risk of stroke.

Stroke Risk Assessment for Atrial Fibrillation[7]

	Criteria		Points	
C	Congestive Heart Failure	☐	Yes	1
		☐	No	0
H	High blood pressure (> 140/90 mmHg on at least 2 occasions or current blood pressure treatment	☐	Yes	1
		☐	No	0
A	Age 75 years or older	☐	Yes	2
		☐	No	0
D	Diabetes mellitus (fasting glucose > 125 mg/dL or treatment with an oral hypoglycemic agent or insulin)	☐	Yes	1
		☐	No	0
S	Stroke or transient ischemic attack (TIA)- both of these involve a loss of blood flow to the brain	☐	Yes	2
		☐	No	0

V	Vascular disease (Prior heart attack, peripheral arterial disease or aortic plaque)	☐	Yes	1
		☐	No	0
A	Age 65 to 74 years old	☐	Yes	1
		☐	No	0
SC	Sex Category female	☐	Yes	1
		☐	No	0
			Total Points:	

STEP 2: Add up the points you earned. Write the answer in the space labeled "Total points" above.

STEP 3: Check to box below that corresponds with how many "Total points" you have. Note what medications are recommended for you.

A. fib. Stroke Risk Score

	Score	Risk
☐	0	Low risk. May not require anticoagulation
☐	1	Low-moderate risk. Should consider anticoagulation

In general, those with a score of 1 should consider full oral anticoagulation instead of aspirin. *** The one exception, however, is in patients who have a score of 1 due to gender alone. In these patients (female < 65 years old without other risk factors), antithrombotic therapy should NOT be given.***

If your score on the stroke risk assessment above indicates you might be a candidate for anticoagulation, you will have the following medications to choose from.

Types of Anticoagulation Used to Treat Atrial Fibrillation[3]

- **Warfarin (Coumadin®)**
- **Apixaban (Eliquis®)**
- **Dabigatran (Pradaxa®)**
- **Rivaroxaban (Xarelto®)**
- **Edoxaban (Savaysa®)**

The newest atrial fibrillation guidelines recommend using apixaban, dabigatran, rivaroxaban, or edoxaban, instead of warfarin when anticoagulation is needed.[3]

Depending on what other health conditions you have, you may find yourself on a combination of the medications described in this chapter. Work closely with your doctor to manage your symptoms and make sure you are getting the most out of your anticoagulation and/or antiarrhythimia medications. A. fib. If you do this, you should find that living with a. fib. has a minimal effect on your day to day activities.

REFERENCES

1. Gregory Y. H. Lip, MD; Amitava Banerjee, MD, DPhil; Giuseppe Boriani, MD, PhD et. al. Antithrombotic Therapy for Atrial Fibrillation. CHEST Guideline and Expert Panel Report CHEST 2018; 154(5):1121-1201

2. Deirdre A. Lane, Gregory Y.H. Lip. Use of the CHA2DS2-VASc and HAS-BLED Scores to Aid Decision Making for Thromboprophylaxis in Nonvalvular Atrial Fibrillation. 14 Aug 2012Circulation. 2012;126:860–865

3. Craig T. January, MD, PhD, FACC, Chair L. Samuel Wann, MD, MACC, FAHA, Vice Chair, et. Al. 2019 AHA/ACC/HRS Focused Update of the 2014 AHA/ACC/HRS Guideline for the Management of Patients With Atrial Fibrillation A Report of the American College of Cardiology/American Heart Association Task Force on Clinical Practice Guidelines and the Heart Rhythm Society Developed in Collaboration With the Society of Thoracic Surgeons

APPENDIX I

2013 ACC/AHA Worksheet for Determining Risk and Dyslipidemia Treatment

Before we begin, please complete each of the following statements:

I have been diagnosed with heart failure	☐ Yes	☐ No
I currently undergo hemodialysis for kidney failure	☐ Yes	☐ No

If you answered 'Yes' to either of the statements above, do not continue. This assessment does not apply. Please consult your doctor to discuss if you should be taking medication to treat dyslipidemia.

STEP 1: Place a check mark to the right of each statement that applies:

1	I have been diagnosed with cardiovascular disease, including angina, previous heart attack, or stroke.	■
2	My LDL-C is 190 mg/dL or above.	■
3	I have type 2 diabetes **AND** am between 40 and 75 years old **AND** my LDL-C 70-189 mg/dL **AND** I do **NOT** have cardiovascular disease.	■
4	I do **NOT** have cardiovascular disease or diabetes **AND** I am 40 to 75 years old **AND** my 10-year risk of heart attack or stroke greater than 7.5% (according to the 2013 risk calculator).	■

If you did not check any of the boxes in STEP 1, congratulations! You do not need to take a statin according to the 2013 guidelines.

If you checked any of the boxes in rows 1, 2, or 3, skip ahead to STEP 3.

If you checked the box in row 4, move on to STEP 2.

STEP 2: Determine your risk using the 2013 ACC/AHA Risk Calculator

Visit: www.cvriskcalculator.com to obtain your risk score. Write your risk score in below for reference.

My CV Risk Score according to the 2013 ACC/AHA Risk Calculator	My Risk Score is _____ %

STEP 3: Determine what statin is right for you

Place checkmarks in any boxes that apply. Tally the number of boxes checked at the bottom of each column.

Moderate-intensity Statins		High-intensity Statins	
☐	Age > 75 years old **AND** have cardiovascular disease (including angina, previous heart attack or stroke)	☐	Age 75 years old or older **AND** have cardiovascular disease (angina, previous heart attack or stroke)
☐	LDL-C < 90 mg/dL **AND** have type 1 or 2 diabetes **AND** age is 40-75 years old **AND**10-year cardiovascular risk less than 7.5%	☐	LDL-C 190 mg/dL or above **AND** I do **NOT** have cardiovascular disease

Moderate-intensity Statins	High-intensity Statins

Moderate-intensity Statins	High-intensity Statins
	☐ Have type 1 or 2 diabetes **AND** am between 40-75 years old **AND** 10-year cardiovascular risk is 7.5% or above according to the 2013 risk calculator
☐ You do **NOT** have diabetes **AND** age is 40-75 years old **AND** LDL-C 190 mg/dL or above **AND** 10-year cardiovascular risk is 7.5% or above (this is not a typo, this statement should occur in both columns)	☐ You do **NOT** have diabetes **AND** age is 40-75 years old **AND** LDL-C 190 mg/dL or above **AND** 10-year cardiovascular risk is 7.5% or above (this is not a typo, this statement should occur in both columns)
Total # Checked Boxes Above: _____	**Total # Checked Boxes Above:** _____

If you have more checkmarks in the moderate-intensity column then consider a moderate-intensity statin on the next page. If you have more checkmarks in the high-intensity column then consider a high-intensity statin.

Moderate-intensity Statins	High-intensity Statins
Lowers LDL-C by 30-50%	Lowers LDL-C by more than 50%
Atorvastatin 10-20 mg	Atorvastatin 40-80 mg
Rosuvastatin 5-10 mg	Rosuvastatin 20-40 mg
Simvastatin 20-40 mg	
Pravastatin 40-80 mg	
Lovastatin 40 mg	
Fluvastatin XL 80 mg	
Fluvastatin 40 mg twice daily	
Pitavastatin 2-4 mg	

FINALLY:

Consider using information from this risk assessment combined with items such as your LDL-P, non-HDL-C, Apo B level, cardiovascular health, weight, and family history to determine if a moderate to high dose statin is for you. Information from this assessment should be discussed with your doctor so that a custom plan of treatment can be outlined for you. Remember that statins carry the risk of certain side effects. Liver dysfunction, nerves problems, and serious muscle conditions are potential side effects of statins.

APPENDIX II

2017 AACE/ACA Worksheet for Determining Risk and Dyslipidemia Treatment

STEP 1: Determine your 10-year risk

Visit one of the following links online to obtain your risk score.

One of the following online calculators may be used*:
• **Framingham Risk Assessment Tool** (https://www.framinghamheartstudy.org/risk-functions/coronary-heart-disease/hard-10-year-risk.php) • **Multi-Ethnic Study of Atherosclerosis (MESA)** 10-year ASCVD Risk with Coronary Artery Calcification Calculator (https://www.mesa-nhlbi. org/MESACHDRisk/MesaRiskScore/RiskScore.aspx) • **Reynolds Risk Score** (http://www.reynoldsriskscore.org) • **United Kingdom Prospective Diabetes Study (UKPDS)** risk engine to calculate ASCVD risk in individuals with T2DM) (https://www.dtu.ox.ac. uk/riskengine)

*Women should use the Reynolds Risk Score or Framingham Risk Assessment.

Write your risk score in below for reference.

My CV Risk Score according to the 2013 ACC/AHA Risk Calculator	My Score is _____ %

STEP 2: Determine your risk factors

Place a check mark to the left of each risk factor that applies:

	High, Very High or Extreme Risk Factors
▪	Type 2 diabetes
▪	Have type 1 diabetes: -duration of more than 15 years **OR...** -with 2 or more of the following (albumin in the urine, stage 3 or 4 chronic kidney disease, initiation of intensive control of blood sugar more than 5 years after diagnosis) **OR...** -poorly controlled hemoglobin A1C **OR...** -insulin resistance with metabolic syndrome

If you checked either box above, move ahead to STEP 3

If you didn't check either box above, move to the table below:

	Major Risk Factors
▪	Age (Men 45 years and older and women 55 years and older)
▪	High LDL-C
▪	High Total cholesterol
▪	High non-HDL-C
▪	Family history of cardiovascular disease
▪	Low HDL-C
▪	Diabetes
▪	High blood pressure
▪	Chronic kidney disease
▪	Cigarette smoking
	Additional Risk Factors
▪	Obesity, abdominal obesity, overweight
	High LDL-P
▪	High Apo B
▪	Presence of small, dense LDL-C (indications include: high TG with low HDL-C, insulin resistance, polycystic ovary syndrome (PCOS), high non-HDL-C, and/or high Apo B)

☐	High TG
☐	Dyslipidemic Triad
☐	Family history of high cholesterol (total, non-HDL-C and/ or LDL-C)
	Non-traditional Risk Factors (all not generally measured)
☐	High lipoprotein (a)
☐	Increased clotting factors
☐	Increased inflammation markers (hsCRP, Lp-PLA2)
☐	Increased homocysteine levels
☐	Increased uric acid
☐	Increased TG-rich remnants (RLP-TG)
___	Total # of risk factors checked

If you have HDL-C > 60 mg/dL, subtract one risk factor. Record your final number of risk factors in the box below:

Number of risk factors	**My Score is _____ risk factors**

STEP 3: Determine your treatment goals

Check the box below that applies to you (if you checked any of the "high, very high, extreme" risk factors boxes in STEP 2, you will fall into the high, very high, or extreme risk categories below. You may want to talk with your doctor about which of the risk category you should consider).

	Risk Category	Risk Factors/ Calculated Risk	TC (mg/dL)	LDL-C (mg/dL)	Non-HDL-C (mg/dL)	Apo B (mg/dL)	TG (mg/dL)	HDL (mg/dL)
	Low	• No risk factors	< 200	< 130	< 160	No recommendation	<150	>40 or as high as possible (>60 is best)
	Moderate	• 2 or less risk factors <u>and</u> calculated 10-year risk < 10%	< 200	< 100	< 130	< 90	<150	>40 or as high as possible (>60 is best)
	High	• Cardiovascular equivalent including diabetes or stage 3 or 4 chronic kidney disease with no other risk factors **OR**... • Individuals with 2 or more risk factors **and** a 10-year risk of 10% - 20%	< 200	< 100	< 130	< 90	<150	>40 or as high as possible (>60 is best)
	Very high risk	• Established or recent hospitalization for acute coronary syndrome (ACS) **OR**... • Coronary, carotid or peripheral vascular disease, diabetes or stage 3 or 4 CKD **with** 1 or more risk factors **OR**... • Calculated 10-year risk greater than 20% or... • Heterozygous familial hypercholesterolemia [HeFH])	< 200	< 70	< 100	< 80	<150	>40 or as high as possible (>60 is best)
	Extreme	• Cardiovascular disease including unstable angina that persists after achieving an LDL-C <70 mg/dL **OR**... • established cardiovascular disease with diabetes, stage 3 or 4 CKD, **and/or** heterozygous familial hypercholesterolemia (HeFH) **OR**... • History of premature cardiovascular disease (<55 years of age for males or <65 years of age for females)	< 200	< 55	< 80	< 70	<150	>40 or as high as possible (>60 is best)

Record which risk category you fall into here:

▉ Low Risk	LDL-C goal is < 130 mg/dL	My LDL-C goal is: ____ (based on my risk category)
▉ Moderate Risk	LDL-C goal is < 100 mg/dL	
▉ High Risk	LDL-C goal is < 100 mg/dL	
▉ Very High Risk	LDL-C goal is < 70 mg/dL	
▉ Extreme Risk	LDL-C goal is < 55 mg/dL	

STEP 4:

Determine how much you need to lower your current LDL-C to achieve your LDL-C goal.

Write in your current, measured LDL-C (you may need to look at your most recent lab report or ask your doctor)

My LDL-C last measurement	**LDL-C is _____ mg/dL**

Write in your LDL-C goal as determined in STEP 3

My LDL-C goal	**LDL-C goal is _____ mg/dL**

Subtract your LDL-C goal from your last LDL-C measurement

Last LDL-C - LDL-C goal	**= _____**
Example: **150 - 100**	**= 50**

Divide your answer by your last LDL-C

Your answer ÷ Last LDL-C	= _____
Example: 50 ÷ 150	= 0.33

Multiply your answer by 100

Your answer X 100	= _____%
Example: 0.33 X 100	= 33%

This is the % you need to reduce your current LDL-C to meet your goal LDL-C.

STEP 5:

Determine which statin will give you the % reduction in LDL-C you need in order to achieve your LDL-C goal

Write down your % reduction from Step 4 here:

% you need to reduce your current LDL-C to meet your goal LDL-C	= _____ %

Choose from the list of statins below based on your % answer:

Low-intensity Statins	Moderate-intensity Statins	High-intensity Statins
Lowers LDL-C by less than 30%	Lowers LDL-C by 30-50%	Lowers LDL-C by more than 50%
Simvastatin 10 mg	Atorvastatin 10-20 mg	Atorvastatin 40-80 mg
Pravastatin 10-20 mg	Rosuvastatin 5-10 mg	Rosuvastatin 20-40 mg
Lovastatin 20 mg	Simvastatin 20-40 mg	
Fluvastatin 20-40 mg	Pravastatin 40-80 mg	
Pitavastatin 1 mg	Lovastatin 40 mg	
	Fluvastatin XL 80 mg	
	Fluvastatin 40 mg twice daily	
	Pitavastatin 2-4 mg	

STEP 6:

Determine if other medications are needed

Talk with your doctor to see if you may need additional medications to lower triglycerides or increase HDL-C

Fibrates
• Gemfibrozil (Lopid®)
• Fenofibrate (Antara®, Lipofen® Lofibra®, Tricor® and Triglide®)
Fish Oil
• Prescription omega 3 fish oil
Niacin
• Niacin
Bile acid sequestrants
• Cholestyramine (Questran®, Prevalite®)
• Colestipol (Colestid®)
• Colesevelam (Welchol®)

Cholesterol absorption inhibitors
• Ezetimibe (Zetia®)
PCSK9 Inhibitors
• Alirocumab (Praluent®)
• Evolocumab (Repatha®)
MTP Inhibitors
• Lomitapide (Juxtapid®)
Antisense Apolipoprotein B Oligonucleotide
• Mipomersen (Kynamro®)

FINALLY:

Consider using information from this risk assessment combined with items such as your LDL-P, non-HDL-C, Apo B level, cardiovascular health, weight, and family history to determine if a statin or other cholesterol medication is for you. Information from this assessment should be discussed with your doctor so that a custom plan of treatment can be outlined for you. Remember that statins and other cholesterol medications carry the risk of certain side effects.

The medications listed above should be used in conjunction with lifestyle modifications like eating healthy, increasing physical activity and quitting tobacco products.

APPENDIX III

Empowered Medicine Guide to Determining High Blood Pressure Goals and Treatment

Remember: Blood pressure can vary throughout the day. Try taking two or three blood pressure readings at least twice a day. Average these numbers to get a more accurate measure of your blood pressure. For example: To find the average systolic blood pressure (**SBP**, also known as 'the top number'), follow these steps:

EXAMPLE: if your readings are 140/90, 155/94, 158/95
1. Add 140 + 155 + 158 (answer is 453)
2. Then divide this number by the number of readings you are looking at (so 453 ÷ 3 readings = 151)
3. So your average SBP would be 151

Use this number in the following steps.

STEP 1: Determine What Stage of High Blood Pressure You May Have

Check which box in the table below applies to your blood pressure

Table 1. **High Blood Pressure Stages***

Check Which Applies to You	Stage	Blood Pressure Reading	
▦	Normal	SBP < 120	DBP < 80
▦	Elevated	SBP 120 - 129	
▦	Stage 1 high blood pressure	SBP 120 - 139	DBP 80 - 89
▦	Stage 2 high blood pressure	SBP > or = to 140	DBP > or = to 90

*SBP = systolic blood pressure (the top number)
 DBP = diastolic blood pressure (the bottom number)

STEP 2: Calculate Your 10-Year Risk of Cardiovascular Disease

If you already have cardiovascular disease, then you can skip to Step 3

If you do not have cardiovascular disease (CVD), then calculate your 10-year cardiovascular (CV) risk using one of the online tools below:

Table 2. **Online Cardiovascular Risk Calculators**

One of the following online calculators may be used:
• **Framingham Risk Assessment Tool** (https://www.framinghamheartstudy.org/risk-functions/ coronary-heart-disease/hard-10-year-risk.php)
• **Multi-Ethnic Study of Atherosclerosis (MESA)** 10-year ASCVD Risk with Coronary Artery Calcification Calculator (https://www.mesa-nhlbi. org/MESACHDRisk/MesaRiskScore/RiskScore.aspx)
• **Reynolds Risk Score** (http://www.reynoldsriskscore.org)
• **United Kingdom Prospective Diabetes Study (UKPDS)** risk engine to calculate ASCVD risk in individuals with T2DM) (https://www.dtu.ox.ac. uk/riskengine)
• **ACC ASCVD Risk Estimator Plus** tool created by the American College of Cardiology (considered by some to be sub-par by some standards as it was not validated prior to putting into practice) (http://tools.acc.org/ASCVD-Risk-Estimator/)

After using one of the online tools above, you will receive a score which will be a percentage. This is the percent chance you have of developing CVD in the next 10 years. This information will be used below to help figure out what your blood pressure treatment goals should be.

Write your risk score in below for reference.

My CV Risk Score according to the Calculator	My Score is _____ %

STEP 3: Discover Your Blood Pressure Goals and When to Treat High Blood Pressure

Check all that apply:

Table 3.**When to Treat and Treatment Goals***[1,4]

Check all that apply	Criteria	JNC 8	ACC/AHA	ACC/AAFP	ASH
▪	Age > 60 years old (without diabetes or chronic kidney disease)	**Treat when:** BP > 150/90		**Treat when:** SBP > 150	**Treat when:** BP > 140/90 unless age is > 80 years old, then consider treating when BP > 150/90
		Goal: BP < 150/90		**Goal:** SBP < 150	**Goal:** BP < 140/90 unless age > 80 years old, then consider goal BP < 150/90

Check all that apply	Criteria	JNC 8	ACC/AHA	ACC/AAFP	ASH
▪	Age 18 to 59 years old (without diabetes or chronic kidney disease)	**Treat when:** BP > 140/90			
		Goal: BP < 140/90			
▪	Age 18 or older with no clinical CVD and 10-year ASCVD risk < 10%		**Treat when:** BP > 140/90		
			Goal: BP < 130/80		
▪	CVD or 10-year ASCVD risk > or = to 10%		**Treat when:** BP > 130/80		
			Goal: BP < 130/80		
▪	Diabetes mellitus	**Treat when:** BP > 140/90	**Treat when:** BP > 130/80		
		Goal: BP < 140/90	**Goal:** BP < 130/80		

398

Check all that apply	Criteria	JNC 8	ACC/AHA	ACC/AAFP	ASH
▪	Chronic kidney disease (includes those with transplant)	**Treat when:** BP > 140/90	**Treat when:** BP > 130/80		
		Goal: BP < 140/90	**Goal:** BP < 130/80		
▪	Age 18 years or older with chronic kidney disease or diabetes	**Treat when:** BP > 140/90			
		Goal: BP < 140/90			**Goal:** Consider BP < 130/80 if there is albumin in the urine
▪	Age > or = to 65 years old, not in assisted living		**Treat when:** BP > 130/80		
			Goal: BP < 130/80		
▪	Heart Failure		**Treat when:** BP > 130/80		
			Goal: BP < 130/80		

Check all that apply	Criteria	JNC 8	ACC/AHA	ACC/AAFP	ASH
■	History of stroke		**Treat when:** BP > 140/90 OR BP > 130/80 if lacunar stroke		
			Goal: BP < 130/80		
■	Peripheral arterial disease		**Treat when:** BP > 130/80		
			Goal: BP < 130/80		

*BP = blood pressure, SBP = systolic blood pressure, DBP = diastolic blood pressure

Note which boxes you checked above. In the box below write in any 'goal blood pressures' that were recommended for you in the table above.

Recommended Blood Pressure Goal(s)	_____, _____, _____

STEP 3: Discover Which Blood Pressure Medications May Be Right to You:

First, take a look at the 4 main classes of medications typically used to treat high blood pressure. You will also find a separate table that lists medications that are less commonly prescribed for high blood pressure.

Table 4. **4 Main Drug Classes Recommended for Initial Treatment of Blood Pressure**

Class of Medications	Examples Recommended by Panel
Thiazide diuretics	Chlorthalidone (Thalitone®), hydrochlorothiazide (Microzide®, Hydrodiuril®), indapamide (Lozol®)
ACEI (angiotensin converting enzyme inhibitors)	Captopril (Capoten®), enalapril (Vasotec®), Lisinopril (Prinivil®, Zestril®, Qbrelis®)
ARB (angiotensin receptor blocker)	Eprosartan (Teveten®), candesartan (Atacad®), losartan (Cozaar®), valsartan (Diovan®), irbesartan (Avapro®)
CCB (calcium channel blocker)	Amlodipine (Norvasc®), diltiazem extended release, verapamil

Table 5. **Other Medications that are Less Commonly Used for High Blood Pressure**

Class of Medications	Examples
Loop Diuretics	bumetanide (Bumex®), furosemide (Lasix®) and torsemide (Demadex®).
Potassium-sparing diuretics	amiloride (Midamor®) and triamterene. Eplerenone (Inspra®) and spironolactone (Aldactone®)
β-blockers (or 'beta blockers')	• Atenolol (Tenormin®), Betaxolol (Kerlone®) • Bisoprolol (Zebeta®) • Metoprolol (Lopressor®, Toprol-XL®) • Nebivolol (Bystolic®) • Nadolol (Corgard®) • Propranolol (Inderal®) • Acebutolol (Sectral®) • Penbutolol (Levatol®) • Pindolol-(Visken®) • Carvedilol (Coreg®) • Labetalol (Normodyne®, Trandate®)
Alpha Blockers	Doxazosin (Cardura®), Prazosin (Minipress®), Terazosin (Hytrin®)
Centrally-acting Drugs	Clonidine (Catapress®), Methyldopa (Aldomet®), Guanfacine (Tenex®)
Vasodilators	Hydralazine (Apresoline®), Minoxidil (Loniten®)
Renin Inhibitors	Aliskiren (Tekturna® and Rasilez®)

As you look over Table 6, checkmark any boxes to the left that may apply to you.

Take this table with you to your next doctor's appointment to discuss which medications you should consider in your blood pressure treatment plan.

Table 6. **Drugs of Choice for High Blood Pressure**[1,4*]

Check all that apply	Population	Drug of Choice	Drugs to Avoid	Comments
■	Non-black population (including those with diabetes)	JNC 8: CCB, thiazide, ACEI or ARB For age < 60 years old ASH recommends: • 1st line: ACEI or ARB • 2nd line: CCB or thiazide • 3rd line: CCB plus ACEI **or** ARB plus thiazide For age > 60 years old ASH recommends: • 1st: CCB or thiazide preferred,	In one study beta blockers resulted in a higher rate of cardiovascular death, heart attack and stroke compared to the use of an ARB. In other studies beta blockers performed similarly to the 4 main classes (thiazides, CCB, ACEI, ARB).	Beta blockers have been shown to decrease the risk of death associated with certain conditions (for example, after a heart attack and in people with heart failure). ***Do not stop taking your beta blocker without consulting your doctor.***

Check all that apply	Population	Drug of Choice	Drugs to Avoid	Comments
		ACEI or ARB ok too • 2nd line: CCB, thiazide, ACEI or ARB • 3rd line: CCB plus ACEI **or** ARB plus thiazide ACC/AHA: • 1st: thiazide • 2nd line: CCB • 3rd line: ACEI or ARB		
▪	Black population (including those with diabetes)	JNC 8: CCB or thiazide ASH recommends: • First line: CCB or thiazide • 2nd line: ACEI or ARB • 3rd line: CCB plus ACEI **or** ARB plus thiazide ACC/AHA: • First line:	ACEI are generally not recommended as a first choice in the black population (***unless the patient has chronic kidney disease***) due to a 51% higher rate of stroke in this population in	CCBs provide better stroke prevention and blood pressure reduction in this population compared to ACEIs. Thiazides reduce stroke risk better than

Check all that apply	Population	Drug of Choice	Drugs to Avoid	Comments
		CCB or thiazide • 2nd line: ACEI or ARB • 3rd line: CCB plus ACEI or ARB plus thiazide	one study compared to CCBs. ACEIs were also less effective at lowering blood pressure in the black population in this study.[1]	ACEIs in this population.
▪	Heart failure	JNC 8 recommends: 1st-Thiazide, 2nd-ACEI (regardless of race) ASH, ACC/AHA: recommends: ACEI or ARB plus beta blocker plus diuretic plus spironolactone regardless of blood pressure. Amlodipine can be added for additional blood pressure	Verapamil and diltiazem should be avoided in patients with systolic heart failure.[4]	

Check all that apply	Population	Drug of Choice	Drugs to Avoid	Comments
		control.		
▪	Age 18 years or older with chronic kidney disease (regardless of race or diabetes status)	JNC 8 recommends: ACEI or ARB (all ages, all races) ASH recommends: • 1st line: ACEI or ARB (ACEI for black population) • 2nd line: CCB or thiazide • 3rd line: CCB or thiazide (whichever hasn't been used yet)		
▪	Age 75 years or older with chronic kidney disease	JNC 8 recommends: ACEI or ARB (all ages, all races) ASH recommends:		

Check all that apply	Population	Drug of Choice	Drugs to Avoid	Comments
		CCBs and thiazide-type diuretic should be used instead of ACEI or ARB due to the risk of high potassium in the blood and further renal impairment		
▪	Coronary artery disease	ASH recommends: • 1st line: beta blocker plus ARB or ACEI • 2nd: add CCB or thiazide • 3rd: CCB or thiazide (whichever hasn't been used yet) ACC/AHA: Beta blocker, ACEI, ARB (depending on other conditions. For example: beta		

Check all that apply	Population	Drug of Choice	Drugs to Avoid	Comments
		blocker for heart attack). Other medications may be added such as dihydropyridine CCB, thiazide, aldosterone antagonist.		
■	Stroke	JNC8: CCB or thiazide is recommended first for the black population with stroke. ASH recommends for non-black population: • 1st line: ACEI or ARB • 2nd line: add CCB or thiazide • 3rd line: CCB or thiazide		

Check all that apply	Population	Drug of Choice	Drugs to Avoid	Comments
		(whichever hasn't been used yet) ACC/AHA: ACEIs are more effective than thiazides or CCBs in lowering BP and preventing stroke in non-black population.		

*CCB = calcium channel blocker, ACEI = angiotensin converting enzyme inhibitors, ARB = angiotensin receptor blockers

STEP 4: Know When to Start One Medication or Two

When discussing the medications listed above, this table may help determine whether you should start out with one or two medications to treat your high blood pressure.

Table 7. **When to Start with More Than One Medication**

	Who	Start With...
■	Adults with stage 1 high blood pressure with a BP goal of 130/80	Start with 1 first line medications. Other agents may be added later if needed
■	Adults with stage 2 high blood pressure with a BP that is more than 20/10 above their BP goal.	Start with 2 first line medications in different classes (thiazides, CCBs, ACEIs, ARBs)

STEP 5: Figure Out When You Should Follow-up With Your Doctor Again

Check the boxes below that apply to you. Take this chart with you to your next doctor's appointment so that you can both decide on a follow-up schedule that works for you.

Table 8. **Recommended High Blood Pressure Montitoring**

	Criteria	Recommended Monitoring
■	Adults with normal BP (BP < 120/80)	Reassess in 1 year
■	Adults with elevated blood pressure (SBP 120-129 or DBP 80) with CVD risk < 10%	Reassess within 3 to 6 months.
■	Adults with Stage 1 high blood pressure (SBP 130-139 or DBP 80-89) with CVD or CVD risk > or = to 10%	If using non-drug therapy, reassess in 3-6 months. If using non-drug and drug therapy, reassess in 1 month (if goal met, follow up in 3-6 months. If goal not met, follow up more often than 3-6 months and consider

		intensifying therapy)
	Adults with Stage 2 high blood pressure (BP > or = to 140/90)	Reassess in 1 month (if goal met, follow up in 3-6 months. If goal not met, follow up more often than 3-6 months and consider intensifying therapy)
	Adults with very high blood pressure (SBP > or = to 180 or DBP > or = to 110)	See your doctor right away or go to the Emergency Room/Urgent Care to be evaluated.

APPENDIX IV

Chronic Obstructive Pulmonary Disease (COPD)

First: we must confirm the diagnosis using spirometry. Then, the next step is to use your answers to some assessment questions to determine which medications may be best for you.

Take note of the different medications used to treat COPD. We will reference these in a moment.

Medications for COPD include:

- **SABAs** (short acting beta agonist)-albuterol, levalbuterol, terbutaline
- **SAMAs** (short acting muscarinic antagonist)-ipratropium
- **LABAs** (long acting beta agonist)-salmeterol, formoterol, arformoterol, indacatrol, olodaterol
- **LAMAs** (long acting muscarinic antagonist)-tiotropium, aclidinlum, glycopyrronium, umeclidinium
- **ICSs** (inhaled corticosteroid)-beclomethasone, budesonide, ciclesonide, flunisolide, fluticasone, mometasone
- **PDE4 Inhibitors**-roflumilast
- **Methylxanthines**-theophylline, aminophylline
- **Mucolytics**-acetylcysteine
- **Opioids**- Morphine, hydrocodone, oxycodone
- **Antibiotics**-azithromycin, erythromycin
- Various combinations of medications in inhalers

STEP 1 Spirometry to Diagnose COPD:

Spirometry is required to make the diagnosis of COPD. :try is a common test done at your doctor's office. Your try results will tell your doctor how your lungs are functioning compared to other people of the same age, height, weight, sex and ethnicity. Your spirometry results will be used to help determine which COPD GOLD group you fall into

STEP 1a: Obtain your FEV1 and FVC from your doctor's office. Write these numbers in below.

My FEV1 is _____
My FVC is _____

STEP 1b: Plug these numbers into the CDC spirometry calculator   at: https://www.cdc.gov/niosh/topics/spirometry/refcalculator.html
Enter this value in the blank below **(this number will be calculated on the CDC online tool so you can just look and write it in here, no math required).**

FEV1/FVC% is _____ **%**

Note: if your FEV1/FVC% is less than 0.7 than your doctor might diagnose you with COPD.

Step 1c: Determine Which GOLD Group You are In

Once you've been diagnosed with COPD, your doctor can use your spirometry results to figure out how to classify your condition. To do this he/she will divide your FEV1 by the predicted FEV1 (from the CDC website).

Your FEV1 ÷ predicted FEV1 (on CDC website) = _____

Then multiply this answer this answer by 100 to get the percent you need.

_____%

You and your doctor will use this percentage to see which GOLD class you fall into.

Mark the box next to the GOLD group that you fit into according to your spirometry results (this helps your doctor determine how severe your COPD is):

Classification of COPD Based on Spirometry Results

☐ **GOLD 1**: Very mild COPD with a FEV1 about 80 percent or more of normal.
☐ **GOLD 2**: Moderate COPD with a FEV1 between 50 and 80 percent of normal.
☐ **GOLD 3**: Severe emphysema with FEV1 between 30 and 50 percent of normal.
☐ **GOLD 4**: Very severe COPD with a lower FEV1 than Stage 3, or those with Stage 3 FEV1 *and* low blood oxygen levels

STEP 2: Assessment Questions About Your Symptoms

Either the Modified British Medical Research Council (mMRC) questionnaire **OR** the COPD Assessment Test (CAT) can be used to help determine how severe your symptoms are.

The Modified British Medical Research Council (mMRC) questionnaire

In the questionnaire below, circle the number next to the box that best describes your symptoms (only circle one number):

Grade	Description of Breathlessness
0	I only get breathless with strenuous exercise.
1	I get short of breath when hurrying on level ground or walking up a slight hill.
2	On level ground, I walk slower than people of the same age because of breathlessness or have to stop for breath when walking at my own pace.
3	I stop for breath after walking about 100 yards or after a few minutes on level ground.
4	I am too breathless to leave the house, or I am breathless when dressing.

COPD Assessment Test (CAT)

In each row below, circle the number that best describes your symptoms:

I never cough	1	2	3	4	5	I cough all the time
I have no phlegm (mucus) in my chest at all	1	2	3	4	5	My chest is full of phlegm
My chest does not feel tight at all	1	2	3	4	5	My chest feels very tight
When I walk up a hill or up one flight of stairs I am not breathless	1	2	3	4	5	When I walk up hill or up one flight of stairs I am very out of breath
I am not limited doing any activities at home	1	2	3	4	5	I am very limited doing any activities at home

I am confident leaving home despite my lung condition	1 2 3 4 5	I am not at all confident leaving home because of my lung condition
I sleep soundly	1 2 3 4 5	I don't sleep soundly because of my lung condition
I have lots of energy	1 2 3 4 5	I have no energy at all

Note your mMRC and/or your CAT test scores here:

My mMRC score is:_____

My CAT score is: _____

STEP 3: Exacerbations and Hospitalizations

The COPD GOLD guidelines recommend that your doctor ask how many COPD exacerbations you've had in the last 12 months and how many of those had resulted in a hospitalization. This information will be combined with the information you provide about your symptoms to determine which ABCD group you fall into for treatment purposes.

Note your exacerbations and hospital admissions information here:

In the last 12 months, I have had _____ number of COPD exacerbations

In the last 12 months, I have had _____ number of hospitalizations due to my COPD

STEP 4: ABCD Scoring

The GOLD COPD "ABCD" grading system is used to figure out which medications may be best for your COPD. The ABCD system combines information you provide about your symptoms, looks at how many exacerbations you've had in the last 12 months and how many of them have landed you in the hospital.

GOLD COPD ABCD Grading System

Exacerbation History

More than 1 exacerbation not requiring a hospital admission OR at least 1 exacerbation requiring hospital admission

| | C
Less symptoms
High Risk | D
More Symptoms
High Risk |

1 or less exacerbations not requiring a hospital admission

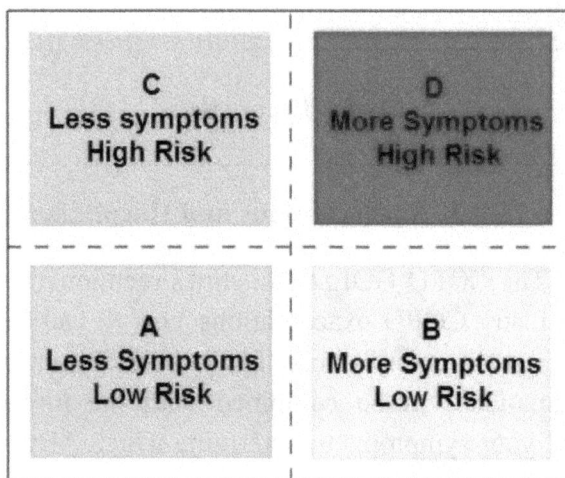

| | A
Less Symptoms
Low Risk | B
More Symptoms
Low Risk |

mMRC score 0-1 OR CAT score less than 10   mMRC score of 2 or more OR CAT score of 10 or more

Symptoms

Your ABCD score will let the doctor know which ABCD group you fall into and which medications may best manage your COPD:

Note your COPD grade here:

My COPD grade is:
☐ Grade A
☐ Grade B
☐ Grade C
☐ Grade D

STEP 5: Determine Which Medications May be Best for You

Using your COPD grade, note which group of medications may be best for you. **Check the box below that applies:**

☐ **Grade A:**
- SABA or SAMA <u>or</u>…
- LABA or LAMA <u>or</u>…
- SABA + SAMA

☐ **Grade B:**
- LABA or LAMA <u>or</u>…
- LABA + LAMA

☐ **Grade C:**
- ICS + LABA + LAMA <u>or</u>…
- LAMA + LABA <u>or</u>…
- LABA + PDE4 inhibitor <u>or</u>…
- LAMA + PDE4 inhibitor

☐ **Grade D:**
- ICS + LABA +/or LAMA <u>or</u>…
- ICS + LABA + LAMA <u>or</u>…
- ICS + LABA + PDE4 inhibitor <u>or</u>…
- LABA + LAMA <u>or</u>…
- LAMA + PDE4 inhibitor

REMEMBER:

•   Proper technique when using an inhaler and/or nebulizer machine helps ensure you receive all of your medication.

•   Proper cleaning and maintenance of your nebulizer machine is very important.

Other Adjunct Therapies:
- Flu shot
- Pneumococcal vaccine
- Oxygen
- Ventilatory support
- Surgical and nonsurgical interventions
- Palliative care and Hospice

If you wish, take the information above with you to your next doctor's appointment to discuss your COPD treatment, especially if your COPD is not controlled. The hope is that the information above will aid in the discussion of your COPD therapy with your doctor.

APPENDIX V

Diabetes

Screening for Prediabetes and diabetes

The ADA recommends people over the age of 45 get screened every 3 years for prediabetes and diabetes. They also recommend using an assessment tool for screening. They offer the ADA risk test for this purpose (located at: www.diabetes.org/socrisktest). **A score of 5 or higher indicates a higher risk for prediabetes or diabetes.**

Testing for prediabetes or diabetes should be considered in adults who are overweight or obese (BMI of 25 kg/m or more, Asian Americans with a BMI greater than 23 kg/m) and have one or more of the risk factors below.

Risk factors for Diabetes

- First degree relative with diabetes
- African American, Latino, Native American, Asian American, Pacific Islander
- History of cardiovascular disease (for example, a history of heart attack)
- High blood pressure (140/90 or more, or are on medication therapy for high blood pressure)
- HDL cholesterol less than 35 mg/dL (0.90 mmol/L) and/or a triglyceride level of 250 mg/dL (2.82 mmol/L) or more.
- Women with polycystic ovary syndrome
- Physical inactivity

STEP 1: If you are over 45 years old and have not been diagnosed with prediabetes or diabetes, take the ADA risk test at the web address above and write your score in below.

My ADA Diabetes Risk Score is = _____

STEP 2: Is this number in step 1 more than 5? If so, contact your health care provider to get tested for prediabetes and diabetes.

I need to be tested for diabetes at my doctor's office	☐ **Yes** (my risk score is more than 5)	☐ **No** (my risk score is less than 5)

Diagnosis of Prediabetes and Diabetes

There are several tests used to test for prediabetes and diabetes.

Tests Used to Test for Prediabetes and Diabetes

Test	What is It?
A1C	A1C is an estimate of your **average blood sugar over the last few months.** This is done by looking at hemoglobin (a protein in the blood that is coated in sugar).
Fasting Blood Glucose (FBG or 'fasting blood sugar')	A blood sugar reading that is taken after at least 8 hours with no food.
Oral Glucose Tolerance Test (OGTT)	An OGTT is a reading of your blood sugar 2 hours after you are given 75 gm of sugar to eat.

Let's look at how these tests can be used to diagnose prediabetes and diabetes.

Diagnosis of Prediabetes and Diabetes*

		A1C	Fasting Blood Sugar (FBG)	Oral Glucose Tolerance Test (OGTT)	Other
☐	**Prediabetes**	A1C of 5.7-6.4%	FBG of 100 mg/dL (5.6 mmol/L) to 125 mg/dL (6.9 mmol/L	Blood glucose of 140 mg/dL (7.8 mmol/L) to 199 mg/dL (11 mmol/L) after a 2-hour OGTT	
☐	**Diabetes**	A1C of 6.5% or more	FBG of 126 mg/dL (7 mmol/L) or greater after no food for at least 8 hours.	Blood glucose of 200 mg/dL (11.1 mmol/L) or more during a 2-hour OGTT test. The test should use 75 gm of glucose dissolved in water	Classic symptoms of high blood sugar with a random blood sugar of 200 mg/dL (11.1 mmol/L) or more.

*NOTE: FBG should be used to diagnose type 1 diabetes (instead of A1C). A panel of autoantibodies may also be ordered.

STEP 3: After visiting your doctor to get tested for prediabetes and type 2 diabetes, circle any symptoms in Table 5 that apply. If you have anything circled in the prediabetes row, check the prediabetes box. If you have anything circled in the type 2 diabetes row, check that box. Did the boxes checked indicate that you may have prediabetes, type 2 diabetes, or neither?

☐ **Prediabetes** ☐ **Type 2 Diabetes** ☐ **Neither**

I've Been Diagnosed with Prediabetes or Diabetes; Now What?

If you've been diagnosed with prediabetes or diabetes it is recommended that your doctor do a complete medical evaluation for you to:

- Confirm the diagnosis
- Check for diabetes complications and other conditions that need to be addressed (like cardiovascular disease or high blood pressure)
- A medical evaluation which may include: medical history, allergies, past side effects, physical exam and lab assessment
- Determine a plan for initial and ongoing care, for the management of your prediabetes or diabetes
- Determine the need for referrals to other doctors, immunizations and other health screenings

STEP 4: Check the appropriate box below when you have set up a complete medical evaluation with your doctor.

I have been diagnosed with prediabetes or diabetes and have scheduled a complete medical evaluation with my doctor	☐ Yes	☐ No

It is recommended that all people with diabetes take part in diabetes self-management education and support (DSMES). The goal of DSMES is to improve health and quality of life through education. It is hoped that through DSMES, people can gain the skills they need to be able to maintain their diabetes care at home.

It is recommended that people with diabetes take part in DSMES at least at these 4 critical times:

5. At diagnosis
6. Every year
7. When problems arise
8. When a change occurs

DSMES programs are offered by various health care professionals. DSMES can be done in a group setting or on an individual basis. It can even be done via technology (via webinars or skype meetings for example). Accredited DSMES programs are generally covered by Medicare and may be covered by most private insurances as well. However, note that **Medicare and private insurances generally cover in-person DSMES visits**. Phone, Skype, or other alternative forms of meeting may not be covered. Check with your insurance.

STEP 5: Contact your doctor's office to find a DSMES program near you. Check the box below when you have made your first DSMES appointment:

My DSMES appoint is scheduled for: _____

Nutrition Therapy

it's recommended that all people with diabetes be offered a referral to a Registered Dietician (RD). RD referrals have been shown to decrease A1C in people with diabetes.

An RD can help you:

7. Learn how to plan your own meals
8. Learn healthful eating patterns
9. Discover how to incorporate a variety of nutritious food into your meal plan
10. Manage your weight
11. Delay or prevent diabetes and its complications
12. Identify your individual nutrition needs

STEP 6: Contact your doctor's office to find a RD near you. Check the box below when you have made your first appointment:

My first RD consultation is scheduled for: _____

What Should My Blood Sugar Goal Be?

You should talk to you doctor about specific blood sugar goals that are right for you. In general, however, it is recommended that one *aim for a goal of 80-130 mg/dL (4.4 to 7.2 mmol/L) right before meals and less than 180 mg/dL (10 mmol/L,) 1 to 2 hours after meals.*

What Should My A1C Goal Be?

The ADA notes that if you are diabetic, your *A1C goal should be less than 7%* (53 mmol/mol) or *eAG less than 154 mg/dL* for most nonpregnant adults. After being diagnosed with diabetes, it is recommended that *people who are meeting their treatment goals test their A1C at least two times a year. People who are not meeting their treatment goals should test every 3 months.*

How Much Insulin Do I Need?

You will need to work with your doctor and your RD to figure out how much insulin you should be taking. Insulin dosing is something that needs to be tailored for each person.

When first starting insulin, most people with type 1 diabetes are started on 0.4 to 1 unit per kilogram of body weight per day (units/kg/day). With type 2 diabetes, it's common to be started at 0.6 to 1 units/kg/day. 50% of this calculated daily dose is typically given as basal insulin (AKA immediate or long-acting insulin). The other 50% is given with meals (divided among the days' meals as rapid, regular or short-acting insulin).

Which Medications Should I Use?

When it comes to figuring out which medications to use, you and your doctor will need to sit down together and figure out which medications may be best for you based on: the considerations above.

The ADA makes the following recommendations for us to use as a guide: Then, below you will find a summary of medications used to treat diabetes.

ADA Recommendations for Choosing Diabetes Treatment

For people with type 1 diabetes:

- Most people with type 1 diabetes should be treated with multiple daily injections of insulin before meals and basal (intermediate or long-acting) insulin or continuous subcutaneous insulin infusion.
- Most people with type 1 diabetes should use rapid-acting insulin
- People with type 1 diabetes should learn to take into consideration one's carbohydrate intake, premeal blood sugar levels, and physical activity.
- People with type 1 diabetes who have been successfully using continuous subcutaneous insulin infusion should have continued access to this therapy after they turn 65 years of age.

People with type 2 diabetes:

☐Metformin is the preferred initial medication that should be used for treatment of type 2 diabetes (as long as it is tolerated and not contraindicated (strong recommendation NOT to use).

☐Long-term use of metformin may be associated with biochemical vitamin B12 deficiency. Vitamin B12 levels should be considered in metformin-treated patients, especially in those with anemia or peripheral neuropathy.

☐Consider initiating insulin therapy (with or without additional agents) in patients with newly diagnosed type 2 diabetes who:

☐Are symptomatic and/or

☐Have A1C ≥10% (86 mmol/mol) and/or

☐Blood glucose levels ≥300 mg/dL (16.7 mmol/L).

☐Patients with newly-diagnosed type 2 diabetes who have A1C ≥9% (75 mmol/mol) may consider starting with two medications (instead of one)

☐In patients without cardiovascular disease, If using one or two medications does not achieve or maintain the A1C goal over 3 months, an additional medication may be used

☐Consideration when choosing a medication to treat diabetes should include efficacy, risk of low blood sugar, history of cardiovascular disease, impact on weight, potential side effects, effects on the kidneys, cost, and how it is given (oral vs. injection)

☐In patients with type 2 diabetes AND established atherosclerotic cardiovascular disease:

☐Medication therapy should begin with lifestyle management and metformin.

☐A medication proven to reduce major adverse cardiovascular events and death from cardiovascular disease should be considered as an additional medication (empagliflozin or liraglutide)

☐After lifestyle management and metformin, canagliflozin may be considered to reduce major adverse cardiovascular events.

☐Continuous reevaluation of the medication regimen and adjustment is recommended

☐For patients with type 2 diabetes who are not achieving their blood sugar goals, drug intensification, including consideration of insulin therapy, should be promptly considered

☐Metformin should be continued when used in combination with other medications, including insulin, if not contraindicated and if tolerated.

Summary of Medications Used to Treat Diabetes

Metformin

Effectiveness: High
Chance of causing low blood sugar: Low
Weight change?: Loss
How to take it; oral

Metformin (Glucophage®, Metformin®, Glumetza®, Riomet®, Fortamet®) is a type of medication called a biguanide. It is a medication that is taken orally. It is available by itself or in a combination product that contain more than two medications:

- Repaglinide and metformin (Prandimet®)
- Metformin and glipizide (Metaglip®)

- Metformin and pioglitazone (ACTOplus Met®)
- Metformin and glyburide (Glucovance®)
- Metformin and rosiglitazone (Avandamet®)
- Metformin and sitagliptin (Janumet®)

Insulin-secretagogues

Effectiveness: High
Chance of causing low blood sugar: Yes (High)
Weight change?: Gain
How to take them: oral

Sulfonylureas

- Glimepiride (Amaryl®)
- Glyburide (DiaBeta®, Micronase®)
- Glipizide (Glucotrol®)
- Chlorpropamide
- Tolazamide (Tolinase®)
- Tolbutamide
- Glipizide and metformin (Metaglip®)
- Glimepiride and rosiglitazone (Avandaryl®)
- Glyburide and metformin (Glucovance®)
- Glimepiride and pioglitazone (Euetact®)

Glinides

- Nateglinide (Starlix®)
- Repaglinide (Prandin®)
- Repaglinide and metformin (Prandimet®)

Pramlintide (Symlin®, SymlinPen®) for type 1 and type 2 diabetes

Effectiveness: High

Chance of causing low blood sugar: Yes
Weight change?: Loss
How to take it; subcutaneous injection

Pramlintide is a medication that you inject subcutaneously (into the fatty under-layer of skin tissue). It has been approved by the Food and Drug Administration (FDA) for the treatment of type 1 and type 2 diabetes in patients who take rapid-acting insulin before meals. It delays emptying of the stomach and enhances the feeling of "feeling full after a meal". Pramlintide is given in fixed doses before meals. It is used in addition to insulin, however, it CANNOT be mixed in the same syringe. Two separate syringes must be used.

It may take some experimenting to find the right dose of pramlintide that works for you. You may want to start out trying it at one meal every day. You can work with your doctor to adjust the dose up or down until you figure out what dose will work for you. Waiting 3 days before increasing the dose may help decrease the amount of nausea you feel.

When you figure out what dose works for you at that meal, then replicate that at other meals (the dose of pramlintide is the same at every meal). Some report that the 'right' dose will produce a 'full feeling' after you eat and/or reduce the spike of insulin that tends to happen after meals. If you do not experience this, you may need to increase your dose.

Pramlintide can cause weight loss and usually decreases the amount of insulin one has to use. Nausea is a common side effect but usually goes away. Other potential side effects include redness at the injection site, stomach pain, tiredness, dizziness, cough, sore throat, and joint pain.

When starting this medication, it's important to work with your doctor on lowering your insulin dose from the start to prevent your

Sodium-glucose Cotransporter 2 Inhibitors (SGLT2)
Effectiveness: Intermediate
Chance of causing low blood sugar: Low

Weight change?: Loss
How to take it: oral
Sodium-glucose Cotransporter 2 Inhibitors (SGLT2) and combination products that contain SGLT2 inhibitors include:

- Canaglifolozin (Invokana®)
- Dapagliflozin (Farxiga®)
- Empagliflozin (Jardiance®)
- Empagliflozin and linagliptin (Glyxambl®)
- Empagliflozin and metformin (Synjardy®)
- Dapagliflozin/metformin (Xigduo XR®)

Thiazolidinediones [TZDs] or "Glitazones"

Effectiveness: High
Chance of causing low blood sugar: No
Weight change?: Gain
How to take them: oral

Examples of thiazolidinediones (TZDs or "glitazones") include:

- Pioglitazone (Actos®)
- Rosiglitazone (Avandia®)
- Rosiglitazone and glimepiride (Avandaryl®)
- Pioglitazone and metformin (ACTOplus Met®)
- Rosiglitazone and metformin (Avandamet®)
- Pioglitazone and glimepiride (Duetact®)

Glucagon-like peptide 1 (GLP1) receptor agonists

Effectiveness: High
Chance of causing low blood sugar: No
Weight change?: Loss
How to take them: subcutaneous injection

Examples of these medications include:

- Exenatide (Byetta® and Bydureon®)
- Liraglutide (Victoza® and Saxenda®)
- Lixisenatide (Lyxumia®)

- Albiglutide (Tanzeum®)
- Dulaglutide (Trulicity®)
- Semaglutide (Ozempic®)

Dipeptidyl peptidase 4 (DPP4) inhibitors (the "gliptins")

Effectiveness: Intermediate
Chance of causing low blood sugar: No
Weight change?: Neutral
How to take them: oral

Examples of peptidyl peptidase 4 (DPP4) inhibitors (AKA the gliptins) include:
- Sitagliptin (Januvia®)
- Saxagliptin (Onglyza®)
- Linagliptin (Tradjenta®)
- Alogliptin (Nesina®)
- Vildagliptin (Galvus®)
- Alogliptin (Nesina®, Vipidia®)
- Metformin and alogliptin (Kazano®)
- Sitagliptin and metformin (Janumet®)

Alpha-glucosidase Inhibitors

Effectiveness: Intermediate
Chance of causing low blood sugar: no
Weight change?: Loss
How to take: oral

Examples of these medications include:
- Acarbose (Precose®)
- Miglitol (Glyset®)

APPENDIX VI

Osteoporosis

STEP 1: Check all of the risk factors that apply:

Risk Factors for Osteoporosis Fractures[9]

☐   **Parental history of hip fracture**
☐   **Smoking**
☐   **Excess alcohol consumption (> 4 drinks per day for men or > 2 drinks per day for women**
☐   **Caffeine intake (> 2.5 cups of coffee per day)**
☐   **Low body weight**
☐   **Woman who is post-menopausal**
☐   **Gonadal hormone deficiency**
     (gonad hormones help with breast development in women, testicular development in men, and pubic hair growth)
☐   **Inadequate activity**
☐   **Increased age**
☐   **Low body weight (< 58 kg (128 lb)**
☐   **Low calcium or vitamin D intake**
☐   **History of fracture**
☐   **White or Asian race**

STEP 2: Next you'll figure out if you need to complete a risk assessment or talk to your doctor about a bone scan. Check the box that applies to you:

☐	I am a woman age 65 or older	Ask your doctor to schedule a bone scan to see if you have osteopenia or osteoporosis
☐	I am a woman younger than 65 and have at least 1 risk factor listed in Table 1	Complete one of the screening tools listed in Table 2. Write your OST score in the box provided
☐	I am a woman younger than 65 and do **NOT** have any of the risk factors listed above	Congratulations! You do not need to have a bone scan at this time
☐	I am a man **over** the age of 70	Consider using the screening tool for men in Table 2
☐	I am a man **under** the age of 70	Congratulations! You do not need to have a bone scan at this time unless your doctor thinks it would be helpful

STEP 3: If in Step 2 it was recommended that you complete a risk assessment, use one of the assessments below to see if you are at high risk for osteoporosis.

Calculators Used to See if One is at Risk for Osteoporosis

Tool	Where to Find It
OST for women	https://reference.medscape.com/calculator/osteoporosis-self-assessment-women
OST for men (optional)	https://reference.medscape.com/calculator/osteoporosis-self-assessment-men

My OST score is:	☐ Low (No DXA scan needed at this time)	☐ Medium (No DXA scan needed at this time)	☐ High (Talk to your doctor about getting a DXA scan)

So, now you should have a pretty good idea if you should have a DXA bone scan, or not. Let's take a closer look at the DXA bone scan results mean.

STEP 4: After you get your DXA scan at the doctor's office, check the box below that applies to you based on your T or Z score. Do you have osteoporosis?

Check one:	Category	T Score from DXA Scan
Women 65 or older, a woman younger than 65 and have at least 1 risk factor listed in Table 1, or man older than 70		
☐	Normal	T score greater than or equal to -1.0
☐	Osteopenia	T score between -1.0 and -2.5
☐	Osteoporosis	T score less than or equal to -2.5
☐	Severe osteoporosis	T score less than or equal to -2.5 with one or more fractures
OR: men younger than 50 years old, children or premenopausal women		
☐	Normal	Z score greater than or equal to -2.0
☐	Suggestive of low bone density	Z score less than -2.0

Do I have osteoporosis, severe osteoporosis or low bone density?	☐ Yes	☐ No

If you answered "Yes" to the question above, read on to see what you can do to treat osteoporosis and other measures you can take to keep it from getting worse. If it was determined that you have 'low bone density' due to your Z score, talk to your doctor to see if he or she thinks you would benefit from osteoporosis therapy.

Other Tests to Find a Cause

It's recommended that patients who are newly diagnosed with osteoporosis have other tests done to see if the cause for osteoporosis can be found. These tests may include[9]:

- serum 25-hydroxyvitamin D
- calcium
- creatinine
- thyroid-stimulating hormone

STEP 5: Check the box below once you have talked with your doctor about screening to see if a secondary cause of osteoporosis can be found

☐	**Yes, I have spoken with my doctor about screening for secondary causes of osteoporosis.**

In additions to the risk factors listed in Table 1, there are medications that you may be taking that can contribute to the development of osteoporosis.

Medications That Can Contribute to Osteoporosis

- Heparin
- Anticonvulsants
- Cyclosporine A
- Tacrolimus
- Barbituates
- Lithium

- Depo-medroxyprogesterone
- Chemotherapy
- Intravenous nutrition
- Glucocorticoids

STEP 6: Check the box below if you are on any of the medications listed in Table 5.

☐	**Yes, I am currently taking medications that may be contributing to osteoporosis. These medications include:** _____ _____ _____

NOTE: Do **NOT** stop taking any the medications listed in Table 5 without talking to your doctor first. Some medications need to be tapered off of slowly. It is also positive that the benefit of using that medications outweighs the risk of osteoporosis.

Non-medication Therapy to Decrease the Risk of Fractures

Remember, all of the medications mentioned below are meant to be used in conjunction with other measures like fall prevention, smoking cessation, decreased caffeine intake, exercise, vitamin D intake, and moderation of alcohol.

Non-medication Therapy to Decrease the Risk of Fractures[9]

- Alcohol and caffeine in moderation
  - o Less than or equal to 4 drinks per day for men or 2 drinks per day for women
  - o Less than or equal to 2.5 cups of coffee or 5 cups of tea per day
- Smoking cessation
- Consider exercise and strength training
- Calcium and Vitamin D supplementation (consider more exposure to sunlight)
- Fall prevention measures

How Much Calcium and Vitamin D Do I Need?

So how much calcium do we need each day? It is important to note that our calcium requirements depend on factors such as age and lactation status. It is important to note that increasing calcium intake beyond these recommendations may put you at risk for kidney stones or cardiovascular disease.[17]

Recommended Daily Allowances for Dietary Calcium[16]

Age	Male	Female
0-6 months	200 mg	200 mg
7-12 months	260 mg	260 mg
1-3 years	700 mg	700 mg
4-8 years	1000 mg	1000 mg
9-13 years	1300 mg	1300 mg
14-18 years	1300 mg	1300 mg
19-50 years	1000 mg	1000 mg
51-70 years	1000 mg	1200 mg
71+ years	1200 mg	1200 mg

Here are some tips on how you can help prevent falls. Falls put you at a higher risk of bone fracture.

Safety Tips to Prevent Falls

- Use a cane, walker, or other assistive device
- If using a cane in an icy region, consider using ice tips at the end to get better grip
- When using a cane or walker, consider suing rubber tips at the tips to get better grip
- Consider using a long-handled gripping device to reach things on the ground
- Avoid walking on slippery surfaces
- Use hand rails when available
- Install handles and rails in the bathroom around the toilet and bath tub
- Consider a plastic shower chair in the shower
- Keep floors inside and outside free of clutter and in good repair
- Be careful when stepping on or off of curbs
- Keep surroundings well-lit. You may consider carrying a small flashlight for times when you might find yourself in dimly lit areas while away from home
- Wear comfortable, low-heeled footwear
- Consider carrying a bag or using a fannypack/backpack to keep your hands free
- Find out which grocery stores and pharmacies in your community deliver to your home
- Consider getting a personal emergency response system to wear in case you fall when you are alone
- For those that are prone to falls, wearing undergarments with hip pad protectors may also help prevent hip fractures.

Falling increases your risk of bone fractures. If you have trouble walking or keeping your balance, there are many types of assistive devices available including:

- Cane

- Offset cane (a cane with a crook in the neck)
- Quadripod cane (a cane with four feet at the bottom)
- Forearm (Lofstrand) crutches
- Standard walker
- Front-wheeled walker
- Four-wheeled walker (also called a rollator)

You'll need to talk to your doctor about which assistive device may be right for you.

Medication for the Treatment of Osteoporosis

Remember in STEP 4, we discussed how the NOF recommends starting medication treatment only in the following groups:

People Who Should Consider Medication Treatment for Osteoporosis[9]

Women 65 or older, a woman younger than 65 and have at least 1 risk factor listed in Table 1, or man older than 70 with:
T score less than or equal to -2.5
OR: men younger than 50 years old, children or premenopausal women with:
Z score less than -2.0

Here is a summary of the medications used to treat or prevent osteoporosis.

Medications for the Prevention and Treatment of Osteoporosis

Class of Medications	Examples of Medications in this Class	Approved for Prevention or Treatment	Fracture Type	How to Take it
Bisphosphonates	Alendronate (Fosamax®)	Prevention Treatment	Hip, vertebral*, nonvertebral**	Oral once daily or weekly
	Alendronate with cholecalciferol (Fosamax plus D®)	Treatment	Hip, vertebral, nonvertebral	Oral once daily or weekly
	Ibandronate (Boniva®)	Prevention Treatment	Vertebral only	Oral once a month
	Risedronate (Actonel®, Atelvia®)	Prevention Treatment	Hip, vertebral, nonvertebral	Different options: Once per day, once per week, once per month, or for 2 days in a row once per month
	Risedronate with calcium (Actonel with calcium®)	Prevention Treatment	Hip, vertebral, nonvertebral	Different options: Once per day, once per week, once per month, or for 2 days in a row once per month
	Zoledronic acid (Reclast®, Zometa®)	Prevention Treatment	Hip, vertebral, nonvertebral	Injection once every 1-2 years
Selective	Raloxifene	Prevention	Vertebral only	Oral daily

Class of Medications	Examples of Medications in this Class	Approved for Prevention or Treatment	Fracture Type	How to Take it
estrogen receptor modulators (SERMs)	(Evista®)	Treatment		
Anabolic Drug	Teriparatide (Forteo®)	Treatment	Vertebral, nonvertebral	Injection once daily
	Denosumab (Prolia®)	Treatment	Hip, vertebral, nonvertebral	Injection every 6 months

*Vertebral: means involving the vertebrae (bones that make up the spine)
**Nonvertebral: means NOT involving the vertebrae (bones that make up the spine)

First line treatment for osteoporosis is to start bisphosphonate therapy. However, people who can't take bisphosphonates or don't respond to them might consider other medications like raloxifene, teriparatide and denosumab.

Remember, all of these medications are meant to be used in conjunction with other measures like fall prevention, smoking cessation, decreased caffeine intake, exercise, vitamin D intake, and moderation of alcohol.

APPENDIX VII

Determining Stroke Risk with Atrial Fibrillation (a. fib.)

Reducing Your Risk of Heart Attack and Stroke if You Have Atrial Fibrillations (a. fib)

A condition called atrial fibrillation (a. fib.) has been associated with an increased risk of stroke. When one has a. fib., their heart beats irregularly. This is due to disorganized electrical signals in the chambers of the heart. This can cause you feel a fast and/or fluttery heartbeat. Sometimes, this allows blood to pool in the chambers of the heart, allowing tiny clots to form. These clots can travel to the brain through the arteries and cause a stroke.

If you have a. fib., you can reduce your risk of stroke. If you meet the criteria, you may be a candidate for aspirin or oral anticoagulation. Anticoagulation medications are drugs that help keep your blood from clotting. They are sometimes called "blood thinners".

The table below is for people who have a. fib. Points are awarded, depending on which risk factors you have. The number of points you have will let you and your doctor know if you should consider aspirin or a blood thinner to decrease your risk of stroke.

STEP 1: Check a box next to each "yes" or "no" answer below.

Stroke Risk Assessment for Atrial Fibrillation

	Criteria		Points	
C	Congestive Heart Failure	☐	Yes	1
		☐	No	0
H	High blood pressure (> 140/90 mmHg on at least 2 occasions or current blood pressure treatment	☐	Yes	1
		☐	No	0
A	Age 75 years or older	☐	Yes	2
		☐	No	0
D	Diabetes mellitus (fasting glucose > 125 mg/dL or treatment with an oral hypoglycemic agent or insulin)	☐	Yes	1
		☐	No	0
S	Stroke or transient ischemic attack (TIA)- both of these involve a loss of blood flow to the brain	☐	Yes	2
		☐	No	0

V	Vascular disease (Prior heart attack, peripheral arterial disease or aortic plaque)	☐ ☐	Yes No	1 0
A	Age 65 to 74 years old	☐ ☐	Yes No	1 0
SC	Sex Category female	☐ ☐	Yes No	1 0
			Total Points:	

STEP 2: Add up the points you earned. Write the answer in the space labeled "Total points" above.

STEP 3: Check to box below that corresponds with how many "Total points" you have. Note what medications are recommended for you.

Table 8: **A. fib. Stroke Risk Score**

	Score	Risk
☐	0	Low risk. May not require anticoagulation
☐	1	Low-moderate risk. Should consider anticoagulation

In general, those with a score of 1 should consider full oral anticoagulation. This means aspirin is probably not potent enough for you and you should choose another medication from Table 3. The one exception, however, is in patients who have a score of 1 due to gender alone. In these patients (female < 65 years old without other risk factors), antithrombotic therapy should NOT be given.

If your score indicates you might be a candidate for anticoagulation, you will have the following medications to choose from (check out the "Medications for the Prevention of Stroke" section toward the end of this chapter to read more about these medications):

Table 9: **Types of Anticoagulation Used to Treat Atrial Fibrillation**

- **Aspirin**
- **Warfarin (Coumadin®)**
- **Apixaban (Eliquis®)**
- **Dabigatran (Pradaxa®)**
- **Rivaroxaban (Xarelto®)**
- **Edoxaban (Savaysa®)**

Work closely with your doctor to manage your symptoms and make sure you are getting the most out of your anticoagulation and/or antiarrhythimia medications. If you do this, you should find that living with a. fib. has a minimal effect on your day to day activities.

About the author

Christi Larson, Pharm. D.

Christi Larson is a pharmacist who is passionate about educating consumers on health care issues, She was inspired at an early age by her paternal grandmother who had a love for medicine. She was intrigued by her grandmother's vast library of medical books, particularly the books about medication. She also credits both sets of grandparents for cultivating her dedication to seniors. Christi earned her Doctor of Pharmacy degree and then completed a one year Pharmacy (PGY1) Residency program. Now, with nearly 20 years in the pharmacy field, she's been a pharmacist, Director, author, speaker and consultant. She's worked in a variety of health care settings including hospital, home care, physician's office, outpatient clinic and retail pharmacy. She continues to be driven by her desire to use what she's learned to ultimately improve patient health, understanding, safety and quality of life.

www.ingramcontent.com/pod-product-compliance
Lightning Source LLC
Chambersburg PA
CBHW071532200326
41519CB00021BB/6458